New Horizons in Pediatric Exercise Science

Cameron J.R. Blimkie, PhD
McMaster University

Oded Bar-Or, MD
Chedoke-McMaster Hospitals

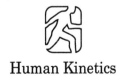

Human Kinetics

Library of Congress Cataloging-in-Publication Data

New horizons in pediatric exercise science / [edited by Cameron J.R.
Blimkie, Oded Bar-Or.
    p.   cm.
"The articles in this book were presented at the first joint
meeting of the European Group of Pediatric Work Physiology (EGPWP)
and the North American Society of Pediatric Exercise Science
(NASPEM) held in September 1993 in Ontario, Canada"--CIP t.p. verso.
    Includes bibliographical references.
    ISBN 0-87322-528-7
    1. Exercise therapy for chiildren--Congresses.   2. Exercise for
children--Congresses.   I. Blimkie, Cameron J.R.   II. Bar-Or, Oded.
III. European Group of Pediatric Work Physiology.   IV. North
American Society of Pediatric Exercise Science.
RJ53.E95N49   1995
618.92--dc20   95-7588
                                                            CIP

ISBN: 0-87322-528-7

Copyright © 1995 by Human Kinetics Publishers, Inc.

The articles in this book were presented at the first joint meeting of the European Group of Pediatric Work Physiology (EGPWP) and the North American Society of Pediatric Exercise Science (NASPEM) held in September 1993 in Ontario, Canada.

Acquisitions Editor: Rik Washburn; **Developmental Editor**: Rodd Whelpley; **Assistant Editors**: Jacqueline Blakley, Karen Bojda, Susan Moore, Kent Reel; **Copyeditor**: Nedra Lambert; **Proofreader**: Pam Johnson; **Typesetting and Text Layout**: Angela K. Snyder; **Text Designer**: Robert Reuther; **Layout Artist**: Tara Welsch; **Cover Designer**: Jack Davis; **Printer**: Braun-Brumfield

Printed in the United States of America   10 9 8 7 6 5 4 3 2 1

Human Kinetics
P.O. Box 5076, Champaign, IL 61825-5076
1-800-747-4457

Canada: Human Kinetics, Box 24040,
Windsor, ON N8Y 4Y9
1-800-465-7301 (in Canada only)

Europe: Human Kinetics,
P.O. Box IW14, Leeds, LS16 6TR, England
(44) 532-781708

Australia: Human Kinetics, 2 Ingrid Street,
Clapham 5062, South Australia
(08) 371 3755

New Zealand: Human Kinetics, P.O. Box 105-231, Auckland 1
(09) 309 2259

Contents

Contributors   v
Preface   vii
Acknowledgments   xi

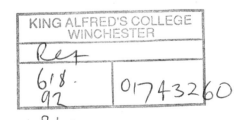

Contributors

Neil Armstrong
P.E.A. Research Center
University of Exeter
Exeter, United Kingdom

Donald A. Bailey
College of Physical Education
University of Saskatchewan
Saskatoon, SK Canada

Gerald Barber
NYU Medical Center
New York, NY USA

Oded Bar-Or
Department of Pediatrics
Chedoke Hospital Division, Evel. Bldg.
Hamilton, ON Canada

Susan I. Barr
University of British Columbia
School of Family and Nutritional
   Sciences
Vancouver, BC Canada

Cameron J.R. Blimkie
McMaster University
Department of Kinesiology
Hamilton, ON Canada

Dan M. Cooper
Torrance, CA USA

Han C.G. Kemper
Department of Health Sciences
Vrije Universiteit
Amsterdam, The Netherlands

Anne B. Loucks
Department of Biological Sciences
Ohio University
Athens, OH USA

Robert M. Malina
Department of Kinesiology and
   Health Education
University of Texas
Austin, TX USA

C. Niemeyer
Department of Health Sciences
Vrije Universiteit
Amsterdam, The Netherlands

Hélène Perrault
Physical Education Department
McGill University
Montreal, PQ Canada

Julio C. Reina
Departments of Physiological Sciences
   and Pediatrics
Universidad del Valle
Cali, Colombia

Andris Rode
School of Physical &
   Health Education
University of Toronto
Toronto, ON Canada

Alan D. Rogol
Department of Pediatrics &
   Pharmacology
University of Virginia
   Health Sciences Center
Charlottesville, VA USA

James F. Sallis
Department of Psychology
San Diego State University
San Diego, CA USA

Roy J. Shephard
School of Physical &
   Health Education
University of Toronto
Toronto, ON Canada

G.B. Spurr
Department of Physiology
Medical College of Wisconsin
Milwaukee, WI USA

Colin E. Webber
Department of Nuclear Medicine
Chedoke-McMaster Hospital
Hamilton, ON Canada

Jack H. Wilmore
Department of Kinesiology and
   Health Education
The University of Texas at Austin
Austin, TX USA

Preface

New Horizons in Pediatric Exercise Science is a compendium of chapters by world authorities on selected topics with a common theme of children and exercise. All chapters were presented as invited lectures at the first joint meeting of the European Group of Pediatric Work Physiology (EGPWP) and the North American Society of Pediatric Exercise Medicine (NASPEM), which was hosted by the Children's Exercise and Nutrition Centre, Chedoke-McMaster Hospitals and McMaster University at the Nottawasaga Inn, Canada, in September 1993.

The European Group of Pediatric Work Physiology is an informally organized yet highly committed group of pediatric clinicians and researchers in exercise physiology, physical education, kinesiology, and rehabilitative medicine. The EGPWP has hosted biennial scientific meetings and published conference proceedings since 1968. Membership in this group is primarily European, and with the exception of a meeting in Israel in 1972 and another in Quebec in 1979, all other meetings have been held in Europe.

The North American Society of Pediatric Exercise Medicine, founded in 1986, is a more formally organized group composed mostly of pediatric exercise physiologists, physicians, and other health care professionals from the USA and Canada. This group has been meeting annually, and abstracts of the conference proceedings are now published in the journal *Pediatric Exercise Science*.

The purpose of the conference at the Nottawasaga Inn was to bring together, for the first time, scholars from both the European and North American groups who have a common interest in children, physical activity, and health. Besides providing an empathic yet specialized presentation forum for young scientists and researchers, the conference also provided the opportunity for the exchange of international perspectives and interdisciplinary dialogue among leading researchers and practitioners in this relatively new, yet rapidly expanding subdiscipline of Pediatric Exercise Science. The conference was also organized to celebrate the 10th anniversary of the Children's Exercise and Nutrition Centre, whose clinical practice and research interests embody the philosophy of both the European and North American groups.

The text is organized into five sections. The introductory chapter by Dan Cooper addresses future research directions and challenges in pediatric exercise research and is dedicated to the memory of Dr. Joseph Rutenfranz, a founding member of the EGPWP, for his contributions to the development of Pediatric Exercise Science in general and the EGPWP in particular. The first section,

"Endocrine Aspects of Pediatric Exercise," includes two chapters. The first chapter, by Anne Loucks, deals with the effects of physical activity on endocrine regulation of the reproductive system in adolescents, and Alan Rogol's chapter, which addresses the role of growth hormone in the regulation of growth in males during puberty, completes out this section.

The second section, entitled "Bone Metabolism, Activity, and Growth," comprises four chapters related to the measurement of bone mineral and the influences of physical activity and nutrition on bone mineral development. In the first chapter, Colin Webber elaborates measurement issues related to the use of dual photon transmission techniques in the assessment of bone mineral content and body composition in children. Han Kemper's chapter addresses the relationship between physical activity and the optimization of bone mass during the developing years. The relationship between the nature of mechanical perturbations to bone and skeletal adaptations during growth are discussed in the third chapter by Don Bailey. In the final chapter, Susan Barr addresses the influence of macro- and micronutrients on bone growth and development during the childhood years.

Part III, entitled "Training and Congenital Heart Disease," is composed of two chapters with clinical and theoretical relevance. In the first chapter, Hélène Perrault presents a physiologist's perspective of theoretical benefits of exercise training after surgical repair of congenital heart disease in young children. In the second chapter, Gerald Barber presents a cardiologist's viewpoint on the role and effectiveness of exercise training in the management of pediatric cardiac patients in general.

The fourth section is entitled "Nutrition and Exercise in Children and Adolescents" and is also composed of two chapters. Gerald Spurr and Julio Reina address the relationship between nutritional status and physical activity in children from a developing country, and the chapter by Jack Wilmore investigates the relationship between nutritional practices and high-level sports competition and training among young females.

The fifth, and last, section of this text is entitled "International Perspectives: Activity, Growth, and Cardiovascular Disease" and contains four chapters. In this section, the relationship between physical activity and cardiorespiratory fitness as childhood antecedents to adult cardiovascular disease risk is presented for selected populations. Neil Armstrong elaborates on the relationship between cardiopulmonary fitness and physical activity patterns in children from selected, developed European countries, whereas Robert Malina deals with the cardiovascular health status of children and youth in developing Latin American countries. James Sallis provides a North American perspective on physical activity research in children and adolescents, and in the final chapter of the text, Roy Shephard and Andris Rode provide a unique perspective on the relationship between lifestyle changes due to social acculturation and cardiovascular disease risk among northern Canadian Inuit children.

The 15 chapters in this text represent only a small, albeit significant component of the scientific exchange that took place at the first joint meeting of the EGPWP and NASPEM. Besides the invited speakers, more than 200 delegates representing

22 countries attended this conference, and many actively participated in presentations of free communications or posters. More than 100 abstracts of these presentations, which comprised the largest part of the scientific activity during this conference, have been published in *Pediatric Exercise Science, 5,* 1993.

Issues in Pediatric Exercise Science is a compilation of state-of-the-art reviews by leading authorities on selected topics of relevance to clinicians, practitioners, and researchers who are interested in the effects of exercise in the growing child. It is not intended as, nor does it pretend to be, a comprehensive treatise of all possible pediatric exercise issues. Nevertheless, this text adds significantly to the body of knowledge in this area and contributes to the further advancement of the still burgeoning subdiscipline of Pediatric Exercise Science.

Acknowledgments

The editors thank Dr. Bruce Alpert and Dr. Brian Wilson for their expert guidance and support as members of the Scientific Planning Committee for the first joint meeting of the European Group of Pediatric Work Physiology and the North American Society of Pediatric Exercise Medicine held at the Nottawasaga Inn, Canada.

The conference would not have been the success it was without the untiring help and tremendous effort from the following members of the Organizing Committee: Marilyn and Tali Bar-Or, Mike Browne, Karen Burrows, Randy Calvert, Alejandro Elorriaga, Wendy Fallis, Gail Frost, Helge Hebestreit, Jennifer Mason, Flavia Meyer, Sandy Schwenger, Eric Small, Lara Smith, Visch Unnithan, Edgar van Mil, Heather Waters, Boguslaw Wilk, and Heather Zurbrigg. Thanks also to Ingrid Ellis for encouragement and expertise in planning and implementing the conference.

A special thanks to the Abstract Review Committee of Bruce Alpert, Frank Galioto, Luc Leger, David Orenstein, Hélène Perrault, Tom Rowland, and Brian Wilson for their effort and time in ensuring the high quality of the scientific presentations. The editors would also like to thank all the chairpersons of both the free communications and symposia for their assistance and support; they are simply too numerous to mention individually. Last, but perhaps more important, the editors would like to provide recognition and extend their appreciation to the following conference supporters. The level and nature of contribution varied amongst supporters, and this is reflected in the various contribution categories. The success of the conference was largely dependent on the combined support from these organizations, and we are greatly indebted to them for their patronage.

Major Sponsors

Health and Welfare Canada; The Dairy Board of Canada; Ironkids Bread; Toddler Bobbler Products, Inc.

Sponsors

Serono Canada, Inc.; Gatorade Sports Science Institute, USA; Mead Johnson Canada; Eli Lilly Canada, Inc.; Taylor Chrysler Dodge Vans; Bell Mobility Cellular Plus Centre; Bionetics Ltd.; Departments of Pediatrics and Kinesiology and Faculties of Health Sciences and Social Sciences, McMaster University.

Exhibitors

Alpine Medical Products; Human Kinetics; Summit Technologies.

Chapter 1

New Horizons in Pediatric Exercise Research

Dan M. Cooper, MD

Introduction

The task set for me by Dr. Bar-Or in convening this meeting is daunting, exciting, and challenging. Daunting because among the participants in this symposium are some of the most original and creative thinkers in the field of developmental exercise physiology; exciting because new advances in biology permit us to probe fundamental aspects of the interrelationship between growth and exercise in ways that were previously unheard of; and challenging because new directions of pediatric exercise research cause us to reevaluate and change some of the fundamental ways that we have traditionally viewed physical activity and the role of exercise testing in children.

The participants in this conference appreciate that children, unlike most adults, naturally engage in spontaneous, vigorous physical activity. We postulate that this phenomenon represents more than mere play; rather, exercise in children is an essential biological process and likely plays a key role in normal growth and development. With this in mind, we know that research on exercise in children need not be limited to questions of competitive or athletic performance, but should include in its scope topics such as the interaction of exercise and tissue growth factors; the molecular biology of the developing skeletal muscle; the maturation of high energy phosphate metabolism; the mathematical analysis of physical activity patterns in children; and many others.

I have developed four topics that I consider to be examples of new horizons in pediatric exercise research:

1. Growth, growth factors, and physical activity
2. Interaction of diet and exercise—implications for growth and development
3. Skeletal muscle adjustments to exercise
4. Assessment of physical activity in children

This text is adapted from the opening lecture of The First Joint Meeting of the European Group of Pediatric Work Physiology and the North American Society of Pediatric Exercise Medicine held September 18-22, 1993, in Alliston, Ontario, Canada.

Growth, Growth Factors, and Physical Activity

Physical activity plays a profound role in tissue anabolism, growth, and development. Yet surprisingly little is understood about the mechanisms that link exercise with muscle hypertrophy (67), increased capillarization and mitochondrial capacity (16), stronger bones (54), changes in body composition (6,10), and improved cardiorespiratory dynamics (23). By identifying common processes responsible for the many *anabolic* effects of physical activity, perhaps we can improve clinical applications of exercise in preventing coronary artery disease (80) and obesity (41,58) and as a rehabilitation tool for children suffering from chronic diseases. Thus the overall aim of research in this area would be to uncover the mechanisms that link physical activity with growth at both the cellular and somatic levels.

Anabolic responses to exercise refer to constructive metabolic processes involved in tissue adaptation to the stress of physical activity. The hypothesis of *central* and *local* components of exercise modulation of growth is presented in Figure 1.1. Central components encompass the mechanisms through which exercise of skeletal muscle groups can seemingly affect cellular growth and function throughout the body [for example, cardiovascular effects or the reduction in body fat stores that accompanies virtually all types of training programs (70)]. Testosterone, estradiol, and growth hormone (GH) likely are involved in the central pathways as well as in circulating insulin-like growth factor-I and II (IGF-I, II), which are potent growth factors and are stimulated by GH in many tissues. Local components encompass those mechanisms that stimulate growth, hypertrophy, and the appearance of new mitochondria and capillaries in the muscle, bone, vascular, and connective tissues involved in the specific exercise. For example,

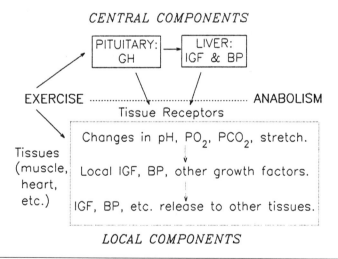

Figure 1.1. Hypothesis of central and local components of exercise anabolism. BP refers to binding proteins. It is likely that the growth factors, their BPs, and tissue receptors contribute to exercise modulation of growth.

IGF-I may be stimulated in tissues independently of GH and may act in both an *autocrine* and *paracrine* manner.

The role of GH in exercise-induced growth is particularly intriguing and not yet well understood. Because exercise stimulates GH secretion (38), and because GH (either directly or in combination with IGF-I) is a potent growth factor for skeletal and heart muscle (7,40,71,76), it is not surprising that many investigations both in humans (29,86) and in other species (19,20,46) indicate that GH plays an important role in the adaptation to exercise. In contrast, there is evidence that exogenous GH administration does not enhance the effect of exercise training on muscle growth or strength in young, well-trained adult males (31,87,88). Additional investigation of the interaction between GH (and its binding proteins and receptors) and physical activity clearly is necessary.

The interaction between physical activity and growth is not limited to individuals engaged in competitive sports and athletics. Disuse atrophy—the reduction in muscle mass and bone density that accompanies bed rest, limb immobilization, or neural injury—occurs even in sedentary individuals (18). This implies that a sizable anabolic stimulus arises from the relatively modest physical activity of daily living. Moreover, the existence of the "training effect"—the ability to improve performance with repeated exercise—suggests a "dose-response" relationship between activity and anabolic effect. Thus, it is not surprising that many of the therapeutic uses of exercise (e.g., respiratory muscle training, treatment of obesity, and cardiac rehabilitation) depend on its anabolic effects.

Current data do not suggest that exercise alone can increase *somatic* growth (e.g., body height) in healthy children. Increased GH stimulation by exercise, might, for example, result in down-regulation of GH receptors with a subsequent reduced effect of GH on IGF-I generation. In addition, there are many instances where an apparent "conflict" for metabolic energy occurs between genetically determined needs of somatic growth and the energy demands of exercise. For example, in marginally nourished but physically active children in developing countries (79), high energy requirements of the physical activity of daily living (conditions imposed by poverty) may result in reduced somatic growth [*infra vide*, Spurr (79)]. In more developed countries where food is abundant, imbalances between energy intake and expenditure also appear often in highly-trained young athletes [particularly females (48,83)]. Recent reports by Jahreis and colleagues (83) demonstrate that highly-trained but functionally malnourished female gymnasts may have a reduced somatic growth potential. Interestingly, circulating IGF-I decreases after only several days of intense training when caloric balance is negative in healthy males (77) and in female gymnasts (48). These observations raise the possibility that the central and local growth factor responses to exercise are not invariably synergistic, particularly when the balance between energy intake and expenditure is impaired.

For developmental biologists, the ways habitual physical activity during childhood can, through anabolic effects on muscles, heart, and blood vessels, beneficially influence health later in life (80) may prove more important than exercise-induced changes of body height or weight.

Little is known about responses to repeated bouts of physical activity in the younger, developing organism where overall body growth is rapid and secretory patterns of growth factors (like GH) are in a state of flux (62). The purpose of a recent set of experiments (25,91) in our laboratory was to determine the role of GH in functional adaptations to exercise during development and to determine the effects of GH suppression and exercise training on somatic growth and circulating IGF-I. We subjected prepubertal female rats to a 4-week period of treadmill exercise training, and we measured growth effects and cardiorespiratory responses to exercise in control rats and in rats with suppressed GH secretory capacity.

The experimental design consisted of training (treadmill exercise) young rats in which normal GH secretion was blocked. Hypophysectomy has been used in the mature rat to obliterate any possible effect of exercise on GH secretion (44,45), but this invasive surgical technique is technically more difficult in younger rats, and it results in reduced spontaneous physical activity and requires the administration of other pituitary hormones to maintain health. As an alternative approach to attenuate GH secretion, we administered anti-GHRH antisera. Wehrenberg and coworkers (85) showed that this markedly inhibits somatic growth, GH, and IGF-I in rats. The treatment was not accompanied by any apparent side effects.

In our study we showed that 4 weeks of treadmill training in young female rats increased $\dot{V}O_2$max, maximal treadmill running time, and hind limb muscle succinate dehydrogenase (SDH) activity (Figures 1.2-1.4). (SDH is a key enzyme of mitochondrial oxidative phosphorylation.) These adaptations occurred even in the GH-suppressed rats (i.e., those treated with anti-GHRH antibodies) in which circulating GH and IGF-I levels were low. The GH-suppressed rats were

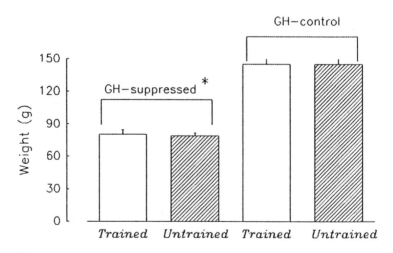

Figure 1.2.   Effect of anti-GHRH antisera on body weight in young female rats (mean + SD). Four weeks of therapy resulted in marked reduction in body weight gain. There was no independent effect of exercise training on body weight (*$p<0.05$, both trained and untrained GH-suppressed rats weighed less than GH control rats).
From Cooper et al. *Pediatr. Res.* 35:223-227, 1994.

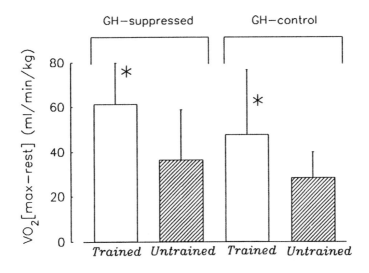

Figure 1.3. Effect of treadmill training on V̇O₂max in GH-suppressed and GH control rats (mean + SD). Training increased V̇O₂max in both the GH-suppressed and GH control groups (*$p<0.05$).
From Cooper et al. *Pediatr. Res.* 35:223-227, 1994.

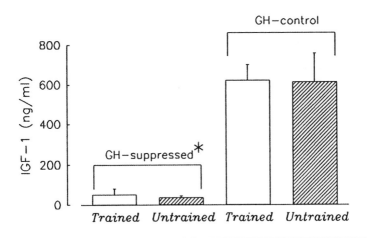

Figure 1.4. Effect of anti-GHRH antisera on circulating IGF-I in trained and untrained rats (mean ± SD). As expected, IGF-I was markedly reduced in GH-suppressed rats. There was no independent effect of exercise training on IGF-I levels (*$p<0.05$, both trained and untrained GH-suppressed rats compared with GH control rats).
From Cooper et al. *Pediatr. Res.* 35:223-227, 1994.

active, required no exogenous hormone replacement (as is the case in surgically hypophysectomized rats), and appeared to suffer no ill effects from the treatment per se. The marked growth retardation (Figure 1.2) and substantially reduced serum levels of IGF-I demonstrated the effectiveness of the anti-GHRH antisera. Our results are consistent with the studies of Goldberg (44) and Gollnick and coworkers (45) who showed that muscle hypertrophy and increases in muscle SDH can occur either as a compensatory mechanism or in response to exercise in mature, hypophysectomized rats.

There are several possible explanations for the apparent discrepancy between our results and previous observations supporting a role for GH in the training effect. First, growth factors such as IGF-I may be less dependent on GH in some tissues than previously thought. DeVol and coworkers (30), for example, demonstrated in rats that compensatory hind limb muscle hypertrophy was accompanied by increases in IGF-I mRNA of the hypertrophied muscle even in hypophysectomized rats. Thus, in addition to possible endocrine effects of circulating IGF-I originating in the liver and stimulated by GH, it appears that IGF-I can be produced in local tissues independently of GH and can result in autocrine or paracrine growth stimulation (57).

Second, gender, particularly in its interaction with puberty, may have played a role in how GH-suppressed rats responded to exercise training. Gender differences in fitness are virtually nonexistent in prepubertal children (27), and MacIntosh and Baldwin (59), whose training protocol we adapted for our current study, noted no gender differences in the effects of exercise on skeletal muscle oxidative capacity in neonatal rats. But gender-related exercise effects become substantial in teenagers, as American girls become progressively less fit than boys (27). In addition, the gender differences that do exist [e.g., differences in heart muscle responses in rats (74) and hemoglobin in humans (82)] are most often noted in mature, postpubertal subjects.

GH secretion increases in puberty (28,39,62), along with marked increases in testosterone in males and estradiol in females. Testosterone appears to contribute to the high amplitude/low baseline pattern of GH secretion observed in mature male rats, and estradiol leads to the low amplitude/high baseline pattern observed in mature female rats (47). While not as dramatic as in the rat, puberty in humans is characterized by greater increase in spontaneous GH pulse frequency and amplitude in males than in females (28,63). Therefore, it is possible that training effects in young females are less GH-dependent than in males. The interaction between hormonal changes associated with puberty and physical activity is not well understood, but our data clearly demonstrate that female rats can respond robustly to exercise training initiated early in life.

Although the GH-suppressed rats had markedly reduced serum concentrations of IGF-I, serum levels alone do not necessarily reflect growth factor responses at the tissue level. The increase in functional adaptations to exercise observed in the GH-suppressed rats suggested the hypothesis that exercise could stimulate *local tissue* increases in IGF-I mRNA and/or protein levels even in the absence of normal pituitary GH activity. To test this hypothesis, we measured IGF-I mRNA and protein levels in the hind limb muscle and liver of trained and untrained, GH control and GH-suppressed rats.

We found that in young female rats with normal pituitary function, improved exercise responses (25) are accompanied by significant increases in both hepatic and skeletal muscle IGF-I mRNA (Figures 1.5-1.7). In rats with suppressed GH, a functional training response also was observed and was accompanied by significant IGF-I mRNA increases in the muscle. We did not observe a significant increase in hepatic IGF-I mRNA following training in the GH-suppressed animals. Numerous studies using different exercise protocols have demonstrated that physical training results in muscle hypertrophy (16,81) and increased capillarization (67). There is much evidence supporting a specific role for IGF-I in the response to training. IGF-I has a mitogenic effect on myoblasts and fibroblasts (8,37); increases net protein accumulation during muscle hypertrophy (8); and stimulates both proliferation and differentiation of muscle satellite cells (1), the precursor cells for muscle growth and hypertrophy in the postnatal organism.

Our study demonstrated a complex interaction among GH suppression, exercise, and IGF-I gene expression. Exercise-induced IGF-I gene stimulation appears to be more GH-dependent in the liver than in the muscle. Moreover, GH suppression leads to an enhancement of the local factors regulating the expression of exon 1 mRNA in skeletal muscle during exercise. Interestingly, there are data supporting a role for the GH-IGF-I axis in the adaptation to exercise, which presumably would involve hepatic production and release of IGF-I into the circulation. There are two independent studies in humans showing that circulating IGF-I is correlated with the degree of physical fitness (52,69), although resistive

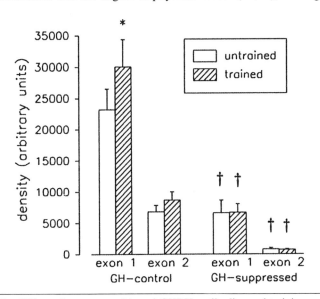

Figure 1.5.   Effect of treatment with anti-GHRH antibodies and training on IGF-I mRNA levels in liver. Liver exon 1 and 2 transcripts were significantly reduced by GH suppression both in untrained and trained animals (†$p<0.0001$). In the GH control rats, training induced a significant increase in exon 1 IGF-I mRNA (*$p<0.05$). From Zanconato et al. *J. Appl. Physiol.* 76:2204-2209, 1994.

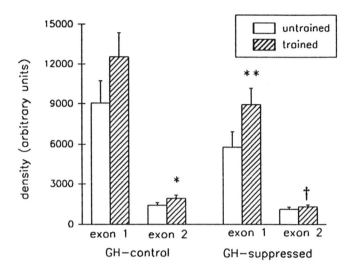

Figure 1.6.   Effect of treatment with anti-GHRH antibodies and training on IGF-I mRNA levels in hind limb muscle. Exon 2 mRNA was significantly reduced by GH suppression in the trained animals (†, $p<0.01$), while in the untrained rats, no significant changes were observed in either exon 1 or 2 mRNAs. In the GH control rats, training induced a significant increase in exon 2 transcripts (*$p<0.05$), while in the GH-suppressed animals, a significant increase was observed for exon 1 mRNA. From Zanconato et al. *J. Appl. Physiol.* 76:2204-2209, 1994.

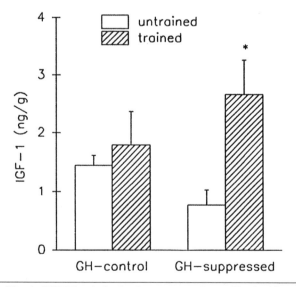

Figure 1.7.   Muscle IGF-I levels in the four groups of rats. No significant changes were observed with GH suppression. In the GH-suppressed group, IGF-I levels were significantly greater in the trained compared to the untrained animals (*$p<0.01$). From Zanconato et al. *J. Appl. Physiol.* 76:2204-2209, 1994.

muscle training seems not to increase circulating IGF-I in *well-trained* subjects (31,88). Weltman et al. (86) found an increased pulse amplitude of *spontaneous* GH secretion in women who had undergone a year of endurance exercise training. Borer and coworkers (21) demonstrated that exercise-induced somatic growth in the hamster was accompanied by increases in spontaneous GH pulse amplitude and frequency.

Physical training induced an increase in liver and muscle IGF-I mRNA in animals with normal GH secretory capacity and a significant increase in IGF-I mRNA and protein in the muscle of GH-suppressed animals. We began the training program in prepubertal female rats, and while we did not perform comparable experiments in more mature rats or in male rats, it is likely that both maturation and gender influence growth factor responses to training in undiscovered ways. We speculate that when GH is suppressed the increase in IGF-I in the working muscles could be sufficient to bring about the functional tissue adaptations to repeated physical activity. In addition, we speculate that the previously shown exercise-induced anabolic effects of physical activity might be mediated at least partially by an increased production of muscle IGF-I, one that appears to be independent of GH. Much work needs to be done to fully elucidate the growth factor response to exercise in the developing organism.

Interaction of Diet and Exercise—
Implications for Growth and Development

There is growing evidence that diet and patterns of physical activity can interact either to benefit or to harm human health. For example, the combination of a diet high in fat with a sedentary lifestyle contributes to obesity, hypercholesterolemia, hypertension, and coronary artery disease (13,56,65). Conversely, appropriate manipulations of diet and exercise may prevent these diseases and may promote cardiorespiratory rehabilitation (12,64). However, the synergistic or antagonistic mechanisms through which diet and physical activity interact are not completely understood. As noted, exercise is a potent physiologic stimulator of GH release in humans, and short exercise bouts (e.g., 10 min) can result in elevated GH for more than an hour (38). We reasoned that one pathway of interaction might be acute influences of diet on the GH response to exercise. Indeed, circulating somatostatin [a powerful inhibitor of GH release (42)] is elevated within 30 minutes of meals high in fat (68). Similarly, elevated concentrations of blood glucose, as occur following meals high in carbohydrates, can inhibit GH release (43). Thus, diet could interact with exercise by influencing the GH response and the consequent effects of GH on body composition and/or the growth of individual tissues.

To test the hypothesis that exercise-induced elevation in GH is acutely affected by diet, we examined GH responses to exercise in healthy young adults after they consumed meals that were high in fat, glucose, or noncaloric placebo (22).

The protocol consisted of a brief period (10 min) of high-intensity exercise, recently demonstrated to elicit a reliable increase in GH (38). In contrast to exercise protocols of 40 or more minutes, often used to examine metabolic and hormonal responses to exercise, shorter periods of exercise may have the advantage of more closely mimicking actual patterns of physical activity in the daily lives of human beings.

We found that exercise-induced GH release can be modulated profoundly by a single meal taken prior to exercise (Figure 1.8). In our study, a high-fat drink attenuated post-exercise peak GH levels and AUC by about 50%. It is worth noting that a typical fast-food meal would likely contain similar calories as fat as our high-fat protocol [e.g., a Big Mac and regular-size french fries contains 446 kcal as fat alone (2)]. We saw an insignificant decrease in the GH response after the ingestion of a high-glucose meal. The increase in metabolic rate and cellular redox state, as judged by the increases in $\dot{V}O_2$ and the lactate-to-pyruvate ratio, were virtually the same following placebo, high-glucose, and high-fat meals. Thus, the reduced GH response to exercise must have resulted from a direct effect of the ingested substrate (i.e., fat) on the hypothalamic pituitary axis or by indirect effects mediated by the hormonal response to the meal itself.

Somatostatin, a major inhibitor of GH secretion, is synthesized in the hypothalamus and other neuronal tissues and throughout the gut, primarily in the upper gastrointestinal tract (17). The structure of extraneural somatostatin has been shown to be identical to that of the hypothalamic hormone (75,78). The precise

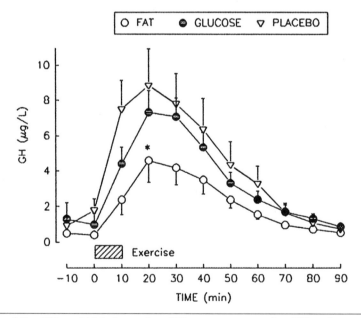

Figure 1.8. Effect of high-fat meal on GH response to exercise. GH peak was significantly reduced only following the high-fat meal (*$p<0.05$).
From Cappon et al. *J. Clin. Endo. Metab.* 76:1418, 1993.

mechanism of somatostatin's negative feedback on GH secretion is complex and incompletely understood, but it involves the close interrelationship at several levels between somatostatin, GH releasing hormone and GH, and their receptors, with probable adrenergic and cholinergic influences as well (50,51).

As in the earlier work of Penman et al. (68), the high-fat liquid meal resulted in a prolonged elevation of circulating somatostatin. The peak response in Penman's study occurred at about 90 minutes (similar to our observations), which is actually *after* the onset of exercise in our protocol. Although somatostatin had not yet reached its maximum, we found that exercise-induced GH levels were lowest following the high-fat meal. While the functional relationship and the physiologic importance of peripheral versus hypothalamic somatostatin in humans is unknown, diet-induced increases in somatostatin remain an intriguing possible mechanism for our observation of a markedly attenuated GH response to exercise following the high-fat meal.

The typical American continues to ingest a high-fat diet (55). Our data suggest a possible mechanism whereby not only the quality and quantity of the caloric intake, but also the hormonal response to a particular diet, may play a role in attenuating the protein-anabolic and lipolytic effects of exercise. We recently reported, for example, that many obese boys have normal and sometimes increased levels of physical fitness (26). Perhaps the prolonged somatostatin response to high-fat meals in these children attenuates the GH response to vigorous activities of daily life and minimizes beneficial lipolytic effects of exercise-induced GH. Whether diet may affect anabolic responses to exercise in other conditions (e.g., diabetes, rehabilitation from heart or lung disease) has yet to be determined.

Skeletal Muscle Adjustments to Exercise

There is increasing evidence suggesting that the metabolic pathways essential for physical activity mature during growth in children. The gas exchange response (measured at the mouth, breath-by-breath) to high intensity exercise in children has been shown to be qualitatively and quantitatively different from that of adults. The oxygen cost of high intensity exercise normalized to the actual work done (O_2/joule) is higher in children, suggesting less dependence on anaerobic metabolism (90) (Figure 1.9). After vigorous exercise, blood and muscle lactate concentrations are lower in children, who also reach lower levels of metabolic acidosis (36,66). Consistent with this is our recent observation that the increase in $\dot{V}O_2$ during constant work rate, high-intensity exercise is smaller in children than it is in adults (4) [the degree to which $\dot{V}O_2$ increases depends on lactate concentrations (72)].

The growth-related differences in the adaptive response to high intensity exercise might be related to maturation of muscle metabolic pathways, but no definitive mechanism has been established. One problem has been the lack of noninvasive methods to study muscle metabolism. The use of phosphorus nuclear magnetic resonance spectroscopy (^{31}P MRS) now provides safe and noninvasive

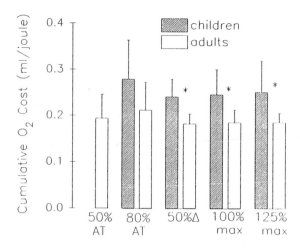

Figure 1.9.   Oxygen cost of 1-minute bouts of constant work rate cycle ergometer exercise. $\dot{V}O_2$ was measured during the exercise and for 10 minutes of recovery. Pre-exercise baseline $\dot{V}O_2$ was subtracted to ensure that the oxygen cost represented the real cost of the work performed. 50% and 80% AT represent the work corresponding to the subject's anaerobic threshold. 50%Δ indicates the work rate representing 50% of the difference between the AT and peak $\dot{V}O_2$.
From Zanconato et al. *J. Appl. Physiol.* 71:993, 1991.

means of monitoring intracellular inorganic phosphate (Pi), phosphocreatine (PCr), and pH (24), that are acceptable for studies in children. These variables, in turn, allow the assessment of muscle oxidative metabolism and intramuscular glycolytic activity (24).

We hypothesized that the growth-related changes in whole-body O_2 uptake and O_2 cost of exercise observed during high-intensity exercise reflect a maturation of the kinetics of high-energy phosphate metabolites in muscle tissue. We tested this hypothesis by examining Pi, PCr, β adenosine triphosphate (βATP), and pH kinetics in calf muscles during progressive incremental exercise. Results obtained from children were compared with results obtained from adults (89).

Our study showed that during progressive exercise, muscle Pi/PCr ratio increases to a smaller extent in children compared with that of adults, even when the data are related to work rate normalized to body weight (Figures 1.10-1.13). In addition, children showed a smaller drop in intramuscular pH. A slow and fast phase of Pi/PCr increase and pH decrease was noted in 75% of the adults and in 50% of the children. The difference in high energy phosphate kinetics we observed between children and adults is limited to the higher intensity range of exercise.

As leg muscle work rate increases, ADP and Pi are released from the breakdown of ATP and PCr. Current theory holds that ADP and Pi regulate the rate of oxidative phosphorylation exactly so that homeostasis of the ATP concentration

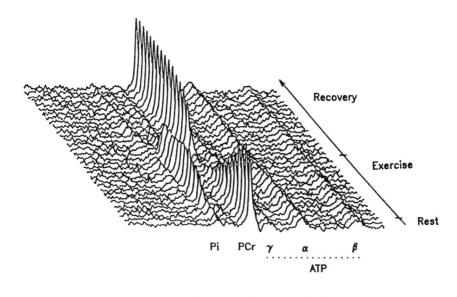

Pi PCr γ   α   β

ATP

Figure 1.10. ^{31}P MRS spectra obtained from the right calf of a 35-year-old man at rest, during incremental plantar flexion to exhaustion, and during recovery. From Zanconato et al. *J. Appl. Physiol.* 74:2214, 1993.

is obtained (24). As ATP hydrolysis approaches the maximal rate of oxidative phosphorylation, glycolysis (similarly activated by ADP and Pi) assumes an increasing proportion of the metabolic burden (24). In healthy adult subjects, the relationship between Pi/PCr and work rate is characterized by an initial linear portion. The slope of Pi/PCr to work rate is directly proportional to the rate of mitochondrial oxidative metabolism. This is followed by a second steeper slope associated with activation of glycolytic processes (24). Production of lactic acid, which is dissociated at physiological pH, results in increasing [H⁺]. Therefore, ^{31}P MRS can indirectly monitor glycolytic activity by measuring intracellular pH.

The initial linear slope was the same in children and adults suggesting a similar rate of mitochondrial oxidative metabolism during low-intensity exercise. But the different response in Pi/PCr ratio and pH during high-intensity exercise indicates growth-related differences in energy metabolism in the high intensity exercise range.

Our data might suggest that children have a higher rate of muscle oxidative phosphorylation during heavy exercise than adults have. Children may use oxygen more efficiently than adults do, children may be less able to facilitate anaerobic pathways, or they may have tissue O_2 requirements during exercise that are not found in adults. A more efficient O_2 utilization could result from factors that influence mitochondrial oxidative ATP resynthesis: delivery of oxygen from the capillary blood; delivery of substrates; or greater density of mitochondrial

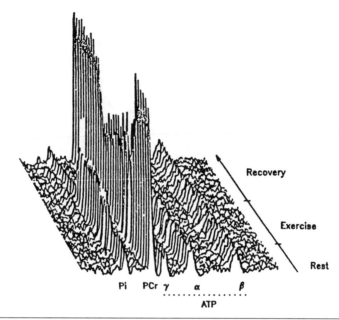

Figure 1.11. ³¹P MRS spectra from the right calf of an 8-year-old boy at rest, during incremental exercise, and during recovery.
From Zanconato et al. *J. Appl. Physiol.* 74:2214, 1993.

population. Each of these factors might be responsible for a greater oxygen-dependent ATP generation, lower Pi/PCr ratio, and higher pH during exercise in children.

But a more efficient oxidative metabolism in children alone should not inhibit the glycolytic capability. As work rate increases, the children, like the adults, would eventually require glycolysis and lactate production as an additional mechanism of ATP rephosphorylation. This phenomenon is observed in trained athletes: Although anaerobic metabolism occurs at higher work rates than in untrained subjects (indicating more efficient aerobic metabolism), lactate levels ultimately achieved are much higher. It is noteworthy that the threshold in the slope of Pi/PCr to work rate occurred at the same relative work rate in children and adults (0.05 psi/kg), an indirect bit of evidence against the idea of greater aerobic efficiency in children. Therefore, it appears that when the work rate exceeds a threshold value, the ability to effect anaerobic metabolism is less in children than it is in adults. And ultimately, the work performed is less in children.

There could be less glycolytic capability in children, so that the rate of the glycolysis may not be sufficient to meet the muscle energy requirements and may result in early muscle exhaustion. The minimal drop in pH seen in children for heavy exercise demonstrates that even after the transition point (i.e., when further energy sources appear to be required), the glycolytic processes play a lesser role. Moreover, the children achieved an end-exercise Pi/PCr value of 0.54

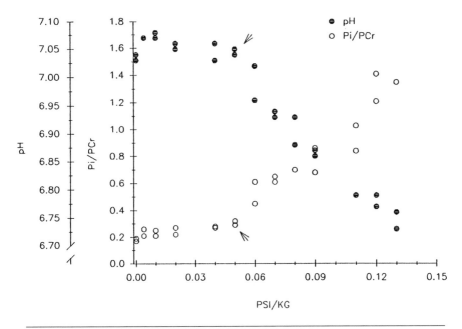

Figure 1.12.   Pi/PCr and pH at rest and during incremental exercise in a 33-year-old man. The arrows indicate the transition points between the slow and fast phases of Pi/PCr increase and pH reduction.
From Zanconato et al. *J. Appl. Physiol.* 74:2214, 1993.

± 0.12 (only 27% of adult values). This indicates that soon after the threshold when the oxidative rate has presumably reached its maximum, children can no longer sustain muscular contraction.

It also could be argued that children do not reach their real maximal work rate because they simply don't try hard enough. Objective criteria for maximal effort are not easy to define even for cycle ergometry, let alone single leg treadle exercise. The children were told that they would be doing a hard exercise and were actively encouraged throughout the test. In addition, a transition in the Pi/PCr to work rate slope (i.e., a critical point in the cellular energy metabolism) was observed in 50% of the children at 62% of the maximal work rate. The same value (62%) was reported for the ratio of anaerobic threshold to $\dot{V}O_2max$ in children of comparable age during maximal cycle ergometer exercise (27).

The results of this study are consistent with previous studies that reported growth related differences in gas exchange response to high-intensity exercise. A higher CO_2-to-O_2 cost ratio (i.e., higher acidosis) for one minute of heavy exercise was observed in adults compared to children (5) (Figure 1.14). Bar-Or reported a lower anaerobic capacity (measured by a supramaximal 30-sec cycle ergometer test—Wingate anaerobic test) in young children compared to that of adolescents and adults (14). In addition, in the few invasive studies that have

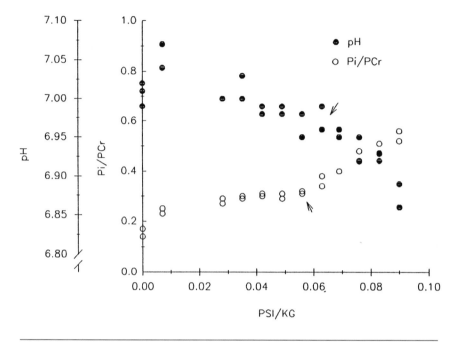

Figure 1.13.   Pi/PCr and pH at rest and during incremental exercise in a 9-year-old girl. The arrows indicate the transition points between the slow and fast phases of Pi/PCr and pH changes.
From Zanconato et al. *J. Appl. Physiol.* 74:2214, 1993.

been done, blood and muscle lactate concentrations at high intensity exercise are lower in children than in adults (36,66).

Our results cannot be explained by a faster lactate removal or subsequent metabolism in children. Because we measured Pi/PCr, we could determine changes in glycolysis independent of changes in pH. If glycolysis had increased with a simultaneous increase in lactate removal, then we ought to have found a more rapid increase in Pi without a parallel drop in pH in children. This was not the case as seen in the relationship between Pi/PCr and pH, which was the same in children and adults.

Both phosphofructokinase (PFK) and glycogen phosphorylase are key regulatory enzymes of glycolysis, but little attention has been paid to a possible maturational pattern of their activity. Eriksson reported a lower muscle concentration of phosphofructokinase in 11- to 13-year-old children compared to adults (35). In addition, studies in rats showed a 17-fold increase in total PFK activity occurring during the first two months of age (equivalent to birth to puberty in humans). This was accompanied by a dramatic decrease in C-type PFK subunit and increase in M-type subunit, the isozyme best suited for glycolysis (34). Finally, low levels of C-type PFK subunit have been shown to promote increased affinity for fructose-6-phosphate and diminished susceptibility to ATP inhibition (32,33).

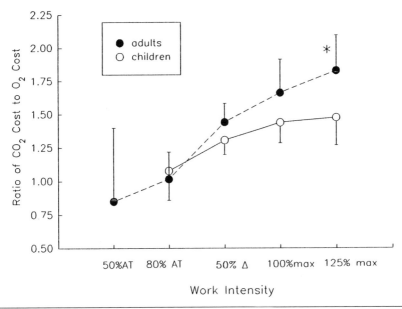

Figure 1.14. Ratio of CO_2 cost to O_2 cost for 1-minute bouts of exercise in adults and children. Data are presented as mean ± SD. In both children and adults, the ratios for above-AT exercise were significantly greater than the below-AT values ($p<0.05$). For the high-intensity exercise, the ratio increased significantly with increasing work intensity from 50%Δ to 100% max and 125% max in adults, but no differences were observed among the ratios in children. At the highest work intensity (125% max), the ratio in adults was significantly greater than the children's value ($p<0.001$). From Armon et al. *Peds. Res.* 29:362, 1991.

We used ^{31}P MRS to study muscle metabolism during exercise in one adult subject with PFK deficiency (3). We observed a normal slope of the initial linear relationship of Pi/PCr to work rate, no drop in pH, and a gradual increase of phosphomonoester levels during exercise. We did not observe a phosphomonoester peak in any of our children. This might reflect a much milder PFK impairment compared to the subject affected by the myopathy.

Maturation of the muscle metabolic response to exercise might be related to the hormonal changes (increase in testosterone, estradiol, growth hormone, and insulin-like growth factor-1) occurring during puberty (61). Little is known about the effect of these hormones on functional and structural muscle growth. Testosterone has been shown to increase sarcotubular and mitochondrial enzymes (73) in mature male subjects. In addition, Kelly et al. demonstrated that testosterone administration stimulated the transition from type IIA (fast oxidative glycolytic) to type IIB (fast glycolytic) fibers in guinea pig temporalis muscles (53).

A maturation of skeletal muscle fiber-type pattern might also account for growth-related differences in the metabolic response to high-intensity exercise. However, several studies examining biopsies of human diaphragm (49) and hind limb muscles (15) demonstrated that fiber-type differentiation occurs relatively early in life and by 6 years of age the skeletal muscle histochemical profile is similar to that of a young adult.

In conclusion, muscle high energy phosphate kinetics during high-intensity exercise is different between children and adults. In this range of work, children seem to rely less on anaerobic glycolytic metabolism than adults do. ^{31}P MRS has proved to be a noninvasive unique technique to gain insight into muscle metabolism during exercise in children. Our results suggest a potentially important role of ^{31}P MRS spectroscopy during exercise in identifying abnormal muscle metabolism and in assessing the value of therapeutic approaches designed to improve exercise tolerance in children with various diseases.

Assessment of Physical Activity in Children

The *pattern* and *intensity* of physical activity in the adult or child may prove to be an important component of exercise-induced growth. For example, it has long been recognized that the naturally occurring pattern of spontaneous GH release in humans is pulsatile. Maiter et al. (60) used the hypophysectomized rat to demonstrate that when exogenous GH was administered in pulses, the resulting serum IGF-I and growth rates were significantly greater than when equivalent doses of GH were given continuously. Activity patterns in children are characterized by short bursts of exercise; perhaps this pattern optimizes the anabolic effects of exercise in the growing child.

Our coinvestigator, Dr. Bailey, has developed a direct observational approach for quantifying patterns of frequency, duration, and intensity of physical activity. Many problems persist in the accurate assessment of energy expenditure, especially in non-laboratory settings under natural conditions. A variety of techniques has been developed for use in the field including self-administered recall, interview administered recall diaries, motion sensors, heart rate monitors, doubly-labeled water, and direct observations. Their advantages and disadvantages have been well reviewed (11,84), and it is clear that there are still limitations to all currently available techniques.

Despite certain drawbacks of direct observational methods (large investment in staff training, possible effects of the observer on physical activity), this approach has distinct advantages over other methods of assessing physical activity in the field. No other technique can precisely quantify the *duration* and *frequency* of specific activity events. For example, the doubly-labeled water technique may be the most accurate method for assessing total energy expenditure over a period of days or weeks, but it will not produce information on the duration or frequency of activity events (not to mention that the isotope is very expensive). Motion sensors may be used to measure intensity of activity, but they cannot be relied upon to measure frequency or duration (9). Heart rate monitors, on the other hand, may be accurate for capturing duration, intensity, and frequency of exercise, but they cannot provide information about the activity events that produced the physiological response. Our ability to precisely quantify and analyze frequency and duration data, along with field estimates of exercise intensity, provide the necessary tools to test our hypotheses relating physical activity with growth factor, gas exchange, and anatomic responses to exercise.

Observations were performed in a wide variety of settings, including in the home, at school, in the car, at friends' homes, at sports events, in the dentist office, in restaurants, and elsewhere throughout the day. The coding system was designed to accurately describe the physical activities of children under free-ranging conditions in such a way as to maximize reliability and replicability of recording.

The level of energy expenditure represented by each activity code was determined after and independently of development of the coding system. Each code was assigned to one of three different levels of energy expenditure intensity (low, moderate, or light) on the basis of laboratory studies of two subjects using indirect calorimetry. Thirty of the 42 different possible activity codes could be replicated in the laboratory. The 30 activities for which energy expenditure data were available were ranked by $\dot{V}O_2$ (ml/min/kg). The remaining 12 activity codes were added to the ranking based on the amount and intensity of movement involved in comparison to the measured activities. Low-intensity activities had $\dot{V}O_2$ values below 10 ml/min/kg, and moderate-intensity activities were between 10 and 20 ml/min/kg. On this basis, most of the high-intensity activities had respiratory exchange ratios above 1.0 (suggesting above-LT exercise).

The direct observations have allowed us to quantify activity intensity, distribution, and duration. Preliminary results of observations from a small group of children have been quite illustrative. For example, in prepubertal children, the median duration of moderate- and high-intensity activities was only about 6 seconds, and the median interval between these short bursts of activity was about 19 seconds.

Most striking about our results is the short duration of activity events, especially those in the high-intensity range. The children we studied engaged in short bursts of intense exercise interspersed with periods of low and moderate exercise. The pattern of the children's activity is one of rapid change from one short activity to another, from one level of intensity to another. In contrast, most standard protocols used to test physiologic responses to exercise in children involve much longer exercise protocols using either progressively increasing or constant work rates. Whether or not these "nonphysiologic" testing procedures are the most effective way to gain insight into exercise capabilities of children has yet to be determined.

It is hoped that tools such as the direct observational approach will yield new insights into the relationship between real-life patterns of activity and anabolic responses to exercise. For example, using the data obtained from the observational studies, we are currently designing protocols in the laboratory to mimic the naturally occurring work rate patterns, and we will test the hypothesis that the naturally occurring patterns optimize the growth factor response to exercise.

Conclusions

Despite the serious budgetary constraints faced by all biomedical researchers, these are exciting times for researchers interested in investigating exercise responses in children. First, there is a growing appreciation that as biomedical scientists we need to increase our efforts to understand the impact of new information on human health. An individual's ability to engage in physical activity is a crucial element of his or her quality of life, and this is particularly important for children. Second, as I have attempted to outline, new tools exist that will allow us to approach the most fundamental questions surrounding physical activity in children, namely, the relationship between growth and exercise and the maturation of exercise responses at the cellular level. These advances suggest a new phase in our efforts to optimize the role of exercise in children as a possible means of preventing disease later in life and to use exercise in a therapeutic manner in the child with chronic disease.

References

1. Allen, R.E.; Boxhorn, K.K. Regulation of skeletal muscle satellite cell proliferation and differentiation by transforming growth factor beta, insulin like growth factor 1, and fibroblast growth factor. J. Cell. Physiol. 138:311-315; 1989.
2. Anonymous. McDonald's food: the facts. Oak Brook, IL: McDonald's Corporation; 1990; 42-55.
3. Argov, Z.; Bank, W.J.; Maris, J.; Leigh, J.S.J.; Chance, B. Muscle energy metabolism in human phosphofructokinase deficiency as recorded by 31-P nuclear magnetic resonance spectroscopy. Ann. Neurol. 22:46-51; 1987.
4. Armon, Y.; Cooper, D.M.; Flores, R.; Zanconato, S.; Barstow, T.J. Oxygen uptake dynamics during high-intensity exercise in children and adults. J. Appl. Physiol. 70:841-848; 1991.
5. Armon, Y.; Cooper, D.M.; Zanconato, S. Maturation of ventilatory responses to one-minute exercise. Pediatr. Res. 29:362-368; 1991.
6. Astrand, P.-O.; Rodahl, K. Textbook of work physiology. New York: McGraw-Hill; 1977, 389-446.
7. Ayling, C.M.; Moreland, B.H.; Zanelli, J.M.; and Schulster, D. Human growth hormone treatment of hypophysectomized rats increases the proportion of type-1 fibres in skeletal muscle. J. Endocrinol. 123:429-435; 1989.
8. Ballard, F.J.; Read, L.C.; Francis, G.L.; Bagley, C.J.; Wallace, J.C. Binding properties and biological potencies of insulin-like growth factors in L6 myoblasts. Biochem. J. 233:223-230; 1986.
9. Ballar, D.L.; Burke, L.M.; Knudson, D.V.; Olson, J.R.; Montoye, H.J. Comparison of three methods of estimating energy expenditure: Caltrac, heart rate, and video analysis. Res. Q. Exerc. Sport 60:362-368; 1989.
10. Ballor, D.L.; Tommerup, L.J.; Smith, D.B.; Thomas, D.P. Body composition, muscle and fat pad changes following two levels of dietary restriction and/or exercise training in male rats. Int. J. Obes. 14:711-722; 1990.
11. Baranowski, T.; Bouchard, C.; Bar-Or, O.; Bricker, T.; Heath, G.; Kimm, S.Y.; Malina, R.; Obarzanek, E.; Pate, R.; Strong, W.B. Assessment, prevalence, and cardiovascular benefits of physical activity and fitness in youth. Med. Sci. Sports Exerc. 24:S237-S247; 1992.
12. Barnard, R.J. Effects of life-style modification on serum lipids. Arch. Intern. Med. 151:1389-1394; 1991.

13. Barnard, R.J.; Ugianskis, E.J.; Martin, D.A.; Inkeles, S.B. Role of diet and exercise in the management of hyperinsulinemia and associated atherosclerotic risk factors. Am. J. Cardiol. 69:440-440; 1992.
14. Bar-Or, O. Pediatric sports medicine for the practitioner. New York: Springer-Verlag; 1983.
15. Bell, R.D.; MacDougall, J.D.; Billeter, R.; Howald, H. Muscle fiber types and morphometric analysis of skeletal muscle in six-year-old children. Med. Sci. Sports. Exerc. 12:28-31; 1980.
16. Blomqvist, C.G.; Saltin, B. Cardiovascular adaptations to physical training. Annu. Rev. Physiol. 45:169-189; 1983.
17. Boden, G.; Shelmet, J.J.; Gastrointestinal hormones and carcinoid tumors and syndrome. In: Felig, P.; Baxter, J.D.; Broadus, A.E.; Frohman, L.A., eds. New York: McGraw-Hill; 1987, 1629-1662.
18. Booth, F.W.; Gollnick, P.D. Effects of disuse on the structure and function of skeletal muscle. Med. Sci. Sport Exerc. 15:415-420; 1983.
19. Borer, K.T. Characteristics of growth-inducing exercise. Physiol. Behav. 24:713-720; 1980.
20. Borer, K.T.; Kuhns, L.R. Radiographic evidence for acceleration of skeletal growth in adult hamsters by exercise. Growth 41:1-13; 1977.
21. Borer, K.T.; Nicoski, D.R.; Owens, V. Alteration of pulsatile growth hormone secretion by growth-inducing exercise: involvement of endogenous opiates and somatostatin. Endocrinol. 118:844-850; 1986.
22. Cappon, J.P.; Ipp, E.; Brasel, J.A.; Cooper, D.M. Acute effects of high-fat and high-glucose meals on the growth hormone response to exercise. J. Clin. Endocrinol. Metab. 76:1418-1422; 1993.
23. Casaburi, R.; Storer, T.W,; Ben-Dov, I.; Wasserman, K. Effect of endurance training on possible determinants of VO_2 during heavy exercise. J. Appl. Physiol. 62:199-207; 1987.
24. Chance, B.; Leigh, J.S.; Kent, J.; McCully, K. Metabolic control principles and 31-P NMR. Federation Proc. 45:2915-2920; 1986.
25. Cooper, D.M.; Moromisato, D.Y.; Zanconato, S.; Moromisato, M.; Jensen, S.; Brasel, J.A. Effect of growth hormone suppression on exercise training and growth responses in young rats. Pediatr. Rats. 35:223-227; 1994.
26. Cooper, D.M.; Poage, J; Barstow, T.J.; Springer, C. Are obese children truly unfit? Minimizing the confounding effect of body size on the exercise response. J. Pediatr. 116:223-230; 1990.
27. Cooper, D.M.; Weiler-Ravell, D.; Whipp, B.J.; Wasserman, K. Aerobic parameters of exercise as a function of body size during growth in children. J. Appl. Physiol. 56:628-634; 1984.
28. Costin, G.; Kaufman, F.R.; Brasel, J. Growth hormone secretory dynamics in subjects with normal stature. J. Pediatr. 115:537-544; 1989.
29. Cuneo, R.C.; Salomon, F.; Wiles, C.M.; Hesp, R.; Sonksen, P.H. Growth hormone treatment in growth hormone-deficient adults. II. Effects on exercise performance. J. Appl. Physiol. 70:695-700; 1991.
30. DeVol, D.L.: Rotwein, P.; Sadow, J.L.; Novakofski, J.; Bechtel, P.J. Activation of insulin-like growth factor gene expression during work-induced skeletal muscle growth. Am. J. Physiol. 259:E89-E95; 1990.
31. Deyssig, R.; Frisch, H.; Blum, W.F.; Waldhor, T. Effect of growth hormone treatment on hormonal parameters, body composition and strength in athletes. Acta Endocrinologica 128:313-316; 1988.
32. Dunaway, G.A.; Kasten, T.P. Physiological implications of the alteration of 6-phosphofructo-1-kinase isozyme pools during brain development and aging. Brain Res. 456:310-316; 1988.
33. Dunaway, G.A.; Kasten, T.P.; Crabtree, S.; Mhaskar, Y. Age-related changes in subunit composition and regulation of hepatic 6-phosphofructo-1-kinase. Biochem. J. 266:823-827; 1990.
34. Dunaway, G.A.; Kasten, T.P.; Nickols, G.A.; Chesky, J.A. Regulation of skeletal muscle 6-phosphofructo-1-kinase during aging and development. Mech. Ageing Dev. 36:13-23; 1986.

35. Eriksson, B.O.; Gollnick, P.B.; Saltin, B. Muscle metabolism and enzyme activity after training in boys 11-13 years old. Acta Physiol. Scand. 87:485-487; 1973.
36. Eriksson, B.O.; Karlsson, J.; Saltin, B. Muscle metabolites during exercise in pubertal boys. Acta Paediat. Scand. 217 (Suppl.):154-157; 1971.
37. Ewton, D.Z.; Falen, S.L.; Florini, J.R. The type 2 insulin-like growth factor (IGF) receptor has low affinity for IGF-I analogs: pleiotypic actions of IGFs on myoblasts are apparently mediated by the type 1 receptor. Endocrinol. 120:115-123; 1987.
38. Felsing, N.E.; Brasel, J.; Cooper, D.M. Effect of low- and high-intensity exercise on circulating growth hormone in men. J. Clin. Endocrinol. Metab. 75:157-162; 1992.
39. Finkelstein, J.W.; Roffwarg, H.P.; Boyar, R.M.; Kream, J.; Hellman, L. Age-related change in the twenty-four hour spontaneous secretion of growth hormone. J. Clin. endocrinol. Metab. 35:665-670; 1972.
40. Flaim, K.E.; Li, J.B.; Jefferson, L.S. Protein turnover in rat skeletal muscle: effects of hypophysectomy and growth hormone. Am. J. Physiol. 234:E38-E43; 1978.
41. Freeman, W.; Weir, D.C.; Whitehead, J.E.; Rogers, D.I.; Sapiano, S.B.; Floyd, C.A.; Kirk, P.M.; Stalker, C.R.; Field, N.J.; Cayton, R.M. Association between risk factors for coronary heart disease in schoolboys and adult mortality rates in the same localities. Arch. Dis. Child. 65:78-83; 1990.
42. Frohman, L.A. The role of hypothalamic hormones in the control of growth hormone secretion and of growth. Acta Paediatr. Scand. Suppl. 343:3-11; 1988.
43. Galbo, H. Endocrinology and metabolism in exercise. Int. J. Sports Med. 2:203-211; 1981.
44. Goldberg, A.L. Work-induced growth of skeletal muscle in normal and hypophysecto-mized rats. Am. J. Physiol. 213:1193-1198; 1967.
45. Gollnick, P.D.; Ianuzzo, C.D. Hormonal deficiencies and the metabolic adaptations of rats to training. Am. J. Physiol. 223:278-282; 1972.
46. Grindeland, R.E.; Roy, R.; Edgerton, V.R.; Grossman, E.; Rudolph, I.; Pierotti, D.; Goldman, B. Exercise and growth hormone have synergistic effects on skeletal muscle and tibias of suspended rats. FASEB J. 5:A1037(abstract); 1991.
47. Hertz, P.; Silbermann, M.; Even, L.; Hochberg, Z. Effects of sex steroids on the response of cultured rat pituitary cells to growth hormone-releasing hormone and somatostatin. Endocrinol. 125:581-585; 1989.
48. Jahreis, G.; Kauf, E.; Frohner, G.; Schmidt, H.E. Influence of intensive exercise on insulin-like growth factor I, thyroid and steroid hormones in female gymnasts. Growth. Regul. 1:95-99; 1991.
49. Keens, T.G.; Bryan, A.C.; Levison, H.; Ianuzzo, C.D. Developmental pattern of muscle fiber types in human ventilatory muscles. J. Appl. Physiol. 44:909-913; 1978.
50. Kelijman, M.; Frohman, L.A. Beta-adrenergic modulation of growth hormone (GH) autofeedback on sleep-associated and pharmacologically induced GH secretion. J. Clin. Endocrinol. Metab. 69:1187-1194; 1989.
51. Kelijman, M.; Frohman, L.A. The role of the cholinergic pathway in growth hormone feedback. J. Clin. Endocrinol. Metab. 72:1081-1087; 1991.
52. Kelley, P.J.; Eisman, J.A.; Stuard, M.C.; Pocock, N.A.; Sambrook, P.N.; Gwinn, T.H. Somatomedin-C, physical fitness, and bone density. J. Clin. Endocrinol. Metab. 70:718-723; 1990.
53. Kelly, A.; Lyons, G.; Gambki, B.; Rubinstein, N. Influence of testosterone on contractile proteins of the guinea pig temporalis muscle. Adv. Exp. Med. Biol. 182:155-168; 1983.
54. Kelly, P.J.; Eisman, J.A.; Stuard, M.C.; Pocock, N.A.; Sambrook, P.N.; Gwinn, T.H. Somatomedin-C, physical fitness, and bone density. J. Clin. Endocrinol. Metab. 70:718-723; 1990.
55. Kristal, A.R.; Shattuck, A.L.; Henry, H.J. Patterns of dietary behavior associated with selecting diets low in fat: reliability and validity of a behavioral approach to dietary assessment. J. Am. Diet. Assoc. 90:214-220; 1990.
56. Leon, A.S. Physical activity levels and coronary heart disease. Med. Clin. Nor. Am. 69:3-20; 1985.

57. LeRoith, D.; Adamo, M.; Werner, H.; Roberts, C.T., Jr., Insulin-like growth factors and their receptors as growth regulators in normal physiology and pathologic states. Trends Endocrinol. Metab. 2:134-139; 1991.

58. Leung, A.K.; Robson, W.L. Childhood obesity. Postgrad. Med. 87:123-130, 133; 1990.

59. MacIntosh, A.M.; Baldwin, K.M. Effects of repetitive exercise on neonatal rat skeletal muscle oxidative capacity. J. Appl. Physiol. 54:530-535; 1983.

60. Maiter, D.; Underwood, L.E.; Maes, M.; Davenport, M.L.; Ketelslegers, J.M. Different effects of intermittent and continuous growth hormone (GH) administration on serum somatomedin-C/insulin-like growth factor I and liver GH receptors in hypophysecto-mized rats. Endocrinol. 123:1053-1059; 1988.

61. Marshall, W.A.; Tanner, J.M. Puberty. In Falkner, F.; Tanner, J.M.; eds. Human growth. New York: Plenum Press; 1986; 171-210.

62. Mauras, N.; Blizzard, R.M.; Link, K.; Johnson, M.L.; Rogol, A.D.; Veldhuis, J.D. Augmentation of growth hormone secretion during puberty: evidence for a pulse amplitude-modulated phenomenon. J. Clin Endocrinol. Metab. 64:596-601; 1987.

63. Miller, J.D.; Tannenbaum, G.S.; Colle, E.; Guyda, H.J. daytime pulsatile growth hormone secretion. J. Clin Endocrinol. Metab. 55:989-994; 1982.

64. Ornish, D.; Brown, S.E.; Scherwitz, L.W.; Billings, J.H.; Armstrong, W.T.; Ports, T.A.; McLanahan, S.M.; Kirkeeide, R.L.; Brand, R.J.; Gould, K.K. Can lifestyle changes reverse coronary heart disease? Lancet 336:129-133; 1990.

65. Paffenbarger, R.S.; Hyde, R.T.; Wing, A.L.; Hsieh, C.C. Physical activity, all-cause mortality, and longevity of college alumni. N. Engl. J. Med. 314:605-613; 1986.

66. Paterson, D.H.; Cunningham, D.A.; Bumstead, L.A. Recovery O_2 and blood lactic acid: longitudinal analysis in boys aged 11 to 15 years. Eur. J. Appl. Physiol. 55:93-99; 1986.

67. Pearson, A.M. Muscle growth and exercise. Crit. Rev. Food Sci. Nutr. 29:167-196; 1990.

68. Penman, E.; Wass, J.A.H.; Medbak, S.; Morgan, L.; Lewis, J.M.; Besser, G.M.; Rees, L.H. Response of circulating immunoreactive somatostatin to nutritional stimuli in normal subjects. Gastroenterology 81:692-699; 1981.

69. Poehlman, E.T.; Copeland, K.C. Influence of physical activity on insulin-like growth factor-I in healthy younger and older men. J. Clin. Endocrinol. Metab. 71:1468-1473; 1990.

70. Pollock, M.L.; Wilmore, J.H. Exercise in health and disease. Philadelphia: W.B. Saunders Company; 1990; 161-182.

71. Rodrigues, E.A.; Caruana, M.P.; Lahiri, A.; Nabarro, J.D.; Jacobs, H.S.; Raftery, E.B. Subclinical cardiac dysfunction in acromegaly: evidence for a specific disease of heart muscle. Br. Heart J. 62:185-194; 1989.

72. Roston, W.L.; Whipp, B.J.; Davis, J.A.; Cunningham, D.A.; Effros, R.M.; Wasserman, K. Oxygen uptake kinetics and lactate concentrations during exercise in humans. Am. Rev. Respir. Dis. 135:1080-1084; 1987.

73. Saborido, A.; Vila, J.; Molano, F.; Megias, A. Effect of anabolic steroids on mitochon-dria and sarcotubular system of skeletal muscle. J. Appl. Physiol. 70:1038-1043; 1991.

74. Schaible, T.F.; Penpargkul, S.; Scheuer, J. Cardiac responses to exercise training in male and female rats. J. Appl. Physiol. 50:112-117; 1981.

75. Schally, A.V.; Dupont, A.; Arimura, A.; Redding, T.W.; Nishi, N.; Linthicum, G.L.; Schleisinger, D.H. Isolation and structure of somatostatin from porcine hypothalami. Biochem. 15:509-514; 1976.

76. Siegel, R.J.; Fishbein, M.C.; Said, J.W; Fealy, M.; Chai, A.; Rubin, S.A.; Melmed, S. Identification of growth hormone at the myocardial cell surface. Am. J. Cardiovasc. Pathol. 2:345-350; 1989.

77. Smith, A.T.; Clemmons, D.R.; Underwood, L.E.; Ben-Ezra, C.; McMurray, R. The effect of exercise on plasma somatomedin-C/insulinlike growth factor I concentrations. Metabolism 36:533-537; 1987.

78. Spiess, J.; Rivier, J.E.; Rodkey, J.A.; Bennet, C.D.; Vale, W. Isolation and characterization of somatostatin from pigeon pancreas. Proc. Natl. Acad. Sci. USA 76:2974-2978; 1979.
79. Spurr, G.B.; Reina, J.C. Patterns of daily energy expenditure in normal and marginally undernourished school-aged Colombian children. Eur. J. Clin. Nutr. 42:819-834; 1988.
80. Strong, W.B. Physical activity and children. Circulation 81:1697-1701; 1990.
81. Takekura, H.; Yoshioka, T. Different metabolic responses to exercise training programmes in single rat muscle fibers. J. Muscle Res. Cell Motil. 11:105-113; 1990.
82. Telford, R.D. and R.B. Cunningham. Sex, sport, and body-size dependency of hematology in highly trained athletes. Med. Sci Sports Exerc. 23:788-794; 1991.
83. Theintz, G.E.; Howald, H.; Weiss, U.; Sizonenko, P.C. Evidence for a reduction of growth potential in adolescent female gymnasts. J. Pediatr. 122:306-313; 1993.
84. Ulijaszek, S.J. Human energetics methods in biological anthropology. Yearbook of Physical Anthropology 35:215-242; 1992.
85. Wehrenberg, W.B.; Bloch, B.; Phillips, B.J. Antibodies to growth hormone-releasing factor inhibit somatic growth. Endocrinology 115:1218-1120; 1984.
86. Weltman, A.; Weltman, J.Y.; Schurrer, R.; Evans, W.S.; Veldhuis, J.D.; Rogol, A.D. Endurance training amplifies the pulsatile release of growth hormone: effects of training intensity. J. Appl. Physiol. 72:2188-2196; 1992.
87. Yarasheski, K.E.; Campbell, J.A.; Smith, K.; Rennie, M.J.; Holloszy, J.O.; Bier, D.M. Effect of growth hormone and resistance exercise on muscle growth in young men. Am. J. Physiol. 262:E261-E267; 1992.
88. Yarasheski, K.E.; Zachwieja, J.J.; Angelopoulos, T.J.; Bier, D.M. Short-term growth hormone treatment does not increase muscle protein synthesis in experienced weight lifters. J. Appl. Physiol. 74:3073-3076; 1993.
89. Zanconato, S.; Buchthal, S.; Barstow, T.J.; Cooper, D.M. 31P-magnetic resonance spectroscopy of leg muscle metabolism during exercise in children and adults. J. Appl. Physiol. 74:2214-2218; 1993.
90. Zanconato, S.; Cooper, D.M.; Armon, Y. Oxygen cost and oxygen uptake dynamics and recovery with one minute of exercise in children and adults. J. Appl. Physiol. 71:993-998; 1991.
91. Zanconato, S.; Moromisato, D.Y.; Moromisato, M.Y.; Woods, J.; Brasel, J.A.; LeRoith, D.; Roberts, Jr., C.T.; Cooper, D.M. Effect of training and growth hormone suppression on insulin-like growth factor-I mRNA in young rats. J. Appl. Physiol. 76:2204-2209; 1994.

Part I

Endocrine Aspects of Pediatric Exercise

Chapter 2

The Reproductive System and Physical Activity in Adolescents

Anne B. Loucks, PhD

Little research has been done on the reproductive endocrinology of adolescents who exercise, and less research has been done on boys than on girls. At present, most of our perspective on the influence of physical activity on the reproductive system in adolescents is extrapolated from information gathered in studies of adults and animals. These extrapolations should be treated with caution because of known and unknown species and age differences in reproductive function. Because of the paucity of data, this review makes no remarks at all about boys.

The cessation of menses (monthly vaginal bleeding episodes) is known as amenorrhea, and it occurs in many physically active women. Amenorrhea is associated with a reduction in estrogen levels, and estrogen is critical for bone health. Consequently, the American Academy of Pediatrics recommends prompt medical intervention after the onset of amenorrhea in physically active girls to preserve normal bone development and to prevent skeletal demineralization (1).

Preliminary results of research performed to date indicate that the factor affecting reproductive function in physically active girls and women is daily energy availability. Energy availability is defined behaviorally as dietary energy intake minus exercise energy expenditure. Humans appear to share this dependence of reproductive function on energy availability with all other mammals (9,34), and females appear to require more energy availability than males (7).

The energy availability hypothesis would be consistent with a higher prevalence of reproductive disorders in endurance rather than explosive sports, in activities in which leanness is perceived to promote success, and whenever dietary energy intake is reduced while exercise energy expenditure is increased. If subsequent research proves the energy availability hypothesis to be true, physically active women and girls may be able to prevent or to reverse reproductive disorders by dietary reform without moderating their exercise regimen.

The Adolescent Reproductive System

Figure 2.1 schematically represents the different states of the female reproductive system during a woman's lifetime. The adulthood state is the only one in which

Reproductive States

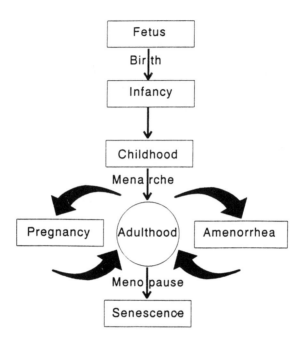

Figure 2.1.   The distinct states in which the reproductive system functions during the human female life cycle. Adulthood is the only state during which regular menses occur. Birth is the only transition that can be explained (by loss of the mother's endocrine environment).

menses occur, but part or all of the reproductive system is highly active in all of the other states except childhood and amenorrhea. We do not yet understand the mechanism that switches the reproductive system from the adulthood to the amenorrhea state, and we do not understand the mechanism of most of the other switches either.

The transition from the childhood to the adulthood state of the reproductive system occurs over several years during adolescence (16,25,31,33). In the population of girls, variation in the average length of the interval between menses decreases markedly during the 5 years after the first menses (menarche) (31). Within individual girls, variation of the length of the interval between menses also decreases markedly over this time (31). Even longer—10 years—is required for the prevalence of anovulatory menstrual cycles (cycles with menses but without the release of an ovum) to decline from over 50% in the first year after menarche to the normal adult prevalence of 5% or less (33). Meanwhile, it takes 12 years for the prevalence of short luteal phase (the interval between the release of an ovum and the next menses) to decline from over 50% to the normal adult prevalence of 10% (33).

These high variabilities in menstrual cycle length and high prevalences of anovulation and short luteal phase (which are normal in adolescence but abnormal in adults) make reproductive research in adolescents especially difficult to control and the effects of experimental treatments especially difficult to distinguish from random variation.

Reproductive Disorders in Adolescent Athletes

Three types of reproductive disorders are of concern in adolescent athletes: delayed menarche, luteal suppression, and amenorrhea.

Delayed Menarche

Retrospective studies have reported that menarche occurred later in athletes than in non-athletes and later in athletes who began training before rather than after menarche (22,30). Such observations have led some researchers to conclude that a young girl's participation in sports delays menarche, and that, therefore, young girls should not participate in sports.

Observational data cannot establish causality, however, and alternative interpretations of the data have been offered. Girls who mature early may be socialized away from athletics, while girls who mature later may continue to participate in athletics because the pre-menarcheal body type favors athletic success (22).

In addition, computer simulation of the retrospective sampling process has shown this process to be inherently biased when it is used to seek associations between events such as the age of menarche and the age at initiation of athletic training (30). Retrospective sampling will find the age of menarche to be later in girls who begin training before rather than after menarche, even in a population of girls among whom there is no relationship whatsoever between these events. Thus, the available observational human data is unconvincing on the question of whether participation in athletics delays menarche.

Controlled animal experiments have provided stronger evidence. Figure 2.2 shows the suppression of luteinizing hormone pulsatility that occurs in rats subjected to periods of prolonged exercise (9,23,24). Such experimental data do not demonstrate that exercise per se delays reproductive development, however, because the delay may have been caused by the means used to induce the animals to exercise. For example, in studies that require animals to exercise for longer and longer periods in order to receive food rewards (23,24), the influence of exercise is confounded by that of diet. Figure 2.3 shows that dietary restriction alone suppresses luteinizing hormone pulsatility and delays the occurrence of the first ovulation in rats, and that this effect is unrelated to body weight (8,9). The data from experiments in which animals exercise for food rewards actually suggest that the factor influencing reproductive development and function may be energy availability, and that exercise itself may have no influence on reproductive function at all beyond its impact on energy availability.

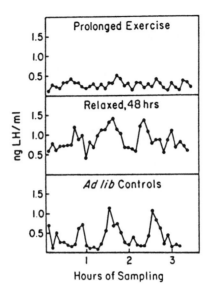

Figure 2.2.   Luteinizing hormone concentrations in female rats. Top: After a prolonged exercise training program (in which animals were required to exercise for longer and longer periods to receive food rewards). Middle: 48 hours after the exercise training requirement for food rewards was relaxed. Bottom: In a matched group of rats who were given free access to running wheels but not forced to run and who ate ad libitum. Luteinizing hormone pulsatility was suppressed in rats subjected to prolonged exercise (from 9).

Luteal Suppression

Many cases of infertility are attributed to an asymptomatic reproductive disorder known as luteal phase deficiency in which there is not enough time after an ovum is released for it to be fertilized and to become implanted into the uterine endometrium before the endometrium is sloughed off in the next menses, or in which progesterone secretion is not adequate for supporting an endometrium receptive to implantation.

Endocrine studies in adults have found luteal phases to be shorter and progesterone levels lower in regularly menstruating competitive (21) and recreational (14) athletes than in regularly menstruating sedentary women (Figure 2.4). Luteal phases were shorter in the athletes even though their menstrual cycles occurred at intervals of approximately 28 days, as did those in the sedentary women, indicating that the luteal suppression was specifically associated with athletics.

Similar data have been presented on adolescent swimmers (4), although these data were confounded by differences in menstrual cycle length. The 21-day menstrual cycles of the four adolescent swimmers were considerably shorter than the 28-day menstrual cycles of their four age-matched controls. We do not know whether the luteal phases of the swimmers were shorter than those in girls with

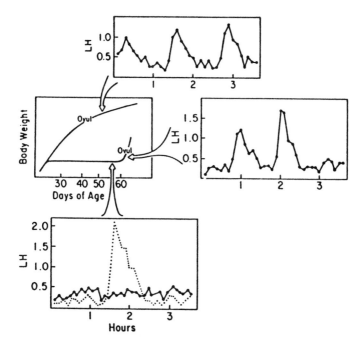

Figure 2.3. Luteinizing hormone concentration in female rats. Left: Body weights in two groups of rats at peripubertal ages. One group ate ad libitum, gained weight, and achieved their first ovulation at approximately 42 days of age. Restricting the diet of the second group until they were more than 60 days of age prevented them from gaining weight or experiencing their first ovulation. Permitting the second group to then eat ad libitum resulted in their experiencing their first ovulation within 12 hours, before their body weight or composition had changed significantly. Top: Luteinizing hormone pulsatility in fully fed rats shortly after their first ovulation. Bottom: Absence of luteinizing hormone pulses in underfed rats more than 10 days after the age at first ovulation in fully fed rats, except immediately after a meal (dotted line). Right: Luteinizing hormone pulsatility in underfed rats between the time they were permitted to eat ad libitum and the occurrence of their first ovulation (from 9).

similar menstrual cycle lengths, or whether the shorter length of the menstrual cycle in the swimmers was caused by their participation in swimming.

Nor do we know whether the prevalence of luteal suppression in adolescent and adult athletes is higher than that in the general population of girls and women, although available data from small studies would suggest that the prevalence among athletes is very high. We also do not know the clinical significance of luteal suppression in athletes. It might be an intermediate condition between menstrual regularity and amenorrhea, which would progress to amenorrhea if training were intensified. This interpretation is unlikely, though, because little difference has been found between the training regimens of regularly menstruating and amenorrheic athletes.

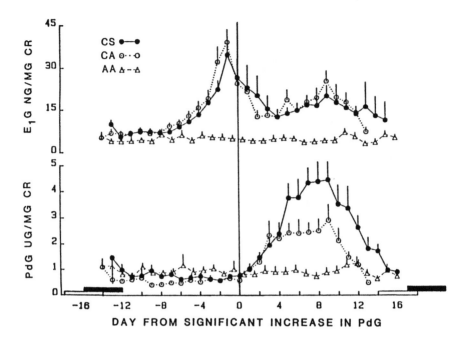

Figure 2.4. Estrone glucuronide (E_1G) and pregnanediol glucuronide (PdG) concentrations over an entire menstrual cycle in regularly menstruating athletes (CA) and sedentary women (CS) and over a period of 30 days in amenorrheic athletes (AA). Menstrual cycles in CA and CS were equal in length, but the luteal phase in CA was shorter and PdG levels lower in CA. The usual cyclic elevations of E_1G and PdG levels were completely suppressed in AA, indicating a complete absence of ovarian follicular development, ovulation, and luteal function (21).

Alternatively, luteal suppression may represent the end point of a successful acclimation to athletic training. Although luteal suppression may be detrimental to the health of athletes, we do not have any data to support that contention. Nothing is known about their fertility.

Another possibility is that some individuals may be genetically more susceptible to reproductive disorders than others, such that the same athletic regimen may lead to amenorrhea in more susceptible and to luteal suppression in less susceptible individuals. Only extensive, well-controlled experiments will resolve this issue.

Amenorrhea

Many surveys have established that the prevalence of amenorrhea is much higher among physically active adult women than in the general population. The prevalence has been reported to be higher than 50% in some groups (35) compared to less than 5% among the general population (2,27,29). Data on the prevalence of amenorrhea among adolescents are lacking, but we have no reason to believe that such data would differ, except in finding a somewhat higher prevalence in the general population of girls than in the general population of women.

Studies in adults have revealed the endocrine alterations in amenorrheic athletes to be extensive. Disruption of the pulsatile secretion of gonadotropin releasing hormone from the hypothalamus of the brain [and thereby of the pulsatile secretion of luteinizing hormone by the pituitary (21,32)] results in the complete suppression of follicular development, ovulation and luteal function, and chronically low estrogen and progesterone levels (21) (Figure 2.4). Prolactin (19) and thyroid hormones (20,26) are also suppressed, while cortisol (21) and melatonin (15) levels are elevated.

Recently, lower estradiol and thyroid hormone levels have been reported in adolescent amenorrheic runners than in regularly menstruating age-matched and weight-matched runners and sedentary girls (3).

Such observational endocrine data suggest that exercise per se is not what disrupts reproductive function in girls and women. Indeed, experiments that have gradually intensified exercise training without controlling dietary intake have not induced amenorrhea in women (5,6,10,28). Amenorrhea has been induced in women, however, when the exercise and dietary regimens are both controlled (11). Furthermore, exercise-induced amenorrhea has been reversed in monkeys by dietary supplementation without moderation of the exercise regimen (12). Thus, an accumulating weight of evidence indicates that the combination of exercise energy expenditure and dietary energy intake is what disrupts reproductive function in physically active girls and women.

Bone Loss in Amenorrheic Athletes

The question of whether athletic amenorrhea is desirable or undesirable and healthy or unhealthy was resolved several years ago with the demonstration that amenorrheic athletes have lower trabecular bone mass than regularly menstruating athletes and sedentary women, and that they are losing bone over time (see 13). As a result, the American Academy of Pediatrics recognizes athletic amenorrhea as a pathology requiring prompt and aggressive treatment, including the administration of low-dose oral contraceptives for steroid supplementation to prevent bone loss (1).

Current Research

Currently, experimental research focuses on two hypotheses about the mechanism of reproductive disorders in physically active women. One hypothesis holds that exercise per se constitutes a stress that, by activating the adrenal axis, disrupts hypothalamic regulation of reproductive function. In this regard, exercise is thought to resemble electroshock. The other current hypothesis is that the expenditure of energy during exercise reduces the amount of energy available for other physiological functions, and that female mammals sacrifice reproductive function whenever a certain critical amount of energy is unavailable on a day-to-day basis.

Until recently, exercise stress and energy availability had been confounded in all human and animal experiments investigating the influence of exercise on reproductive function. Figure 2.5 illustrates an experimental design recently employed to independently control exercise stress and energy availability in a study of thyroid metabolism in regularly menstruating women. The results shown in Figure 2.6 demonstrate that exercise per se has no influence upon thyroid metabolism beyond its influence on energy availability (17). Related studies have found the suppression of thyroid metabolism occurs at a particular threshold of energy availability in exercising women (18). Effects on other metabolic hormones are similar (data not yet published). Studies of the effects of energy availability on reproductive hormones in exercising women are ongoing. Such controlled prospective experiments for distinguishing the independent effects of exercise and energy availability on the development and regulation of the adolescent reproductive system have not been performed to date.

EXPERIMENTAL DESIGN

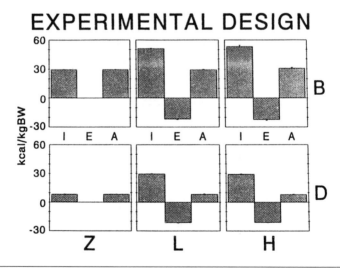

Figure 2.5. An experiment design for independently controlling exercise and energy availability. Six groups performed combinations of no (Z), 40% VO₂max (L), or 70% VO₂max (H) aerobic exercise and received an energy availability that was either balanced (B) or deprived (D). Energy availability (in kilocalories per kilogram of body weight) (A) was defined as dietary energy intake (I) minus exercise energy expenditure (E). The high degree of control on the administered I and E and on the resulting A is reflected by the small standard error bars in each histogram (17).

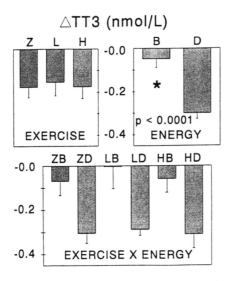

Figure 2.6.   Changes in serum triiodothyronine (TT_3) in regularly menstruating women resulting from 4 days of the treatments shown in Figure 2.5. Dietary supplementation prevented the suppressive effect of exercise energy expenditure on TT_3 levels. Bottom: Reductions in TT_3 in each treatment combination. Top left: Reductions in TT_3 were similar regardless of whether subjects exercised at a high intensity (H), low intensity (L), or not at all (Z). Top right: Reductions in TT_3 occurred selectively in the groups with inadequate energy availability (17).

References

1. American Academy of Pediatrics Committee on Sports Medicine. Amenorrhea in adolescent athletes. Pediatrics 84:394-395; 1989.
2. Bachman, G.A.; Kemmann, E. Prevalence of oligomenorrhea and amenorrhea in a college population. Am. J. Obstet. Gynecol. 144:98-102; 1982.
3. Baer, J.T. Endocrine parameters in amenorrheic and eumenorrheic adolescent female runners. Int. J. Sports Med. 14:191-195; 1993.
4. Bonen, A.; Belcastro, A.N.; Ling, W.Y.; Simpson, A.A. Profiles of selected hormones during menstrual cycles of teenage athletes. J. Appl. Physiol.: Respirat. Environ. Exercise Physiol. 50:545-551; 1981.
5. Bonen, A. Recreational exercise does not impair menstrual cycles: a prospective study. Int. J. Sports Med. 13:110-120, 1992.
6. Boyden T.W.; Pamenter, P.W.; Stanforth, P.R.; Rotkis, T.C.; Wilmore, J.H. Impaired gonadotropin responses to gonadotropin-releasing hormone stimulation in endurance-trained women. Fertil. Steril. 41:359-363; 1984.
7. Bronson, F.H. Mammalian reproduction: an ecological perspective. Biol. Reprod. 32:1-26; 1985.
8. Bronson, F.H. Food-restricted, prepubertal, female rats: rapid recovery of luteinizing hormone pulsing with excess food, and full recovery of pubertal development with gonadotropin-releasing hormone. Endocrinology 118:2483-2487; 1986.
9. Bronson, F.H.; Manning, J. Food consumption, prolonged exercise, and LH secretion in the peripubertal female rat. In: Pirke, K.M.; Wuttke, W.; Schweiger, U., eds. The

menstrual cycle and its disorders: influences of nutrition, exercise and neurotransmitters. Berlin: Springer-Verlag; 1989; 42-49.

10. Bullen, B.A.; Skrinar, G.S.; Beitins, I.Z.; Carr, D.B.; Reppert, S.M.; Dotson, C.O.; Fencl, M.de M.; Gervino, E.V.; McArthur, J.W. Endurance training effects on plasma hormonal responsiveness and sex hormone excretion. J. Appl. Physiol.: Respirat. Environ. Exercise Physiol. 56:1453-1463; 1984.

11. Bullen, B.A.; Skrinar, G.S.; Beitins, I.Z.; von Mering, G.; Turnbull, B.A.; McArthur, J.W. Induction of menstrual disorders by strenuous exercise in untrained women. N. Engl. J. Med. 312:1349-1353; 1985.

12. Cameron, J.L.; Nosbisch, C.; Helmreich, D.L.; Parfitt, D.B. Reversal of exercise-induced amenorrhea in female cynomolgus monkeys (Macaca fascicularis) by increasing food intake. Proceedings of The Endocrine Society 72nd Annual Meeting; 1990; 285; Abstract 1042.

13. Drinkwater, B.L. Amenorrhea, body weight, and osteoporosis. In: Brownell, K.D.; Rodin, J.; Wilmore, J.H., eds. Eating, body weight and performance in athletes. Philadelphia: Lea & Febiger; 1992: 235-247.

14. Ellison, P.T.; Lager, C. Moderate recreational running is associated with lowered salivary progesterone profiles in women. Am. J. Obstet. Gyneco. 154:1000-1003; 1986.

15. Laughlin, G.A., Loucks, A.B.; Yen, S.S.C. Marked augmentation of nocturnal melatonin secretion in amenorrheic athletes but not in cycling athletes: unaltered by opioidergic or dopaminergic blockade. J. Clin. Endocrinol. Metab. 73:1321-1326; 1991.

16. Loucks, A.B. Athletics and menstrual dysfunction in young women. In: Gisolfi, C.V.; Lamb, D.R., eds. Perspectives in exercise science and sports medicine. Volume 2: Youth, Exercise, and Sport. Indianapolis: Benchmark Press; 1989: 513-538.

17. Loucks, A.B.; Callister, R. Induction and prevention of low-T_3 syndrome in exercising women. Am. J. Physiol. 264 (Regulatory Integrative Comp. Physiol. 33):R924-R930; 1993.

18. Loucks, A.B.; Heath, E.M. Induction of low-T_3 syndrome in exercising women occurs at a threshold of energy availability. Am. J. Physiol. 266 (Regulatory Integrative Comp. Physiol. 35):R817-R823, 1994.

19. Loucks, A.B.; Laughlin, G.L. Hypoprolactinemia in amenorrheic athletes: 24-hour profiles and responses to thyrotropin-releasing hormone and metoclopramide. Proceedings of the 1992 Endocrine Society Meeting; 1992; 67; Abstract #61.

20. Loucks, A.B.; Laughlin, G.A.; Mortola, J.F.; Girton, L.; Nelson, J.C.; Yen, S.S.C. Hypothalamic-pituitary-thyroidal function in eumenorrheic and amenorrheic athletes. J. Clin. Endocrinol. Metab. 75:514-518; 1992.

21. Loucks, A.B.; Mortola, J.F.; Girton, L.; Yen, S.S.C. Alterations in the hypothalamic-pituitary-ovarian and hypothalamic-pituitary-adrenal axes in athletic women. J. Clin. Endocrinol. Metab. 68:402-411; 1989.

22. Malina, R.M. Menarche in athletes: a synthesis and hypothesis. Ann. Hum. Biol. 10:1-24; 1983.

23. Manning, J.M.; Bronson, F.H. Effects of prolonged exercise on puberty and luteinizing hormone secretion in female rats. Am. J. Physiol. 257 (Regulatory Integrative Comp. Physiol. 26):R1359-R1364; 1989.

24. Manning, J.M.; Bronson, F.H. Suppression of puberty in rats by exercise: effects on hormone levels and reversal with GnRH infusion. Am. J. Physiol. 260 (Regulatory Integrative Comp. Physiol. 29):R717-R723; 1991.

25. Metcalf, M.G.; Skidmore, D.S.; Lowry, G.F.; Mackenzie, J.A. Incidence of ovulation in the years after menarche. J. Endocr. 97:213-219; 1983.

26. Myerson, M.; Gutin, B.; Warren, M.P.; May, M.T.; Contento, I.; Lee, M.; Pi-Sunyer, F.X.; Pierson, R.N. Jr.; Brooks-Gunn, J. Resting metabolic rate and energy balance in amenorrheic and eumenorrheic runners. Med. Sci. Sports Exerc. 23:15-22; 1991.

27. Pettersson, F.; Fries, H.; Nillius, S.J. Epidemiology of secondary amenorrhea. I. Incidence and prevalence rates. Am. J. Obstet. Gynecol. 117:80-86; 1973.

28. Rogol, A.D.; Weltman, A.; Weltman, J.Y.; Seip, R.L.; Snead, D.B.; Levine, S.; Haskvitz, E.M.; Thompson, D.L.; Schurrer, R.; Dowling, E.; Walberg-Rankin, J.; Evans, W.S.; Veldhuis, J.D. Durability of the reproductive axis in eumenorrheic women during 1 yr of endurance training. J. Appl. Physiol. 72:1571-1580; 1992.
29. Singh, K.B. Menstrual disorders in college students. Am. J. Obstet. Gynecol. 140:299-302; 1981.
30. Stager, J.M.; Wigglesworth, J.K.; Hatler, L.K. Interpreting the relationship between age of menarche and prepubertal training. Med. Sci. Sports Exerc. 22:54-58; 1990.
31. Treolar, A.E.; Boynton, R.E.; Behn, B.G.; Brown, B.W. Variation of human menstrual cycle through reproductive life. Int. J. Fertil. 12:77-126; 1967.
32. Veldhuis, J.D.; Evans, W.S.; Demers, L.M.; Thorner, M.O.; Wakat, D.; Rogol, A.D. Altered neuroendocrine regulation of gonadotropin secretion in women distance runners. J. Clin. Endocrinol. Metab. 61:557-563, 1985.
33. Vollman, R.F. The menstrual cycle. In: Friedman, E.A., ed. Major problems in obstetrics and gynecology. Vol. 7. Philadelphia: W.B. Saunders; 1977.
34. Wade, G.N.; Schneider, J.E. Metabolic fuels and reproduction in female mammals. Neurosci. Biobehav. Rev. 16:235-272; 1992.
35. Warren, M.P.; Brooks-Gunn, J.; Hamilton, L.H.; Warren, L.F.; Hamilton, W.G. Scoliosis and fractures in young ballet dancers. N. Engl. J. Med. 314:1348-1353; 1986.

Chapter 3

Growth and Growth Hormone Secretion at Puberty in Males

Alan D. Rogol, MD, PhD

Introduction

Continued growth of a child is generally considered a sign of health and well-being. How the child compares with his/her peers can be derived by comparing that child with the normal group represented on a standard growth chart. By definition, *normal* (physiologic) growth encompasses the 95% confidence interval for a specific group of subjects. A majority of children with a normal growth pattern, but who remain below the lower 2.5 percentile (approximately −2 SD), also will be otherwise normal; however, the farther below the −2 SD level, the more likely the child has a condition that is keeping him/her from reaching the genetically defined final height.

Normal Growth

Normal variants of growth were found in 82% of children with height less than the third percentile and in 50% of children whose height was more than 3 SD below the mean for chronologic age in a population study from Newcastle-upon-Tyne (6). Even at a university referral service virtually one-half of children evaluated for height SD score below −2 SD had a physiologic variant as the "explanation" for their short stature (3). On the other hand, growth failure at any point other than full maturity must be considered pathologic, no matter what point on the growth curve a particular child has achieved. Any single point on the growth chart is not very informative. When several growth points are plotted, however, it should become apparent whether the child's growth is average, a variant of normal, or pathologic. The point at which a child is placed at any given time can be related to the *height age*—the age at which the child's height would be at the 50th percentile. The height age is obtained from the growth chart by drawing a line parallel to the chronological age axis from the child's plotted point to the 50th percentile. The height age then is determined along the chronological age scale at the intersection of the drawn line and the 50th percentile. It is an indication of the mean age of children of that height. Most children who have abnormalities of growth will have retarded height age compared to chronological age, although a few will demonstrate accelerated growth.

The skeletal or dental maturation may be used to assess a child's developmental status. The method of Greulich and Pyle (2) has proved to be a convenient screening procedure. A single radiograph of the left hand and wrist is obtained, and the developmental maturation (bone age) is compared to that of children of normal stature by using an atlas. Because girls are more developmentally advanced at any chronological age than boys are, there are separate standards for girls and boys.

The normal growth curve is characterized by rapid fetal growth with a peak intrauterine growth velocity at 4 mo gestational age, followed by marked deceleration of growth after birth and then a period of relatively slow but constant growth during childhood and a rapid growth spurt at puberty falling to zero velocity as the epiphyses close. Rough guidelines for normal growth are 25 cm, but always at a decreasing rate during the first year of life, 12.5 cm the second year, and from the end of the second year until the onset of puberty, the normal child typically grows between 5 and 7.5 cm per year.

A small percentage of normal children will grow at a rate of approximately 4 cm per year, but the minimal normal growth velocity is generally accepted as 5 cm per year. Although size at birth is correlated to intrauterine environment as well as genetic (polygenic) factors, between birth and 2 years of age infants make adjustments for these maternal factors and increase or decrease the growth velocity in relationship to the norm to reach the genetically-determined growth potential (16). After 2 years of age, children tend to follow this growth channel. Any deviation from this percentile on the growth curve may indicate a pathologic process interfering with normal growth. A simple rule of thumb is that a child grows 10 inches (25 cm) in the first year, half that (5 inches, 12.5 cm) in the second year, and half that (2-1/2 inches, 6.4 cm) each year thereafter until puberty. An average newborn measures 20 inches (51 cm); an average 1-year-old measures 30 inches (76 cm); a 2-year-old, 35 inches (89 cm); a 4-year-old, 40 inches (102 cm); and an 8-year-old, 50 inches (127 cm). The nadir in growth rate, the so-called preadolescent "dip," is often exaggerated in teenagers with delayed puberty. The growth rate may decelerate to below 4 cm per year, occurring just before the beginning of the adolescent growth spurt at the appropriate biological (skeletal) age.

Growth Hormone

Growth hormone is released in an episodic, burst-like (pulsatile) manner throughout the day, but especially following the onset of slow-wave sleep (stages 3 and 4). Its secretion is controlled by two hypothalamic peptide hormones: growth hormone releasing hormone (GHRH) and growth hormone release inhibiting hormone (somatostatin). Additional loci of control include brain neurotransmitters and neuropeptides, insulin-like growth factor-I [IGF-I (long-loop feedback)],

GH itself (short-loop feedback), and GH RH and somatostatin (ultra short-loop feedback). In addition, metabolic substrates (e.g., glucose and fatty acids) take part in the regulation of growth hormone secretion. It is the quantity and pattern of circulating GH that ultimately permits the animal to grow, although genetic, disease, and especially nutritional factors may override any straightforward relationship between GH secretion and linear growth.

Control of Growth Hormone Release

Central Neurotransmitters

Virtually all of the known (classical) neurotransmitters including the catecholamines, the cholinergic, serotoninergic, opiatergic, and γ-aminobutyric acid systems have been implicated in the control of GH synthesis and release. Few act directly at the pituitary to effect GH synthesis or release, but they generally act indirectly, especially at the hypothalamus, to modulate GHRH and somatostatin synthesis or release.

Growth Hormone Releasing Hormones, Somatostatin, and Growth Hormone Releasing Peptide

Growth hormone releasing hormone, long postulated but only recently discovered, has been isolated, purified, and sequenced. The majority of GHRH-containing neurons are located in the ventral medial and arcuate nuclei of the medial basal hypothalamus. Fibers from these nuclei project to the hypophysiotropic area of the median eminence.

Somatostatin is a 14 amino acid cyclic peptide that inhibits TSH as well as GH secretion from the pituitary and has a great number of other effects on the brain, the endocrine and exocrine pancreas and, especially, the rest of the gastrointestinal tract. Its major site of synthesis (for control of the anterior pituitary) is the periventricular nucleus, although it is widely distributed in other brain areas. Growth hormone enhances the expression of the structural gene for somatostatin and thus affects the synthesis as well as the release of this neurohormone.

The episodic secretion of GH depends upon the specific rhythms of GHRH and somatostatin. The release of these neurohormones is virtually 180° out of phase. A pulse of GH is produced when somatostatin tone is low while GHRH is released (12a). Such reciprocal changes are responsible for the ultradian pattern of GH secretion. The data are consistent with the hypothesis that somatostatin secretion sets the timing (frequency and duration) and GHRH sets the magnitude of GH release.

Growth hormone releasing peptide (GHRP), the synthetic hexapeptide: his-D Trp-Ala-Trp-D Phe-Lys-NH$_2$, specifically stimulates GH release in children and adults when administered by the intravenous, subcutaneous, intranasal, and oral routes. It appears to be synergistic with the GHRH and may act as a functional antagonist to somatostatin.

Pituitary

Growth hormone participates in its own feedback control of release. An auto-feedback mechanism had been proposed for many years, but it is only recently that some of the details of this mechanism have been amenable to testing. Growth hormone administration to humans and animals has been followed within several hours (but not less) by blunted serum GH responses to provocative stimuli, diminished pulsatile GH release, or diminished pituitary GH content. Since circulating levels of IGF-I were also increased, the precise mechanism, long-loop versus short-loop feedback, could not be determined. The mode of delivery of GH also may be a critical parameter. The pulsatile intravenous administration of GH is more efficacious than continuous administration of the same quantity to raise IGF-I mRNA levels in skeletal tissues (e.g., skeletal muscle and rib growth plates). The liver reacted differently, however, in that both continuous and pulsatile GH infusion elevated the amount of IGF-I mRNA in an indistinguishable manner. The pituitary expresses the IGF-I gene, suggesting that IGF-I may regulate GH secretion by an autocrine/paracrine mechanism as well as in the usual endocrine manner. Many metabolic substrates also are altered by GH administration. Short- and long-term studies have suggested different mechanisms. At present it appears that in the longer time (i.e., more than 12h), GH inhibits its own synthesis and release by augmenting circulating IGF-I concentrations acting to decrease GHRH secretion and increase somatostatin release. Shorter-term inhibition is probably mediated by such metabolic substrates as glucose and free fatty acids. However, alterations in adenylate cyclase activity (GHRH activates adenylate cyclase via G_s and somatostatin inhibits this enzyme via G_i), calcium fluxes, and phosphatidylinositol turnover interact strongly with these substrates.

Peripheral Feedback Signals

Insulin-like growth factor-I substantially inhibits GH synthesis and release by the long-loop feedback mechanism noted previously. IGF-I specifically inhibits GH mRNA synthesis and GH release both in the basal state and after stimulation with GHRH. In animals, antibodies against IGF-I receptors can block the growth-promoting actions of GH on its target cells, strongly suggesting an indirect role for GH in growth. IGF-I circulates bound to several carrier proteins, which prolong the half-life of this growth factor. The predominant 150-kD form is GH dependent. The physiologic role of these various proteins has not been clarified fully: They may be relatively unimportant because of extensive local growth factor synthesis, or they may represent a storage depot or a clearance pathway.

Free fatty acids and glucose interact with other modulators to augment or inhibit GH secretion. Administration of free fatty acids or the increase in free fatty acids following GH administration reduce the subsequent GH response to GHRH, catecholamines, physical exercise, and other stimuli.

Other nutritional factors doubtlessly are involved. Amino acids serve not only as building blocks for muscle protein (anabolic action of GH), but also as precursors for the synthesis of some of the neurotransmitters that control the synthesis and release of GHRH and somatostatin. In adult volunteers, fasting quickly causes an increase in GH concentrations and a decrease in IGF-I levels. Refeeding is associated with a return to normal of both GH and IGF-I levels. The nitrogen and energy contents of the refeeding diet influence the return to physiologic circulating GH and IGF-I levels. Physical and psychological stress elevate GH levels in humans, but the detailed mechanisms have not been described, especially for the latter. Insulin-like growth factor-I levels rise two- to threefold with the more advanced pubertal stages in boys and girls before diminishing again to adult levels. The pubertal rise is well-correlated with the sex-hormone-mediated augmentation of GH secretion and accelerated growth in the later stages of puberty. Individuals over age 50 have declining levels of IGF-I. There is, however, the intriguing possibility of interplay between the endocrine actions of circulating GH and IGF-I and the paracrine/autocrine actions consistent with the dual effector hypothesis of GH action. The local effects are probably more important in those tissues with high local IGF-I gene expression (mainly mesenchymal). These nutritionally, stress, and sex-hormone mediated effects probably are linked at multiple hierarchical levels permitting interactions among them in addition to their individual effects.

Growth Hormone Secretory Dynamics: Developmental Aspects

At all ages—fetal through adult—growth hormone is secreted in an intermittent, pulsatile pattern. During childhood there are apparently no differences between boys and girls, although several investigators have noted a significant positive correlation between physical stature and circulating levels for GH, or between the amount of GH secreted per day and the height of the children (1). In addition, Hindmarsh and colleagues (2a) reported a relationship between height velocity and mean 24h growth levels in short prepubertal children. When Kerrigan and colleagues (4,5) investigated this issue in more detail in short boys, they found no significant differences in pulsatile GH release between normally growing prepubertal boys and the short subjects; however, a subset of short prepubertal boys with significantly delayed bone age had subnormal GH release as indicated by low sum of GH pulse areas and sum of GH pulse amplitudes. The finding of significant correlation in all subjects between growth velocity and the sum of GH pulse amplitudes is important, because the results are compatible with the hypothesis that alterations of amplitude-modulated GH release underlie the pathophysiology of suboptimal growth in some short, prepubertal children.

Variability in Growth Hormone Secretion

Reliability of Physiologic Monitoring of Growth Hormone Release

This axis can be evaluated physiologically (daily secretory pattern, exercise) or pharmacologically (GH response to neurotransmitters, certain amino acids, insulin-induced hypoglycemia, etc.). For the present purpose I shall focus on the daily secretory pattern. The method of sampling (continuous vs. intermittent), its frequency, methods of assay, and especially analysis of the profiles are critical, but will not be discussed here. The assessment of hormone secretory profiles has been used to determine alterations within the physiologic range or as evidence for the effects of pharmacologic intervention. The comparison of individual hormone concentration profiles, however, is based upon the assumption of strict reliability. For GH we have assessed the reliability of the concentration versus time profiles in children (two more 12h or 24h profiles in the same state of sexual development) and adult women (two 12h or 24h profiles during the early follicular phase of the menstrual cycle). For the 12h profiles (21 pairs) or 24h profiles (18 pairs) in the women, no significant mean differences were observed between studies for any parameter of pulsatile release (Weltman et al., unpublished observations); however, the reliability as indicated by the correlation coefficients for specific parameters of pulsatile release varied from $r=0.25$ (nadir concentration) and 0.36 for peak frequency to $r=0.66$ (integrated concentration) and $r=0.71$ (incremental peak amplitude). These data suggest a large degree of biologic variability at least over short (24h) sampling intervals for some of the parameters of pulsatile GH release (e.g., number of peaks), but moderate to good stability in others (e.g., incremental peak increase and integrated concentration). The amount of GH released per day is more stable than the mode by which it is released. Thus, one must take into account this natural variation before one can point to a pathologic condition or pharmacologic intervention as etiologic for the alteration in a specific parameter of pulsatile release (for example, GH pulse frequency).

Prepuberty

There is marked between-subject variability in physiologic GH release in normally growing boys and girls, even before the effects of gonadal steroid hormones are noted (9,13). Attempts to correlate absolute values (e.g., mean 12h or 24h GH level) with growth rate are difficult because of the confounding effects of the GH binding proteins, IGF-I and the IGF-binding proteins, and those derivatives of intermediary metabolism and body composition that regulate them. These factors preclude a simple relationship between circulating mean GH levels and linear growth velocity. Thus, it may be impossible to predict growth velocity or, for that matter, growth hormone *sufficiency* for an individual from mean GH levels or from the pulsatile pattern of circulating GH. The existing data suggest that *normality* is most appropriately defined individually.

To better study the effects of gonadal steroid hormones on GH production at adolescence, we initially investigated the quantitative aspects of variable GH release in normal prepubertal boys. We evaluated nine boys. Each had at least three consecutive 24h study periods (venous sampling every 20 min for 24h at 4-month intervals) before the onset of any pubertal sexual development. The within subject variability for the mean range of GH concentration for a group of 11 prepubertal boys evaluated three to six times, as well as the entire range of values for mean 24h GH concentrations of the complete group, are shown in Figure 3.1. Note the much lower variability within individual subjects compared to the group of subjects.

To gain additional insight into the neuroendocrine events giving rise to the GH concentration profiles, we chose to employ deconvolution analysis (17,18) and compare daily secretory rate, secretory burst amplitude (maximal secretory rate), burst frequency, GH mass per burst, and half-life of disappearance. Although there were no differences when analyzed at half-year intervals from 9.5 to 11 years, it was clear that there is far greater variability between subjects than within subjects for all parameters as shown in Table 3.1. The variability found between subjects agrees well with the data obtained from the prepubertal boys in our previous cross-sectional study (8). These results suggest that between-subject differences in these normally growing boys arise more from differences in the

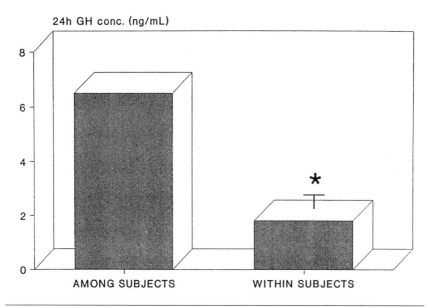

Figure 3.1. Variability of mean 24h growth hormone concentration; comparison of among subject (left) and within subject (right) variability (*n* = 11). Vertical axis represents mean 24h GH concentration, ng/mL.

Table 3.1   Growth hormone secretion in late prepubertal boys[a]

	Inter-subject CV[b] (%)	Intra-subject CV[b] (%)
Daily secretory rate	44	23 ± 4[d]
Burst frequency	18	11 ± 2[c]
Mass per burst	46	24 ± 5[d]
Half-time of disappearance	30	23 ± 4[c]

[a]$n = 11$
[b]coefficient of variation
[c]$P < 0.05$
[d]$P < 0.001$

amount of GH released during a secretory episode than from the frequency of these events. It is difficult to precisely define the factor(s) responsible for the relatively wide between-subject variability; however, the quantity of GH secreted correlated inversely with the mean intrasubject body mass index [BMI-SDS (a surrogate for relative fatness); BMI=weight/(height)^2], 24h production rate ($r= -0.67$, $P=0.049$), and GH secretory burst amplitude ($r=-0.73$, $P=0.026$). The 24h GH burst frequency did not correlate significantly with the BMI-SDS.

Puberty

Puberty is characterized by the onset of development of the secondary sexual characteristics and the impressive acceleration of linear growth. The secondary sexual characteristics are a result of androgen production from the adrenals in both sexes (adrenarche) and testosterone from the testes in males and estrogens from the ovaries in females (gonadarche). Although the rapid growth spurt had previously been attributed directly to the rising concentrations of gonadal steroid hormones, an indirect effect mediated through growth hormone and the IGFs is now considered extremely important. During early childhood, linear growth velocity steadily decreases from its initially rapid rate to reach a steady state of approximately 5.5 cm/year. As puberty approaches, the rate of growth slows slightly before its sudden acceleration to reach a peak during mid-adolescence. This peak occurs later in boys than in girls. It then diminishes toward zero as epiphyseal fusion approaches. At the zenith of the pubertal growth spurt, the growth velocity often rises to rates greater than at any other time since early infancy. There appears to be little doubt that the neuroendocrine axis affecting the growth hormone secretory system plays a pivotal role because an adequate pubertal growth spurt cannot occur without sufficient quantities of growth hormone (1a). However, growth hormone alone apparently is not sufficient, because an important physiological synergism exists between the gonadal and somatotropic axes coincident with normal pubertal development. Thus, the combined growth-promoting effect of concerted activation of these axes is required for normal pubertal development to proceed.

We initially sought to determine the role of androgens (testosterone) in the pubertal elevation of circulating IGF-I concentrations. Parker and colleagues (12) showed that testosterone administered intramuscularly would stimulate IGF-I production in prepubertal boys who could release growth hormone, but not in boys who were growth hormone deficient (Table 3.2). These findings were more fully developed by investigating the alterations in the pulsatile release of growth hormone as boys enter and progress through pubertal development (see Table 3.3 and Figure 3.2). Investigations by Link and coworkers (7), Mauras et al. (11), and Martha and colleagues (9) indicate that concomitant with a rise in IGF-I concentrations, mean circulating growth hormone levels increase during puberty around the time of the mid-pubertal growth spurt in normal boys and in delayed pubertal boys administered testosterone therapy. The mode of this increase is through an augmentation in the size (amplitude and pulse area), rather than the number, of detectable growth hormone pulses.

An increase in growth hormone pulse increment over baseline is the primary mechanism producing the increase in mean 24h GH concentration. Changes in pulse width (duration) contribute little. Shortly after cessation of linear growth, the 24h pattern of growth hormone secretion returns toward prepubertal levels (9) with the result that concentration profiles in young men are remarkably similar

Table 3.2   Insulin-like growth factor-I in concentrations in prepubertal boys[a]

GH sufficient (*n* = 4)			
Control[b]	GH Rx[c]	T Rx[d]	GH + T Rx
0.64 ± 0.13	—	1.81 ± 0.09	—
GH deficient[e] (*n* = 6)			
0.16 ± 0.05	0.84 ± 0.34	0.25 ± 0.09	0.87 ± 0.46

[a] U/mL
[b] GH 0.05 u/kg · day×7 days
[c] GH therapy had been discontinued for at least 30 days
[d] testosterone therapy; testosterone propionate 25 mg/day, IM × 7 days
[e] GH sufficient group of boys with constitutional delay of growth and adolescence (control before start of therapy, long-term therapy employed was testosterone enanthate) (revised from Parker et al., 1984)

Table 3.3   Analysis of growth hormone concentration series at puberty

Group	Mean GH concentration (µg/L)	No. of GH pulses (pulses/24h)	Amplitude[a] GH pulses (µg/L)
Group A			
Prepubertal (n = 10)	2.7 ± 0.5	5.5 ± 0.4	8.6 ± 1.7
Late pubertal (n = 5)	5.4 ± 0.7[b]	5.4 ± 0.7[c]	17.1 ± 2.6[d]
Group B			
Constitutional delay	before 2.3 ± 0.8	6.6 ± 0.9	6.8 ± 1.6
Administered testosterone (n = 5)	after 6.4 ± 1.1[e]	7.6 ± 0.5[e]	15.4 ± 2.4[f]

[a]amplitude = mean peak height
[b]P = 0.01 vs. Group A
[c]P<0.05 vs. Group A
[d]P<0.02 vs. Group A
[e]P<0.05 vs. Group C before therapy
[f]P<0.05 vs. Group C before therapy
From Mauras et al., 1987

to those in prepubertal boys, but greater than those in older men, despite a continued rise in serum testosterone concentration.

To investigate the mechanisms by which androgens increase mean circulating growth hormone concentrations in pubertal boys, we applied a multiple-parameter deconvolution model of circulating growth hormone concentration versus time profiles from 48 normal boys (8). The 24h growth hormone profiles were characterized by 10.7 ± 0.5 (mean ± SE) discrete pituitary secretory bursts with a mean secretion half duration of 35.6 ± 1.4 min and mass of growth hormone secreted per burst of 25.5 ± 2.4 ng/mL. Values for total 24h growth hormone production rate according to the subjects' stage of pubertal development are presented in Table 3.4.

Estrogens also may affect pubertal growth and growth hormone secretion. They are considered to have a biphasic effect—first stimulating, and then in larger doses inhibiting, linear growth. Mean GH levels were found to be significantly increased at breast stages 2 through 4 by Rose and colleagues (14). Pulse frequency and percentage of GH values below the detection limit did not change significantly with pubertal stage. The percentage of GH values below the detection limit, however, was significantly lower in stage 4 girls than in boys, possibly indicating an alteration in somatostatin secretion or action. Mean pulse amplitude was increased significantly at all advanced stages of puberty as compared with that in the younger, prepubertal girls. Mean nighttime GH level correlated inversely with body mass index, even in the girls of normal height and weight, indicating

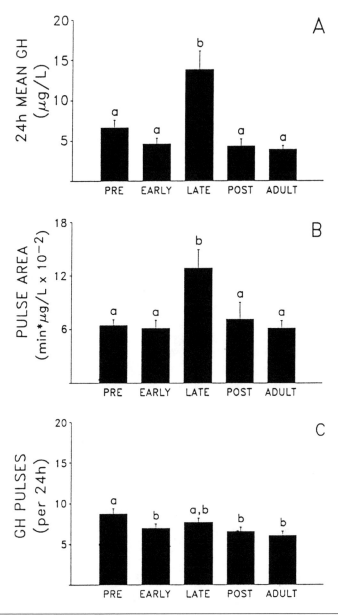

Figure 3.2.   A. The mean (±SE) 24h concentrations of growth hormone for the five study groups are illustrated. B. The mean (±SE) area under the growth hormone concentration versus time curve for individual growth hormone pulses, as identified by the Cluster pulse detection algorithm, is presented. C. The number of growth hormone pulses (mean ± SE), as detected by the Cluster algorithm, in the 24h growth hormone concentration profiles for subjects in the five study groups are graphed. In each panel, any two *vertical bars* not identified by the same letter represent statistically different values ($p<0.05$); *bars* sharing a common letter represent statistically indistinguishable values ($p>0.05$).
From Martha et al. with permission (J. Clin. Endocrinol. Metab. 1989; 69:563-570).

Table 3.4   Daily growth hormone production rate in boys at different pubertal stages (n = 54)

	PR[a,b] (μg/24h)
Prepubertal	24 ± 2
Early puberty	18 ± 3[c]
Late puberty	31 ± 5
Post puberty	13 ± 5[c]
Adult	14 ± 2[c]

[a]Production rate per kilogram body weight (±SE)
[b]Assuming a distribution volume of 7.9%
[c]Statistically different from late pubertal, $P < 0.05$

a complex relationship that includes body composition (14). Similar correlation analysis revealed that the 24h GH secretory rate in boys varied inversely with the subject's body mass index SD-score [$r=-0.65$, $p<0.01$ (8)].

Levine-Ross and colleagues introduced the concept that low doses of ethinyl estradiol (100 ng/kg•d) could enhance linear growth without unduly advancing skeletal maturation and suggested such therapy for hypogonadal girls with Turner's syndrome (15). The physiological actions of such low doses of estrogen have not been defined clearly. Mauras and colleagues studied the possible alterations in endogenous GH secretion in such young girls (10). There were consistent and significant increases in mean GH concentration and mean GH pulse amplitude without a detectable change in GH pulse frequency in seven patients with Turner's syndrome following 5 weeks of low dose (100 ng/kg•d) ethinyl estradiol therapy (Figure 3.3). These findings were not accompanied by any significant changes in plasma IGF-I concentration, serum estradiol concentration, or urinary cytological maturational indexes. Thus, this hypogonadal model, which presumably applies to normal prepubertal girls, demonstrates exquisite somatotrope sensitivity to low dose estrogen action.

Summary

The growth rate at puberty is greater than at any time since early infancy. The precise mechanisms underlying the explosive change in velocity have not been determined with precision, but undoubtedly involve a major interaction between the hypothalamic-pituitary axes for growth hormone and the gonads, given adequate nutrition and the absence of significant disease process. The pattern of pubertal growth and the alterations in growth hormone secretory dynamics are significantly less variable than the timing and tempo of the pubertal process. Adult height is

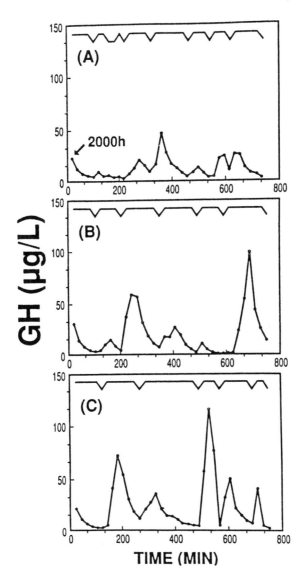

Figure 3.3.   Twelve-hour profile of serum GH concentrations in a patient (no. 3.) before (A) and after 1 week (B) and 5 weeks (C) of low dose EE therapy. Blood was drawn every 20 minutes for 12 hours. Deflections on *top* represent pulses detected by Cluster analysis.

From Mauras et al. with permission (J. Clin. Endocrinol. Metab. 1989; 69:1053-1058).

reached at the end of this process with its variability primarily due to genetic influences rather than the various hormonal systems.

Acknowledgments

I am indebted to my colleagues, Robert M. Blizzard, Michael L. Johnson, Paul M. Martha, Jr., and Johannes D. Veldhuis, and to our two research coordinators, Margaret Ball and Melanie Harlowe. A number of pediatric endocrine fellows have contributed to patient care and have been responsible for some aspects of the data: Mark Parker, Kathleen Link, Nelly Mauras, James Kerrigan, and Francesco Nievas-Rivera. Sandra Jackson and her staff of the General Clinical Research Center at the University of Virginia Health Sciences Center have continued to provide excellent patient care. Ginger Bauler and Catherine Kern provided expert laboratory assistance.

References

1. Albertsson-Wikland, K.; Rosberg, S.; Libre, E.; Lundberg, L-O.; Groth, T. Growth hormone secretory rates in children as estimated by deconvolution analysis of 24-h plasma concentration profiled. Am. J. Physiol. 257 (Endocrinol. Metab. 20):E809; 1989.
1a. Aynsley-Green, A.; Zachmann, M.; Prader, A. Interrelationship of the therapeutic effects of growth hormone and testosterone on growth in hypopituitarism. J. Pediatr. 89:992-999; 1976.
2. Greulich, W.W.; Pyle, S.I. Radiographic atlas of skeletal development of the hand and wrist (2nd ed.). Stanford, CA: Stanford University Press; 1959.
2a. Hindmarsh, P.; Smith, P.J.; Brook, C.G.D.; Matthews, D.R. The relationship between height velocity and growth hormone secretion in short prepubertal children. Clin. Endocrinol. (Oxf). 27: 1987.
3. Horner, J.M.; Thorsen, A.V.; Hintz, R.L. Growth deceleration patterns in children with constitutional short stature: an aid to diagnosis. Pediatrics. 62:529-534; 1978.
4. Kerrigan, J.R.; Martha, P.M. Jr.; Blizzard, R.M.; Christie, C.M.; Rogol, A.D. Variations of pulsatile growth hormone release in healthy short prepubertal boys. Pediatr. Res. 28:11-14; July 1990.
5. Kerrigan, J.R.; Martha, P.M. Jr.; Veldhuis, J.D.; Blizzard, R.M.; Rogol, A.D. Altered growth hormone secretory dynamics in prepubertal males with constitutional delay of growth. Pediatr. Res. 33:278-283; 1993.
6. Lacey, K.A.; Parker, J.M. The normal short child: community study of children in New Castle-upon-Tyne. Arch. Dis. Child. 49:417-424, 1974.
7. Link, K.; Blizzard, R.M.; Evans, W.S.; Kaiser, D.L.; Parker, M.W.; Rogol, A.D. The effect of androgens on the pulsatile release and the twenty-four hour mean concentration of growth hormone in peripubertal males. J. Clin. Endocrinol. Metab. 62:159-164; 1986.
8. Martha, P.M. Jr.; Gorman, K.M.; Blizzard, R.M.; Rogol, A.D.; Veldhuis, J.D. Endogenous growth hormone secretion and clearance rates in normal boys, as determined by deconvolution analysis: relationship to age, pubertal status, and body mass. J. Clin. Endocrinol. Metab. 74:336-344; 1992.

9. Martha, P.M. Jr.; Rogol, A.D.; Veldhuis, J.D.; Kerrigan, J.R.; Goodman, D.W.; Blizzard, R.M. Alterations in the pulsatile properties of circulating growth hormone concentrations during puberty in boys. J. Clin. Endocrinol. Metab. 69:563-570; 1989.

10. Mauras, N.; Rogol, A.D.; Veldhuis, J.D. Specific, time-dependent actions of low-dose ethinyl estradiol administration on the episodic release of growth hormone, follicle-stimulating hormone, and luteinizing hormone in prepubertal girls with Turner's syndrome. J. Clin. Endocrinol. Metab. 69:1053-1058; 1989.

11. Mauras, N.; Blizzard, R.M.; Link, K.; Johnson, M.L.; Rogol, A.D.; Veldhuis, J.D. Augmentation of growth hormone secretion during puberty: evidence for a pulse amplitude-modulated phenomenon. J. Clin. Endocrinol. Metab. 64:596-601; 1987.

12. Parker, M.W.; Johanson, A.J.; Rogol, A.D.; Kaiser, D.L.; Blizzard, R.M. Effect of testosterone on somatomedin-C concentrations in prepubertal boys. J. Clin. Endocrinol. Metab. 58:87-90; 1984.

12a. Plotsky, P.M.; Vale, W. Patterns of growth hormone-releasing factor and somatostatin secretion into the hypophyseal portal circulation in the rat. Science. 230:461; 1985.

13. Rose, S.R.; Municchi, G.; Barnes, K.M.; Kamp, G.A.; Uriarte, M.M.; Ross, J.L.; Cassorla, F.; Cutler, G.B. Jr. Spontaneous growth hormone secretion increases during puberty in normal girls and boys. J. Clin. Endocrinol. Metab. 73:428-435; 1991.

14. Rose, S.R.; Municchi, G.; Barnes, K.M.; Kamp, G.A.; Uriarte, M.M.; Ross, J.L.; Cassorla, F.; Butler, G.B. Jr. Spontaneous growth hormone secretion increases during puberty in normal girls and boys. J. Clin. Endocrinol. Metab. 73:428-435; 1991.

15. Ross, J.L.; Cassorla, F.G.; Carpenter, G.; Long, L.M.; Royster, M.S.; Loriaux, D.L.; Cutler, G.B. Jr. The effect of short term treatment with growth hormone and ethinyl estradiol on lower leg growth rate in girls with Turner's syndrome. J. Clin. Endocrinol. Metab. 67:515-518; 1988.

16. Smith, D.W.; Truog, W.; Rogers, J.E.; et al. Shifting linear growth during infancy: illustration of genetic factors in growth from fetal life through infancy. J. Pediatr. 89:225; 1976.

17. Veldhuis, J.D.; Johnson, M.L. Deconvolution analyses of hormone data. Meth. Enzymol. 210:539-575; 1992.

18. Veldhuis, J.D.; Faria, A.; Vance, M.L.; Evans, W.S.; Thorner, M.O.; Johnson, M.L. Contemporary tools for the analysis of episodic growth hormone secretion and clearance in vivo. Acta. Paediart. Scand. 347:63-82; 1988.

Part II
Bone Metabolism, Activity, and Growth

Chapter 4

Dual Photon Transmission Measurements of Bone Mass and Body Composition During Growth

Colin E. Webber, PhD

Introduction

Wilhelm Conrad Roentgen is credited with the discovery of X rays in November 1895. One of the first exercises he undertook just one month later was to x-ray his wife's hand. The picture showed bones, soft tissue, and two rings. So 98 years ago researchers could distinguish materials of different density and composition by looking at the products of X-ray interactions. To use such interactions to measure the amounts of different materials present in an object, however, took many years, first to develop the equipment necessary to detect and quantitate numbers of photons and second, to understand the various interaction processes to optimize the developed equipment. The purpose of this article is to review dual photon absorptiometry, a technique that has emerged during the last 2 decades as an important diagnostic tool in the investigation of metabolic bone disease. The fundamental physics governing the proper application and the limitations of the technique are outlined. This is followed by a review of the results obtained from dual photon absorptiometry measurements of bone mass and body composition during growth.

Theoretical Foundation of Dual Photon Absorptiometry

When a photon interacts with body tissues, it can either be absorbed or scattered. The only absorption process of concern is photoelectric absorption in which a photon interacts with an inner shell electron of an atom. The photon disappears and the electron is ejected from the atom. The electron vacancy is filled by an outer shell electron and a characteristic X ray is emitted. Since this X ray is characteristic of low atomic number atoms such as H, C, O, N, Ca, and P, it will be a low energy X ray. Hence the energy carried by the incident photon is transferred to the local tissue by an atomic electron and a characteristic X ray, both of which have short path lengths in tissue.

One of two scattering processes can occur when a photon interacts with tissue. In coherent scattering the photon interacts with a whole atom. The incident photon does not lose any energy but its direction is altered. The other scattering process is Compton scattering where the incident photon interacts with a loosely bound or free electron. A portion of the photon's energy is transferred to the electron, and the direction of the photon is changed.

The fundamental parameters describing the likelihood of these particular processes taking place are the atomic cross sections, σ_{photo}, σ_{coh}, and σ_{Com}. These cross sections have units of cm^2atom^{-1} and can be thought of as a target, the area of which represents the probability of that interaction taking place. Each atomic cross section varies in a different way as a function of the interacting photon's energy and with the material's atomic composition. These dependencies dictate the optimum conditions required for the in vivo measurement of bone mass and soft tissue composition. For example, Figure 4.1 shows the dependence of the photoelectric atomic cross section upon atomic number for photons of energy 40 and 100 keV.

Clearly, if we wished to propose a mechanism that was particularly sensitive to the presence of calcium (atomic number 20) but not to the presence of carbon

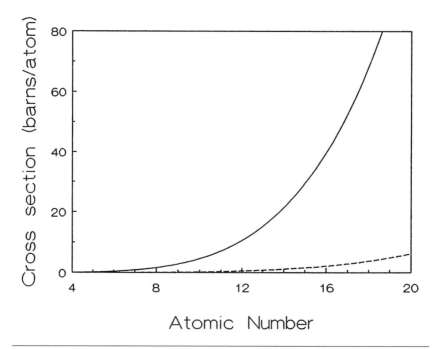

Figure 4.1. The dependence of the atomic cross section for photoelectric absorption upon element atomic number for photons of 40 keV (—) and 100 keV (- -).

(atomic number 6), we would measure the ratio of photoelectric interactions at 40 keV to those at 100 keV. A similar presentation of the Compton atomic cross section is given in Figure 4.2. Photons at each energy scatter in the same manner from different elements. To complete the picture, Figure 4.3 shows the dependence of the coherent atomic cross section upon atomic number for the two photon energies. Some dependency upon atomic number is evident, but not to the extent seen with photoelectric absorption. These fundamental properties of photon interactions mean that if conditions are adjusted to ensure that photoelectric absorption will occur, then we will have the basis of a system that will distinguish bone mineral from soft tissue due principally to atomic number differences.

To convert atomic cross sections into bulk properties of an object, we must introduce the atomic density (N_0/A). That is

$$\mu_{photo} = \sigma_{photo} \ (N_0/A) \tag{1}$$

where N_0/A is Avogadro's number (atom/mole) divided by the atomic mass (g/mole), and μ is the partial attenuation coefficient for the photoelectric effect in the object and has units of cm^2g^{-1}. Similar expressions could be written for μ_{Com} and μ_{coh}. Because each of the three interaction processes acts independently of the other two, partial coefficients can be summed to give a total mass attenuation coefficient, μ, which will describe the probability of interaction for a photon within an object.

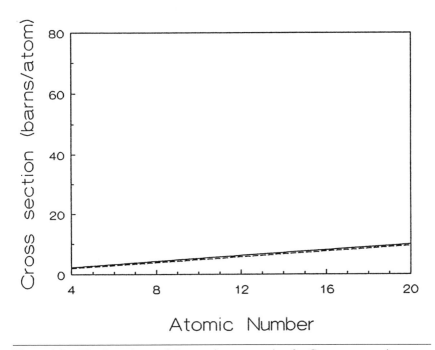

Figure 4.2. The dependence of the atomic cross section for Compton scattering upon element atomic number for photons of 40 keV (—) and 100 keV (- -).

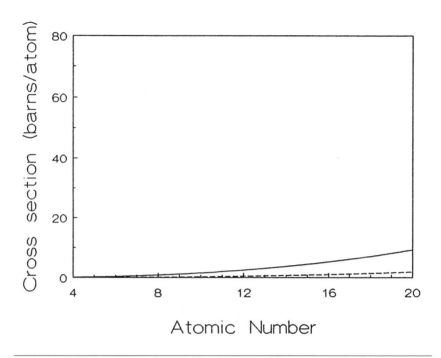

Figure 4.3.   The dependence of the atomic cross section for coherent scattering upon element atomic number for photons of 40 keV (—) and 100 keV (- -).

Imagine a well collimated beam of photons incident upon a detector with an intensity of I_0. We then introduce an object that reduces the intensity of the photon beam to I. The exponential nature of attenuation of electromagnetic radiation means that these two intensities are related by

$$I = I_0 e^{-\mu m} \tag{2}$$

where m is the mass of material in the beam in units of gcm^{-2}. This equation states that any photon that interacts in the object, whether by photoelectric absorption or by Compton or coherent scattering, is removed from the beam and is not detected. This immediately imposes the condition that the detector has to be well collimated so that scattered photons, even those scattered through small angles, are unlikely to reach the detector. If we impose this narrow beam geometry on our equipment, then we can use Equation 2 to measure the mass of an object from a knowledge of I, I_0, and μ.

The use of a single value of μ in Equation 2 implies not only that just a single material is present in the object, but also that all photons have the same energy. For a two component object the corresponding expression would be

$$I = I_0 e^{-(\mu_1 m_1 + \mu_2 m_2)} \tag{3}$$

where the subscripts refer to two different components. This equation does not contain sufficient information to allow a measurement of either m_1 or m_2. If the measurement is repeated at another photon energy, however, we can write the following two equations:

$$I_H = I_{0,H}e^{-(\mu_{1,H}m_1 + \mu_{2,H}m_2)} \tag{4}$$

and

$$I_L = I_{0,L}e^{-(\mu_{1,L}m_1 + \mu_{2,L}m_2)} \tag{5}$$

where the additional subscripts H and L refer to high and low energy photons respectively. Provided these two equations are independent of each other, we can eliminate the mass of one component to give the mass of the other. That is

$$m_1 = \frac{\mu_{2,H}\ln\left(I_{0,L}/I_L\right) - \mu_{2,L}\ln(I_{0,H}/I_H)}{(\mu_{1,L}\,\mu_{2,H} - \mu_{1,H}\,\mu_{2,L})} \tag{6}$$

Equations 4 and 5 are independent if the dependence of μ_1 upon energy is different from the dependence of μ_2 upon energy, otherwise the denominator of Equation 6 would be zero. The value m_1 is the mass of component 1 present between the source and the detector, and because no information is obtained about the distribution of mass in the direction of the photon beam, m_1 can be expressed only in gram per unit area. This is the technique of dual photon absorptiometry (DPA). The source of photons may be a radioisotope source or an X-ray tube. In either case, the principles of measurement are identical although the latter is given the acronym DXA. Normally, Equation 6 is expressed in the form

$$m_1 = \frac{\ln\left(I_{0,L}/I_L\right) - R_{ST}\ln\left(I_{0,H}/I_H\right)}{(\mu_{1,L} - R_{ST}\mu_{1,H})} \tag{7}$$

where R_{ST} is given by $\mu_{2,L}/\mu_{2,H}$ and is dependent on the composition of soft tissue. Equation 7 states that the mass of one component can be obtained from measurements of the appropriate intensities listed in the numerator and by inserting appropriate values for the mass attenuation coefficients. If bone and soft tissue are the two components of the object, then the measured intensities are related to bone and soft tissue mass by means of calibration. A bone densitometer is calibrated from transmission measurements using a phantom constructed from known masses of materials which mimic the attenuation coefficients of bone and soft tissue at each energy. Aluminum and lucite have been used for this purpose. Bone mineral area mass is normally referred to as bone mineral density, although it is not truly a density measurement, and is given the acronym BMD. The product of BMD and the projected bone area gives the bone mineral content or BMC.

Equations 4 and 5 assume that the compositions of both bone mineral and soft tissue are universal constants. That is, the same values of μ_1 and μ_2 can be used for the phantom and for all subjects. For practical purposes, it is true that bone mineral has a constant composition and density. However, the assumption is certainly not true for soft tissue where the mass attenuation coefficient is determined in large part by the fat to lean ratio. Consequently, soft tissue composition must be measured for each subject. Mathematically this is equivalent to measuring R_{ST} from Equation 7 when m_1 is equal to zero. That is,

$$m_1 = \frac{\ln (I_{0,L}/I_L) - R_{ST}\ln (I_{0,H}/I_H)}{(\mu_{1,L} - R_{ST}\mu_{1,H})} = 0 \qquad (8)$$

or

$$\ln (I_{0,L}/I_L) = R_{ST}\ln (I_{0,H}/I_H) \qquad (9)$$

This equation states that a value for R_{ST} can be derived from transmission measurements through soft tissue. This value is then applied to the bone mass analysis using Equation 7. It has been assumed that, physically, the fat fraction for soft tissue lateral to the spine is the same as that of soft tissue anterior and posterior to the spine. Thus, dual photon measurements of bone mass must include transmission measurements through soft tissue sites as well as sites containing mineral and soft tissue.

When we scan the total body we obtain a measurement of total body bone mass and total body soft tissue mass. In addition, we obtain the total body bone mineral area density. R_{ST} values are measured for all sites containing only soft tissue (approximately 6,000 of 10,000 pixels). A weighted mean R_{ST} ratio will allow division of the soft tissue mass into total body fat and total body lean mass. The ratio is related to a fat to lean composition by means of a factory installed calibration using materials that simulate the attenuation properties of fat and lean. Such materials as ethanol and water, polyoxymethylene and water, or stearic acid and 0.6% NaCl have been utilized for this purpose (18,20).

Some Problems and Difficulties

This theoretical description of dual photon absorptiometry appears deceptively simple. It suggests that with a suitable source to provide photons at two distinct energies and with a radiation detector, we can measure bone mass and body composition. However, there are several pitfalls to overcome. First, a transmitted photon can be detected only if it interacts with the sodium iodide crystal normally used in commercial densitometers. When a photon is totally absorbed by the crystal, the signal processed by the electronics corresponds to the full energy of the detected photon. Unfortunately a significant fraction of photons is not completely absorbed, and these photons deposit less than their full energy in the crystal. This leads to a signal which appears to correspond to the absorption of a photon of lower energy. Thus, it is possible for a high energy photon to appear in the energy region corresponding to a low energy photon. This factor is termed crossover. Any high energy photon that scatters in the object also will lose energy.

Consequently, scattered photons not rejected by collimation or photons that scatter more than once in the object and are then detected, can also contribute to crossover.

A second difficulty is the requirement for linearity between the measured count rate and the intensity of photons incident upon the detector. The detector should respond linearly to photons transmitted from the source through air ($I_{0,H}$ and $I_{0,L}$) and also to photons transmitted through the subject (I_H and I_L), count rates which may differ by 3 orders of magnitude. Each pulse requires a finite length of time for processing, and the electronics cannot respond to a second pulse during this interval. This is termed dead time and at higher count rates, count rate losses can occur introducing non-linearities between the apparent count rate and the true photon intensities.

Another fundamental difficulty is that the equations assume all high energy photons have the same single high energy and that all low energy photons have the same single low energy. Even if the radioisotope ^{153}Gd is used as a source of photons and especially when an X-ray tube provides the incident beam, a range of photon energies exists within both the high and low energy beams. This means that because lower energy photons are preferentially absorbed as the beams penetrate tissue, the mean energy of each beam gradually increases or the beam hardens. This in turn means that the values of the mass attenuation coefficients change, and a dependency upon object thickness is introduced (3).

As with all measurement techniques involving radiation, the statistics of radiation detection must be considered. For example, consider the problem of measuring the count rate for radiation transmitted through a small object. If the difference between the intensity of photons transmitted through the object and the intensity of photons incident upon the object is little more than the statistical fluctuation in either rate, then large errors are inevitable.

Corrections for the effects of crossover, dead time, beam hardening, and object thickness are made within software algorithms. Another problem already alluded to is calibration, particularly for fat and lean tissue mass. It is not a trivial matter to construct a calibration object that faithfully reflects the properties of bone mineral, muscle, and fat at the required photon energies. An evaluation of the appropriateness of a number of calibration standards has been performed (20). It was concluded that various materials could be used for calibration, provided correct values for the fat equivalents are known and provided the thickness dependence of each densitometer is evaluated.

One additional patient dependent factor which can affect the accuracy of an in vivo measurement of bone mass is the evaluation of soft tissue composition adjacent to the spine. Any non-uniformity of fat distribution at the measurement site could lead to an error. The extent of this effect in lumbar spine bone mass measurement has been disputed (14,43,46), but the weight of the evidence suggests that errors of up to 10% are possible due to fat non-uniformities (50).

All of the factors cited affect the accuracy of a measurement. Experimentally, it is difficult to make assessments of accuracy. For bone mass measurements, either isolated bones submerged in water are measured and compared with ash weights, or measurements are made in cadavers again followed by ashing of excised bones. The former experiments usually show errors of less than 3%, increasing to only about 7% for ash weights below 3g (5), whereas the latter indicate that errors of up to about 10% may be present (13,27). For normal size individuals, however, the accuracy error is small compared to the variation of values observed in normal subjects.

Clinically, the important parameter is precision rather than accuracy. The significant clinical questions relate to the detection of differences between two measurements on the same subject rather than the distinction of a single result from an expected normal range. If the reproducibility of a measurement is 2%, then the variance of the difference between 2 measurements is $(2^2 + 2^2)^{1/2}$ or 2.8%. This means that even if no real change in bone mass occurred between 2 measurements, there is a 95% probability that the measured difference will lie anywhere between −5.6% and +5.6% (24). This example justifies continued efforts to improve precision of measurements. Reproducibility is critically dependent upon technique and quality assurance. Reported values for equipment used in bone research centers are generally about 2% (38,40). In routine clinical operation it is unlikely that reproducibilities of such quality are achieved. It is to the credit of the software designers and the instrument manufacturers that results of excellent precision can be obtained with the equipment available today, particularly with respect to bone densitometry.

Dual Photon Measurements of Bone Mass During Growth

Figure 4.4 shows an example of the type of study performed with dual photon absorptiometry to establish the pattern of growth in bone mass. Lumbar spine BMD was measured in 129 males and 107 females between the ages of 3 and 30 (21).

The results suggest that in males, growth during puberty contributes little to peak bone mass. It would seem for females that approximately half of peak bone mass accumulates at the time of puberty and that bone mass does not increase after the early teenage years. However, these conclusions must be tempered with caution. The inherent properties of cross-sectional studies limit their ability to detect subtle age dependent changes in bone mass. The variation in such data includes a component due to the measurement technique and another contribution from the biological variation between individuals. Even though the measurements in Figure 4.4 were obtained using the less precise ^{153}Gd based DPA, the differences between individuals is the dominant source of variance and is about 5 times the machine variance. To eliminate population variance, sequential studies that will include only technical variation must be performed. Even though sequential studies are much more difficult and expensive, the confidence placed in conclusions based on sequential data will be much greater than that derived from cross-sectional studies. Figure 4.5 shows the results of 3 measurements separated by

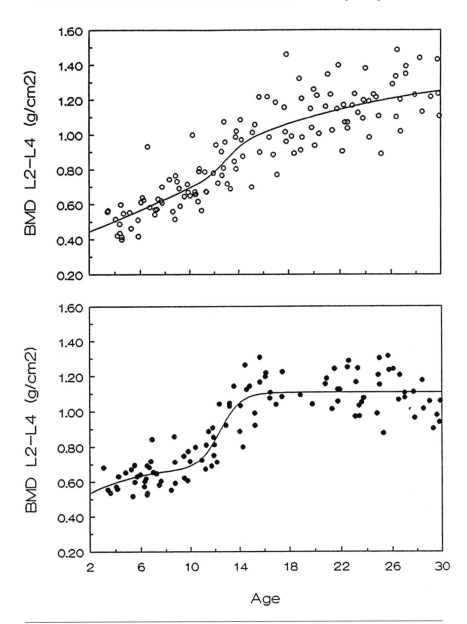

Figure 4.4.   Lumbar spine bone mineral density as a function of age in males (O) and females (●). The solid line is the non-linear least squares fit to the data.
From "The contribution of growth and puberty to peak bone mass" by C.L. Gordon, J.M. Halton, S.A. Atkinson, and C.E. Webber, *Growth, Development and Aging*, 1991, *55*, 257-262. Copyright 1991 by Growth Publishing Co. Inc. Reprinted with permission.

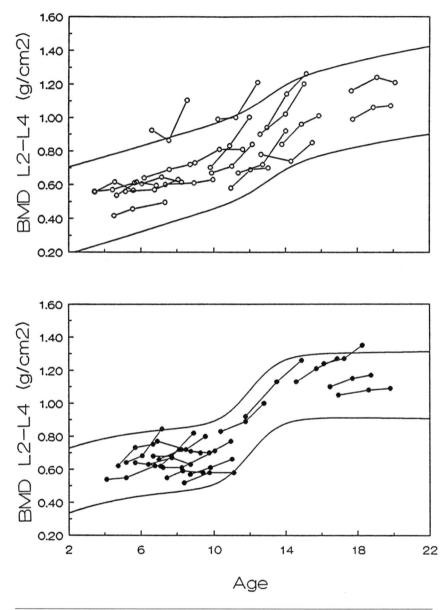

Figure 4.5.   Sequential measurements of lumbar spine bone mineral density in 21 males (○) and 19 females (●). The solid lines are the 95% confidence limits for the population shown in Figure 4.4.

1 year intervals in each of a number of males and females using the same [153]Gd based instrument that was used to obtain the data shown in Figure 4.4. The solid lines are the 95% confidence limits derived from the cross-sectional data. The rate of change for each subject is similar to that which would be predicted from the cross-sectional measurements. However, each of the four teenage girls who returned for repeat measurements demonstrated an increasing bone mass.

Another important factor in studies of BMD during growth is the ratio of trabecular to cortical bone at the measurement site. Age dependent changes in the rate of mineral accumulation by cortical and trabecular bone are different. Therefore, the pattern in Figure 4.4 will be influenced by the high proportion of trabecular bone in the lumbar spine (12), and one can expect that patterns measured at predominantly cortical bone sites such as the radius and proximal femur will be different (31). Indeed, the pattern of change expected from lumbar spine vertebral body measurements using lateral X-ray based dual photon absorptiometry could be quite different from lumbar spine measurements using antero-posterior scanning, because the latter will include both the trabecular bone of the vertebral body and the predominantly cortical bone of the posterior processes. One can expect that even lateral DXA measurements will be different from CT measurements because the latter will reflect entirely trabecular bone from within the vertebral body (17). One should also remember that BMD measurements are not independent of body size. About half the changes in BMD shown in Figure 4.4 will be due to bone size changes instead of changes in bone mineralization (30).

Of particular importance in maintaining skeletal integrity in later life is to attain the maximum bone mass allowed genetically. That is, the risk of suffering a hip fracture in old age is probably inversely related to the peak bone mass reached during growth. To illustrate this point consider the BMD values of $1.3 \mathrm{gcm}^{-2}$ and $0.9 \mathrm{gcm}^{-2}$, both results obtained from normal women and included within the young adult normal range in Figure 4.4. The normal rate of loss of BMD during aging is about $0.01 \mathrm{gcm}^{-2} \mathrm{y}^{-1}$. Consequently after 40 years, the first woman would have a BMD of $0.9 \mathrm{gcm}^{-2}$, a result still within the normal young adult range. The second woman would have a BMD of about $0.5 \mathrm{gcm}^{-2}$, a grossly abnormal result associated with a dramatic increase in fracture risk of about 20. This argument may well explain the lower incidence of osteoporotic fracture in black women because black girls achieve a higher peak bone mass than white girls (2,34).

In Vivo Studies of Bone Mass During Growth

Lumbar spine BMD was measured by DXA in a cross-sectional study of 65 girls and 70 boys between the ages of 1 and 15 (19). BMD was not different between males and females except at age 12 when BMD was greater for girls. In another study of 96 females and 106 males between the ages of 3 and 25, no gender based differences in lumbar spine BMD were found before puberty (16). As in the previous study, BMD for females was greater peri-puberty. Post-puberty

BMD was similar between the sexes, and maximum BMD was reached between 16 and 20 years. Lumbar spine and femoral neck BMD were measured in 98 females and 109 males between the ages of 9 and 18 (4). Lumbar spine BMD increased earlier with respect to age in females, but not with respect to pubertal development. There were no detectable differences between the sexes for spine BMD, although 15-year-old females had reached adult reference values for both the spine and femoral neck. When Tanner staging and body weight were controlled in another cross-sectional study involving 134 girls and 84 boys between the ages of 1 and 19, there were no significant influences of age, sex, race, physical activity, and diet upon bone mass (47). Although these studies are consistent, they provide no answer to the question of the age of attainment of peak bone mass. If it is assumed that from person to person this age can vary between 15 and 30, and if it also is assumed that after peak bone mass has been reached bone loss commences, it may be expected that population studies would show a constant BMD from early teenage years to the end of the third decade. Theintz et al. (49) made sequential measurements of bone mass using DPX in 198 adolescents ages 9 to 19. They found that in females the rate of increase at the spine fell toward zero after age 16 but was still positive at age 18. However, there was no change in proximal femur bone mass after age 16. In males, rates of increase were positive throughout the teenage years.

Other studies using dual photon absorptiometry have not focused on growth patterns, but have explored correlations between BMD and independent predictor variables such as weight, height, pubertal stage, grip strength, calcium intake, and physical activity (11,33,37,41). Generally, BMD is highly correlated with weight, height, and age, but body weight accounts for the greatest fraction of the variance in BMD.

The strongest evidence that peak bone mass can be optimized comes from the longitudinal prospective study by Recker et al. (44). They showed in a group of 156 female college students from professional schools a median gain of lumbar spine BMD of 6.8% during the third decade. The rate of spine BMD increase was negatively correlated with age and positively correlated with the Ca/protein intake ratio and with physical activity, suggesting that lifestyle modifications of improving calcium intake and increasing levels of physical activity could produce beneficial effects on lumbar spine bone mass. Their results suggested that mineral acquisition ceased in this population between 28.3 and 29.5 years, and the study supported the results of earlier work based on cross-sectional measurements, which suggested that axial and appendicular peak bone mass could be modified in women ages 25 to 34 by altering calcium intake and levels of activity (29). Barden and Mazess (1), however, were unable to detect any changes in axial or appendicular BMD following repeated measurements in women ages 20 to 39. In addition, quantitated computed tomography measurements of lumbar spine trabecular bone have shown that androgen and estrogen levels may ultimately determine lumbar spine trabecular bone mass (7).

Dual Photon Measurements of
Body Composition During Growth

Total body dual photon scans measure total body bone mineral mass and soft tissue mass. The weighted mean value of the R_{ST} ratios determined at each measurement site containing only soft tissue allows an estimation of the fat to lean ratio. Thus, soft tissue mass can be divided into fat mass and lean body mass and particularly with DXA, results of useful precision can be obtained (36). With dual photon absorptiometry all three components are measured directly, and no assumptions about tissue density or composition need to be invoked (39). Another feature is that muscle, fat, and mineral mass can be measured for such regions as the arms, trunk, pelvis, and legs (26). However, the inherent similarity between the attenuation properties of lean tissue and fat and the requirement in a whole body scan of measuring attenuation through a considerable range of tissue thicknesses, introduce considerable challenges to the technology. In the following section, studies relevant to this issue are reviewed.

Assessments of In Vivo Measurements

To illustrate the improvements in reliability that have followed technological progress in dual photon absorptiometry measurements of body composition and also to demonstrate some of the difficulties which might remain, I believe it is worthwhile to compare performance evaluations of earlier and later instruments. The body size dependence of original radioisotope based equipment produced considerable errors in fat mass measurements for subjects with unusual body thicknesses. That is, negative values were obtained in infants, small animals, and lean subjects, while falsely raised values were obtained in obese subjects. At the same time, accurate results were obtained for subjects of normal body thickness (22). In another assessment of accuracy it was shown that although changes in fluid volume could be measured accurately as changes in soft tissue mass (32), the changes could not be assigned correctly as a change in lean or fat tissue mass. These errors were due to the similarity of muscle and fat attenuation coefficients, the less sophisticated algorithms available in the past, and the lower number of photons delivered from a radioisotope source.

The most stringent test of body composition measurements is the accurate and precise assessment of fat and lean mass in infants. Such measurements have been made in newborns, and the values obtained are similar to published body composition data obtained using other techniques (51). Other work using phantoms to simulate the neonate/infant showed that while excellent correlations can be obtained between known and measured masses of fat and lean tissues, the slopes of the regression lines were not always equal to 1 (8).

When total body composition is measured in small pigs weighing about 1.5 kg and true composition is measured by chemical analysis of the carcass, the correct sum of mineral plus soft tissue mass is obtained (6). However, when the

DXA measured bone mineral mass is compared with total ash weight, BMC is underestimated. Reasonable values are obtained for DXA measured lean tissue mass but fat mass is overestimated. When similar measurements are made in larger pigs of around 5 kg, better results are obtained. Again, total mass is measured with only a small error. Bone mineral, lean mass, and fat mass estimates are improved, although there is still a systematic overestimate of fat mass (6). The measurement of body composition in pigs weighing between 35 and 95 kg showed that fat mass and lean mass did not differ significantly from the chemically determined masses (48).

With the latest technology it is possible to correctly identify changes in adult body composition following either addition or removal of fluid from the appropriate body compartments (28). Not only are the expected total body changes observed, but the correct regional assignments also are made. However, other work (45) shows that the problem of locating sufficient mineral-free pixels in the trunk region can lead to an underestimation of body fat for that region. Another obvious inherent difficulty in regional body composition measurements is that it is not possible to obtain mineral free measurements in the head. Finally the reproducibility of body composition measurements using DXA is better than 2%, although for regional measurements of composition the coefficients of variation are between 2% and 8% (9,25).

In Vivo Studies of Body Composition During Growth

An example of the application of dual photon body composition measurements during growth in children and adolescents is shown in Figure 4.6, where total body mineral mass and density, as well as lean body mass and total body fat mass, are given for 76 females between the ages of 8 and 26 (23).

It is worth noting the similarity between the age dependent patterns of increase in BMC and lean body mass. The impact of growth in different body regions is shown for the same subjects in Figure 4.7. In measurements on 234 children, Faulkner et al. (15) also identified a strong relationship between lean mass and bone mineral density for the whole body and for regions within the body. Geusens et al. (16) have shown by regional analysis of whole body scans that bone growth is not homogeneous throughout the skeleton, is different between the sexes, and is different between cortical and trabecular bone.

Radiation Dose

One of the most important considerations in the use of photon absorptiometry in growing children is that the subject is exposed to ionizing radiation, and it is imperative that the risks involved in the measurement be considered. Clearly, the total amount of energy deposited during a dual photon scan will be greatest when the whole body is scanned for a body composition measurement. The first point to make is that because the radiation dose is so small it is very difficult to measure. Using the best available dosimeter techniques, researchers can show

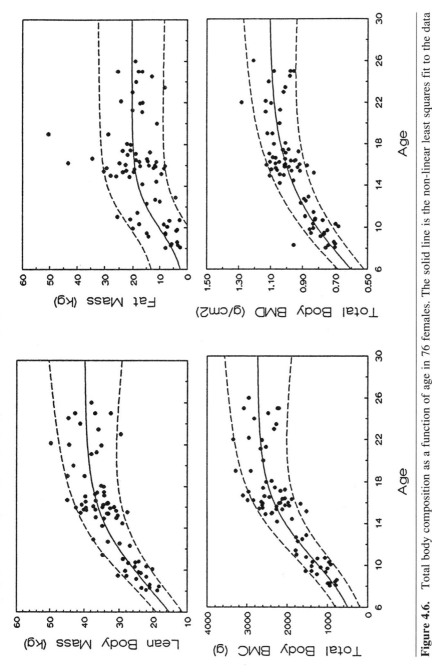

Figure 4.6. Total body composition as a function of age in 76 females. The solid line is the non-linear least squares fit to the data and the dashed lines indicate the 95% confidence limits for the sample.

From "Body composition and bone mineral distribution during growth in females" by C.L. Gordon and C.E. Webber, *Canadian Association of Radiologists Journal*, 1993, *44*, 112-116. Copyright 1993 by the Canadian Medical Association. Reprinted with permission.

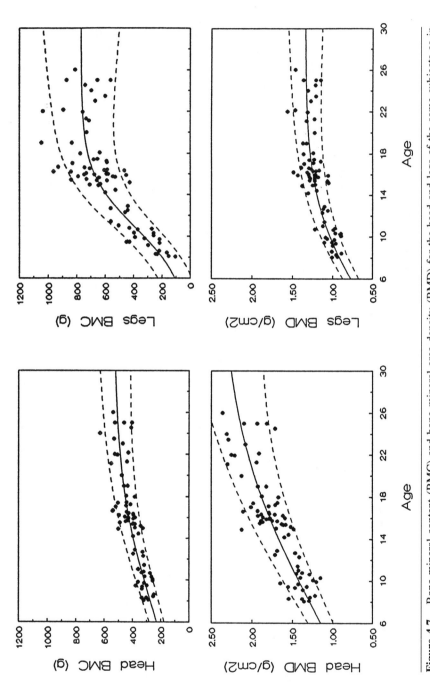

Figure 4.7. Bone mineral content (BMC) and bone mineral area density (BMD) for the head and legs of the same subjects as in Figure 4.6.

that the absorbed dose to the subject is less than 40 μGy (42,52). Such a dose is roughly equivalent to the whole body exposure received from natural radiation and radioactivity during 5 days of normal living. Radiation doses can also be expressed in terms of the effective dose equivalent which allows comparison of the health effects of the absorbed dose to the health effects associated with other activities. For example, the health detriment associated with smoking one cigarette is about equal to that associated with six whole body dual photon scans (10). The loss of life expectancy associated with obesity can be expressed as a health detriment and can be related to the health detriment associated with radiation. Such calculations predict that the risk associated with eating a calorie rich dessert could be equivalent to that associated with one person having about 34 whole body dual photon scans (10). The risks associated with lumbar spine and femoral neck bone densitometry will be even smaller because of the limited volume of tissue irradiated. These comparisons show that whole body dual photon scanning is a low risk procedure that can be used for sequential in vivo measurements.

Conclusion

Dual photon absorptiometry can provide safe, accurate, and precise measurements of bone mass and body composition in the majority of in vivo applications. The technology has allowed improved estimates of fracture risk and treatment evaluation in patients suffering from osteoporosis and has permitted the age dependent patterns of attainment of peak bone mass to be studied. Dual photon absorptiometry has been recommended as a reference technique for assessing changes in body composition in children and adults (35). It is the only technique that provides simultaneous, independent, direct estimates of lean body mass, fat mass, total body bone mineral mass, and total body mineral area density. The fat mass measured by dual photon absorptiometry represents the sum of all fat-like elements, while the lean mass is the sum of all fat-free, non-mineral tissue elements. With the latest instrumentation, accuracy errors may be present only for the extremes of body size such as the premature infant and grossly obese subjects, where the difficulties in measuring photon attenuation correctly for unusual tissue path lengths may be present. Dual photon absorptiometry should be considered as a first choice technique for the non-invasive measurement of body composition during growth.

Acknowledgments

It is a pleasure to acknowledge the work of Tom Farrell, Chris Gordon, and Lesley Beaumont, who each contributed much to the results reported here. This work was partially funded by the Medical Research Council of Canada.

References

1. Barden, H.S.; Mazess, R.B. Longitudinal study of bone mineral density in premenopausal women. J. Bone Min. Res. 5 Supp 2:S180; 1990.
2. Bell, N.H.; Shary, J.; Stevens, J.; Garza, M.; Gordon, L.; Edwards, J. Demonstration that bone mass is greater in black than in white children. J. Bone Min. Res. 6:719-723; 1991.
3. Blake, G.M.; McKeeney, D.B.; Chhaya, S.C.; Ryan, P.J.; Fogelman, I. Dual energy X-ray absorptiometry: the effects of beam hardening on bone density measurements. Med. Phys. 19:459-465; 1992.
4. Bonjour, J.P.; Theintz, G.; Buchs, B.; Slosman, D.; Rizzoli, R. Critical years and stages of puberty for spinal and femoral bone mass accumulation during adolescence. J. Clin. Endocrin. Metab. 73:555-563; 1991.
5. Braillon, P.M.; Salle, B.L.; Brunet, J.; Glorieux, F.H.; Delmas, P.D.; Meunier, P.J. Dual energy X-ray absorptiometry measurement of bone mineral content in newborns: validation of the technique. Ped. Res. 32:77-80; 1992.
6. Brunton, J.A.; Bayley, H.S.; Atkinson, S.A. Validation and application of dual energy X-ray absorptiometry (DXA) to measure bone mass and body composition in small infants. Amer. J. Clin. Nut. 58:839-845; 1993.
7. Buchanan, J.R.; Myers, C.; Lloyd, T.; Leuenberger, P.; Deners, L.M. Determinants of peak trabecular bone density in women: the role of androgens, estrogen and exercise. J. Bone Min. Res. 3:673-680; 1988.
8. Chan, G.M. Performance of dual-energy X-ray absorptiometry in evaluating bone, lean body mass, and fat in pediatric subjects. J. Bone Min. Res. 7:369-374; 1992.
9. Chilibeck, P.D.; Calder, A.; Sale, D.; and Webber, C. Reproducibility of dual energy X-ray absorptiometry. Can. Assoc. Radiol. J. 45:297-302; 1994.
10. Cohen, B.L.; Lee, I.S. A catalog of risks. Health Phys. 36:707-722; 1979.
11. DeSchepper, J.; Derde, M.P.; Van den Broeck, M.; Piepsz, A.; Jonckheer, M.H. Normative data for lumbar spine bone mineral content in children; influence of age, height, weight and pubertal stage. J. Nucl. Med. 32:216-220; 1991.
12. Eastell, R.; Mosekilde, L.; Hodgson, S.F.; Riggs, B.L. Proportion of human vertebral body bone that is cancellous. J. Bone Min. Res. 5:1237-1241; 1990.
13. Farrell, T.J.; Webber, C.E. The error due to fat inhomogeneity in lumbar spine bone mineral measurements. Clin. Phys. Physiol. Meas. 10:57-64; 1989.
14. Farrell, T.J.; Webber, C.E. Spine densitometry-further comments on errors. Clin. Phys. Physiol. Meas. 11:254-256; 1990.
15. Faulkner, R.A.; Bailey, D.A.; Drinkwater, D.T.; Wilkinson, A.A.; Houston, C.S.; McKay, H.A. Regional and total body bone mineral content, bone mineral density and total body tissue composition in children 8-16 years of age. Calc. Tiss. Int. 53:7-13; 1993.
16. Geusens, P.; Cantatore, F.; Nijs, J.; Proesmans, W.; Emma, F.; Dequeker, J. Heterogeneity of growth of bone in children at the spine, radius and total skeleton. Growth Develop. Aging. 55:249-256; 1991.
17. Gilsanz, V.; Gibbens, D.T.; Roe, T.F.; Carlson, M.; Senac, M.O.; Boechat, M.I.; Huang, H.K.; Schulz, E.E.; Libanati, C.R.; Cann, C.E. Vertebral bone density in children: effect of puberty. Radiol. 166:847-850; 1988.
18. Gingold, E.L.; Hasegawa, B.H. Systematic bias in basis material decomposition applied to quantitative dual-energy x-ray imaging. Med. Phys. 19:25-33; 1992.
19. Glastre, G.; Braillon, P.; David, L.; Cochat, P.; Meunier, P.J.; Delmas, P.D. Measurement of bone mineral content of the lumbar spine by dual energy X-ray absorptiometry in normal children: correlations with growth parameters. J. Clin. Endocrin. Metab. 70:1330-1333; 1990.

20. Goodsitt, M.M. Evaluation of a new set of calibration standards for the measurement of fat content via DPA and DXA. Med. Phys. 19:35-44; 1992.
21. Gordon, C.L.; Halton, J.M.; Atkinson, S.A.; Webber, C.E. The contributions of growth and puberty to peak bone mass. Growth Devel. Aging. 55:257-262; 1991.
22. Gordon, C.L. The accuracy of dual photon absorptiometry measurements of soft tissue composition. M.Sc. thesis, McMaster University, April, 1992.
23. Gordon, C.L.; Webber, C.E. Body composition and bone mineral distribution during growth in females. Can. Assoc. Radiol. J. 44:112-116; 1993.
24. Heaney, R.P. En recherche de la différence (P<0.05). Bone Min. 1:99-114; 1986.
25. Herd, R.J.M.; Blake, G.M.; Parker, J.C.; Ryan, P.J.; Fogelman, I. Total body studies in normal British women using dual energy X-ray absorptiometry. Brit. J. Radiol. 66:303-308; 1993.
26. Heymsfield, S.B.; Smith, R.; Aulet, M.; Bensen, B.; Lichtman, S.; Wang, J.; Pierson, R.N. Appendicular skeletal muscle mass: measurement by dual photon absorptiometry. Am. J. Clin. Nutr. 52:214-218; 1990.
27. Ho, C.P.; Kim, R.W.; Scaffler, M.B.; Sartoris, D.J. Accuracy of dual energy radiographic absorptiometry of the lumbar spine: cadaver study. Radiol. 176:171-173; 1990.
28. Horber, F.F.; Thomi, F.; Casez, J.P.; Fonteille, J.; Jaeger, P. Impact of hydration status on body composition as measured by dual energy X-ray absorptiometry in normal volunteers and patients on haemodialysis. Brit. J. Radiol. 65:895-900; 1992.
29. Kanders, B.; Dempster, D.W.; Lindsay, R. Interaction of calcium nutrition and physical activity on bone mass in young women. J. Bone Min. Res. 3:145-149; 1988.
30. Katzman, D.K.; Bachrach, L.K.; Carter, D.R.; Marcus, R. Clinical and anthropometric correlates of bone mineral acquisition in healthy adolescent girls. J. Clin. Endocrin. Metab. 73:1332-1339; 1991.
31. Kröger, H.; Kotaniemi, A.; Vainio, P.; Alhava, E. Bone densitometry of the spine and femur in children by dual-energy X-ray absorptiometry. Bone Min. 17:75-85; 1992.
32. Lands, L.C.; Heigenhauser, G.J.F.; Gordon, C.; Jones, N.L.; Webber, C.E. Accuracy of measurements of small changes in soft tissue mass by use of dual-photon absorptiometry. J. App. Physiol. 71:698-702; 1991.
33. Lloyd, T.; Rollings, N.; Andon, M.B.; Demers, L.M.; Eggli, D.F.; Kieselhorst, K.; Kulin, H.; Landis, J.R.; Martel, J.K.; Orr, G.; Smith, P. Determinants of bone density in young women. 1. Relationships among pubertal development, total body bone mass, and total body bone density in premenarchal females. J. Clin. Endocrin. Metab. 75:383-387; 1992.
34. Luckey, M.M.; Meier, D.E.; Mandell, J.P.; DaCosta, M.C.; Hubbard, M.L.; Goldsmith, S.J. Radial and vertebral bone density in white and black women: evidence for racial differences in premenopausal bone homeostasis. J. Clin. Endocrin. Metab. 69:762-770; 1989.
35. Lukaski, H.C. Soft tissue composition and bone mineral status: evaluation by dual-energy X-ray absorptiometry. J. Nutr. 123:438-443; 1993.
36. Mazess, R.B.; Barden, H.S.; Bisek, J.P.; Hanson, J. Dual energy X-ray absorptiometry for total body and regional bone-mineral and soft tissue composition. Am. J. Clin. Nutr. 51:1106-1112; 1990.
37. McCormick, D.P.; Ponder, S.W.; Fawcett, H.D.; Palmer, J.L. Spinal bone mineral density in 335 normal and obese children and adolescents: evidence for ethnic and sex differences. J. Bone Min. Res. 6:507-513; 1991.
38. Nilas, L.; Borg, J.; Gotfredsen, A.; Christiansen, C. Comparison of single- and dual-photon absorptiometry in postmenopausal bone mineral loss. J. Nucl. Med. 26:1257-1262; 1985.
39. Ortiz, O.; Russell, M.; Daley, T.L.; Baumgartner, R.N.; Waki, M.; Lichtman, S.; Wang, J.; Pierson, R.N.; Heymsfield, S.B. Differences in skeletal muscle and bone mineral mass between black and white females and their relevance to estimates of body composition. Amer. J. Clin. Nut. 55:8-13; 1992.

40. Orwoll, E.S.; Oviatt, S.K. Longitudinal precision of dual energy X-ray absorptiometry in a multicenter study. J. Bone Min. Res. 6:191-197; 1991.
41. Ponder, S.W.; McCormick, D.P.; Fawcett, H.D.; Palmer, J.L.; McKernan, M.G.; Brouhard, B.H. Spinal bone mineral density in children aged 5.00 through 11.99 years. Am. J. Dis. Child. 144:1346-1348; 1990.
42. Pye, D.W.; Hannan, W.J.; Hesp, R. Effective dose equivalent in dual X-ray absorptiometry. Brit. J. Radiol. 63:149; 1990.
43. Pye, D.W. Estimation of the magnitude of the error in bone mineral measurement due to fat: the effect of machine calibration. Clin. Phys. Physiol. Meas. 12:87-91; 1991.
44. Recker, R.R.; Davies, M.; Hinders, S.M.; Heaney, R.P.; Stegman, M.R.; Kimmel, D.B. Bone gain in young adult women. JAMA. 268:2403-2408; 1992.
45. Snead, D.B.; Birge, S.J.; Kohrt, W.M. Age-related differences in body composition by hydrodensitometry and dual-energy x-ray absorptiometry. J. App. Physiol. 74:770-775; 1993.
46. Sorenson, J.A. Spine densitometry—further comments on errors. Clin. Phys. Physiol. Meas. 11:251-253; 1990.
47. Southard, R.N.; Morris, J.D.; Mahan, J.D.; Hayes, J.R.; Torch, M.A.; Sommer, A.; Zipf, W.B. Bone mass in healthy children: measurement with quantitative DXA. Radiol. 179:735-738; 1991.
48. Svendsen, O.L.; Haarbo, J.; Hassager, C.; Christiansen, C. Accuracy of measurements of body composition by dual-energy x-ray absorptiometry in vivo. Am. J. Clin. Nutr. 57:605-608; 1993.
49. Theintz, G.; Buchs, B.; Rizzoli, R.; Slosman, D.; Clavien, H.; Sizonenko, P.C.; Bonjour, J.P. Longitudinal monitoring of bone mass accumulation in healthy adolescents: evidence for a marked reduction after 16 years of age at the levels of lumbar spine and femoral neck in female subjects. J. Clin. Endocrin. Metab. 75:1060-1065; 1992.
50. Tothill, P.; Pye, D.W. Errors due to non-uniform distribution of fat in dual X-ray absorptiometry of the lumbar spine. Brit. J. Radiol. 65:807-813; 1992.
51. Venkataraman, P.S.; Ahluwalia, B.W. Total bone mineral content and body composition by X-ray densitometry in newborns. Pediatrics. 90:767-770; 1992.
52. Waker, A.J.; Oldroyd, B.; Marco, M. The application of microdosimetry in clinical bone densitometry using a dual-photon absorptiometer. Brit. J. Radiol. 65:523-527; 1992.

Chapter 5

The Importance of a Physically Active Lifestyle During Youth for Peak Bone Mass

A Review With Emphasis on Methodological Constraints and Preventive Strategies

Han C.G. Kemper, PhD, and C. Niemeyer, MSc

Introduction

In this review we evaluate the recent scientific literature with respect to the importance of physical activity for the development of bone mass. The focus is on the methodological constraints of most of the investigations and their limitations to prove cause and effect relationships of the effects of physical activity on the bone mass. In the reviewed studies, bone mass is measured by different methods (single photon absorptiometry, dual photon absorptiometry, dual energy X-ray absorptiometry, and quantitative computed tomography) to establish the bone mineral density (BMD in gram per square cm) in different parts of the human skeleton (arm, hip, spine, and heel) and that of animals (rat, turkey, and sheep). These details will be mentioned only if necessary and if they have important consequences for the interpretation of the results. Most of the research is aimed at prevention and retardation of bone loss in postmenopausal women. The question remains whether it is also possible to increase the bone mass during the growing years to attain higher maximal bone mass at young adult age (Figure 5.1).

Because we know little about the natural development of bone mass during youth, the literature is reviewed on the changes in bone mass during pre- and postpubertal growth, the differences in bone development in boys and girls, and the point in time the maximal amount of bone mass (the so-called peak bone mineral density) is reached. The last part of this paper is devoted to the results of a longitudinal study in males and females whose physical activity pattern was monitored from age 13 to age 27 (40). When the subjects reached age 27, bone mineral density in the lumbar spine was measured, and the effects of differences in the amount of weight-bearing activities in the previous years was investigated.

PREVENTIVE STRATEGY

increasing peak BMD

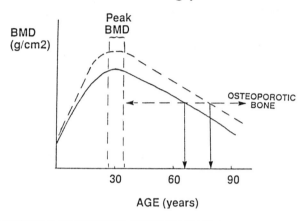

Figure 5.1.   Schematic illustration of a strategy to prevent osteoporosis by increasing peak bone mass during youth.

Mechanisms of Bone Formation

Bone mass seems to be dependent on centrally regulated hormonal factors, locally determined mechanical factors, and the interaction between both (73).

(1) The hormonal system is aimed at maintaining the calcium concentration in serum via the parathyroid hormone, the vitamin D content, calcitonin, and gonadal hormones.

(2) The two most important forces acting on the bones are muscle contractions and gravitational forces. Depending on the daily pattern of these forces, the bone is adapting and remodeling its functional structure. The supposed mechanisms are the following:

• During flexion the bone's behavior acts like a piezo-electric crystal while accumulating calcium at the concave (=negative loaded) side (6).
• Micro-fractions, occurring by overload, stimulate the osteoclasts in removing the damaged structures, and at the same time the osteoblasts repair the structure of the bone matrix. In the case of a too strong or too often damaged bone, the process of repairing falls behind the process of removal (12a). When the mechanical load falls below the fracture intensity, remodeling activities are stimulated and result in bone hypertrophy (14). In animal experiments, remodeling of the bone after a change in mechanical load by weight-bearing activities [including experiments with added extra weights, (82)] has been proved in a great number of animals (87). Moreover, in some

of these experiments it is shown that the effects are proportional to the intensity of the (extra) load. The amount of hypertrophy seems also to depend on the difference of the extra load compared to the before experienced daily load on the bone in question (39).

(3) Not much is known about the interaction between central-hormonal and local-mechanical factors. Physical activity leads to an increase of serum estrogen levels; this diminishes the sensitivity for the bone of the parathyroid hormone and the activity of the osteoclasts. When bone mass increases more calcium (Ca) and phosphorus (P) are resorbed from the blood; this lowering of Ca- and P-concentrations in the blood stimulates the parathyroid hormone. The latter inhibits the vitamin D production, stimulates calcium absorption, and decreases calcium secretion.

Methodological Problems

To prove that there is a cause and effect relationship between the amount of physical activity and bone mass, longitudinal studies are necessary to study the change of the development over time. In addition, an intervention with extra physical activities has to be given to an experimental group and compared with a control group not submitted to such a regimen of extra exercise. If both experimental group and control group are chosen randomly, all confounding factors are under control and the differences in bone mass at the end of follow-up can be ascribed to the intervention of physical activity.

Such an experimental longitudinal investigation, however, is seldom performed and can only be executed with several limitations in human subjects. Most of these investigations are done in elderly women over a maximal period of four years.

Several other possibilities are used in the literature:

- Cross-sectional studies, which compare differences in bone mass of subjects with different physical activity patterns on one point of time (such as sporting and non-sporting people)
- Effects of diminished activities that are caused in subjects by injuries or total immobilization of bed rest due to hospitalization
- Effects of extremely long and intensive training and competition in endurance athletes

In all these designs it is not possible to deduct cause-effect relationships about the effects of physical activity on the bone mass under study, because these effects also could be caused by other confounding factors such as self-selection and differences in genetics between the groups that are compared.

In the following pages we will review the main results obtained from the different designs.

Cross-sectional Studies

Comparisons of sporting people with non-sporting people are problematic because other possible intervening factors can explain the differences found in bone mass (e.g., differences in genetic background, nutrition, self-selection, compliance, activity level, and body composition). Correlations between muscle mass (68,52), body weight (56), and muscle force (19,32,33,85) with bone mass can partly be explained by these confounders (47).

Comparison Within Subjects

This problem of confounding can be partly overcome by within-subjects comparisons. To avoid genetic confounding, Jones et al. (37) measured the density of cortical bone of the humerus of professional tennis players and compared their playing arm with their non-playing arm: In men and women the cortical density of the playing arm appeared ca 35% and 28% higher than of the non-playing arm respectively. In older tennis players (>55 years) comparable results were found, although they are less pronounced: Montoye et al. (1950) and Huddleston et al. (34) observed in the radius and the humerus of the dominant arm respectively 13% and 8 to 13% more bone mass than in the non-dominant arm. Krolner et al. (42) studied women with arm fractures (mean age 60 years) who played tennis for one hour twice a week for an 8-month period. They showed an increase in bone mass in the injured arm and a decrease in the contra-lateral arm.

Comparisons Between Active and Inactive Subjects

In general, sporting activities in which the body weight is carried create forces on the lower back and legs sufficient to stimulate hypertrophy of the bones. Therefore, highest bone density can be found in weight lifters, followed by athletic throwers (shot put, discus, javelin), runners, and soccer players (53).

Swimming seems to have a beneficial influence on the arm, wrist, and hand (radius and metatarsalia), but not on the trunk and legs (vertebra and femur) (36). This specific effect can be explained by the swimming activities: 80% of propulsion in swimming is generated by the arms. The trunk and legs are less involved, and gravitational forces have less influence on the trunk because of the horizontal position of the body in the water. Comparison of cross-country runners with controls of the same age of seven locations (including os calcaneus) revealed a 10 to 20% higher bone mass in the runners (6).

Comparisons between physically active women and inactive women at all ages always indicate a higher bone mineral density in the active women (36,38,55). Brewer et al. (9) reported higher bone density at two of the four measured locations in middle-aged female endurance athletes with a training history of at least five years, than in age matched, untrained controls. Bailey et al. (4) compared the bone density in the os calcis (containing much trabecular and little cortical bone) with computed tomography of female students whose activity patterns varied between inactive to top sport. Analysis of variance resulted in significantly higher bone density in the four different activity groups (inactive, active, very active, and top sport) that was proportional with the amount of physical activity. Stillman et al. (76) found comparable results in the bone mineral content of the radius of women in age groups of 35, 45, 55, 65, and 70+. Yano et al. (88) found significant correlations between the amount of bone mass in the radius, ulna, and os calcis and the daily physical activity pattern of U.S. citizens of Japanese ancestry. This correlation was more apparent in men than in women, because, the authors explain, on average the males had a higher physical activity pattern than the females.

Talmage and Anderson (77) and Talmage et al. (78) showed, in a population of 1,200 females ranging in age from 18 to 98 years, the following results:

- The ones who were active in their youth had a higher bone density at age 25 than their inactive counterparts.
- The ones who remained active throughout adulthood showed more bone mass and a lower relative risk for osteoporosis compared to the inactive women.
- The expected decrease in bone mineral density of the radius in the 124 very active sporting women (1 hour, 3 times per week, 9 months per year for at least 5 years) did not occur as it did in the case of the 1,105 non-active women.

Studies to date show that physical activity in women with anorexia nervosa (63) has a protecting function on the bone density and counterbalances the prevalent estrogen deficiency.

Longitudinal Studies

Follow-up studies are necessary to demonstrate if a change in physical activity influences the bone mass. The effects of physical exercise on bone mass can be hypothesized on the basis of the forces and movements that are generated by the muscle contractions and the gravitational forces of parts of the body mass. These stimulate the function of the osteoblasts and, consequently, total muscle mass and total bone mass demonstrate a high correlation (61).

Effects of Bed Rest

Bone atrophy is clearly demonstrated by immobilization such as bed rest, plastering of limbs, and denervation. The atrophic effects are bone specific. Even one night of sleep initiates a negative calcium balance. Plastering after sport injuries results in an 18% loss of bone mass. Also, patients with polio and spinal cord lesions lose bone mass rapidly due to the diminished weight-bearing activities. During long-term bed rest, the absence of gravitational forces and muscle activity leads to bone resorption and diminished remodeling of the bone (3). During bed rest, the decalcification takes place predominantly in the lumbar spine, the sacrum, and the femur, but far less in the skeleton of the arm, the wrist, and the hand. In young people, the regeneration after bed rest is greater than in elderly people; this may stipulate the importance of remaining active during the entire course of life. Investigations from Issekutz et al. (35) on the effects of bed rest on the calcium metabolism have indicated that the increased calcium excretion in urine is not caused by the inactivity of the subjects per se, but is more closely related to the absence of the pressures in the longitudinal direction of the long bones: Increased calcium excretion was apparent during both supine cycling exercise (1-4 hours per day) and during passive sitting in a wheelchair (8 hours per day). On the contrary, 3 hours per day of standing caused a significant decrease of the calcium excretion to normal values. However, when subjects were placed in the supine position by means of a harness at the feet and at the shoulder for 3 hours per day and a force was applied equal to the force of the body mass in the standing position, this compression resulted in normal calcium excretion rates in the urine (Figure 5.2).

If the calcium excretion is a valid measure of bone mineralization, these elegant experiments suggest that the mechanical load on the bone is essential for a normal healthy bone mineralization. The results of these older experiments are supported by recent investigations by astronauts. During a 3-week period of weightlessness in the space lab, astronauts were found to have significantly elevated calcium excretion in the urine (43).

According to the studies, the effectiveness of physical activity for the structure of bone mass is more dependent on the biomechanics of the activity than on the

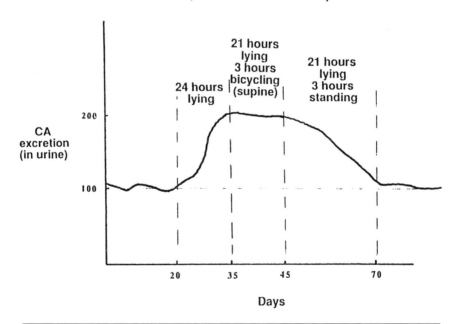

Figure 5.2.   Effects of biomechanical loading of the body on calcium excretion in urine.
After Issekutz et al., 1966.

energetics. Weight-bearing exercises such as walking, running, stair climbing, and dancing can—because of the accompanying longitudinal pressure on the long bones of the legs and vertebrae—have a better protective effect on the bone mineralization than weight-supporting exercises such as swimming and cycling, even if they result in the same energy expenditure (74).

More than a decade ago the German scientist Julius Wolff proposed a theory about adaptation of biological material. His theory is known nowadays as Wolff's Law: Any living cell or tissue is able, within certain limits, to adapt itself in structure and function, depending on the environmental constraints laid upon it. The same may hold for bone tissue: It changes its structure preferably on the forces that act on it.

Although not all underlying mechanisms are understood, it is probable that the density of trabecular bone will be influenced by the daily load experienced in the previous period (including intensity, duration, and frequency). In addition, it is also probable that the magnitude of the forces is more effective than the number of repetitions (46). In this respect, two recent publications concerning postmenopausal women are of importance. Cavanagh and Cann (13) found that a 1-year training at walking pace could not prevent trabecular bone loss in the lumbar spine. Dalsky et al. (17), on the other hand, proved that a heavy resistance training resulted in an increase of the lumbar bone mineral density: It seems that weight lifting, characterized by a high power and a low repetition, is more effective than walking or jogging (high repetition and low power). The effects of mechanical loading have been more systematically and extensively studied in animals such as sheep (54), turkeys (66), and rats (83).

Influence of Extra Physical Activity

Longitudinal studies that include interventions with extra physical activity are indispensable to prove that the bone mass can be influenced by the daily physical activity pattern of the subjects involved. These investigations are relatively seldom found in the literature. Of the 21 studies found, only 1 is done in males; 17 of the studies are with subjects older than 45 years; and in 8 of the studies the follow-up was over a relatively short period (less than one year).

Taking into account the quality of the research designs used, we found only a few studies acceptable for review. We only describe the results of longitudinal studies that are methodologically acceptable according to the following nine criteria:

1. Selection of a homogeneous population
2. Minimal number of 10 subjects in each group
3. Presence of a control group
4. Adequate data presentation and data analysis
5. Adequate randomization
6. At least six months of follow-up
7. Measurement of relevant effect parameters
8. Information about nutritional and physical activity patterns
9. Compliance of subjects of at least 60%

Effects in Older Women. Aloia et al. (1) and Chow et al. (15) found that in older women a 1-year period of exercise consisting of a combination of calisthenics, stretching, and dance for 30 to 60 minutes three times per week resulted in significant increases in the bone mineral density of the radius compared to non-exercising control groups.

Smith et al. (70) showed a significant increase in the bone mass of the radius of 20 elderly women, who during a period of 3 years (three times per week for half an hour each time) participated in calisthenics on a chair, compared to controls. Three other investigations from Smith et al. (71, 72, 74) give further support to the hypothesis that physical activity can enhance the bone density in elderly women.

(1) Women (n=12) with a mean age of 81 years performed special exercises for elderly. The intensity was 2 to 3 times basal metabolic rate, two times per week for 30 minutes over a period of 3 years. The intervention group showed a 2% increase in bone density of the radius, while the control group (n=18) showed a concomitant decrease of 3%, which is comparable with the tendency of the general population.

(2) For 3 years, 86 women (mean age 50 years) exercised three times a week for 45 minutes each time. In the first year the exercises were predominantly weight-bearing. After the first year, nevertheless, both the intervention group and the control group lost bone in their forearms: The intervention group lost 4% of their bone density in the radius and 6% in the ulna, and the control group (n=62) ca 2% and ca 3% respectively. These results can be explained by the exercises that were not specially aimed at the upper body. In the second and third year this was changed. Consequently, bone density increased in the intervention group in both ulna (ca 4%) and radius (1.5%), while the control group continued to lose bone.

(3) After a continued intervention over a total period of 4 years, the bone loss in ulna and radius of both pre- and postmenopausal women was significantly less than in the controls.

The importance of weight-bearing activities such as walking, jogging, and stair climbing for the maintenance of bone mass of postmenopausal women is demonstrated by Dalsky et al. (17) and Sandler et al. (67). Dalsky et al. found significantly higher lumbar bone mass after training periods of 9 and 22 months; after 13 months of cessation of the training, however, the bone density returned to the pre-training level. Sandler et al. (67) also demonstrated system effects as measured by significant increase of the cross section of the (not loaded) radius in female subjects who participated in a walking exercise (3.6 km, two times per week for 3 years). This effect was present only in the females who had a relatively strong isometric handgrip force.

In all eight studies, bone mineral density in both lumbar spine and arms of older pre- and postmenopausal women increased significantly more than in the controls when the extra physical activity included weight-bearing activities.

Effects in Young Men and Women. Studies in young subjects are scarce: of five studies only one was done with males (48). Margulies et al. trained 268 18 to 21-year-old military recruits very intensively (8 hours per day, 6 days per week) for 14 weeks. A significant increase of 5 to 11% was observed in bone mineral density of both legs. However, there was no control group, the period was relatively short, and, most important, 110 of the subjects could not comply because of stress fractures. Therefore, no evidence is available about the effects of extra physical activity on the bone density in young males.

Of the four remaining studies in young women, only the studies of Blake-Gleeson (29) and Blimkie et al. (7) are valid for review. Blake-Gleeson et al. set up a weight training program for 34 women ages 24 to 46. The women trained for one-half hour three times per week for 1 year at an intensity of 60% of their one repetition maximum. Bone density in lumbar spine and calcaneus in the 34 women were compared to that in 38 controls. No changes were found in either group. Blimkie et al. also found no significant changes in younger girls (14-18 years) over a period of 26 weeks.

These studies concluded that in females age 14 to 46, the effects of weight training do not influence the bone density. No valid data on males are available.

Influence of Extremely High Physical Activity

Up to now we have focused on the prevention of bone loss. Not much is known about the effects on people who are subjected to very hard and long physical work or heavy endurance sports training. In general, male marathon and cross-country runners have a higher bone density than do non-runners (2,16). But these cross-sectional observations are less valid.

In endurance trained female athletes, a high prevalence of secondary amenorrhea is apparent, varying from 5 to 40%. It is believed that these athletes will lose bone mass because of a too low estrogen concentration (12). On the other hand, we can assume that with the high training activity this (hormonal caused) bone loss will compensate or even will reverse in an (mechanical related) increase.

Several authors have found that female endurance athletes with absence of or irregular menses have lower bone mineral density than females with a regular menstruation pattern (23,24,44,51). Marcus et al. (45) found in female endurance runners that amenorrheics had lower lumbar bone mass than eumenorrheics. However, the lumbar bone mass in these athletes was significantly higher than in females with secondary amenorrhea who were not physically active.

Drinkwater et al. (20,21) performed two studies in female marathon runners. Two groups of 25-year-old amenorrheic ($n=14$) and eumenorrheic ($n=14$) females were compared. The only difference between the groups was the amount of training: The amenorrheic runners covered 60 km/week and the eumenorrheic runners 40 km/week. The results showed that the athletes with amenorrhea had significantly lower bone density in the lumbar spine and significantly lower estrogen levels than did the athletes who were eumenorrheic. Drinkwater et al. (21) continued to follow these female athletes. Return of menses in seven of these former amenorrheic runners was accompanied with a 6% increase in their lumbar bone mass. The runners who remained amenorrheic showed a continuation of bone loss in lumbar vertebrae of 3%. It seems, therefore, that in female athletes the estrogen level plays an important role (18a) and is more important in causing the decrease in bone mass than the physical activity. It also explains why male endurance athletes do not have the same bone loss.

We can conclude that the bone loss in female endurance athletes is not caused primarily by the extremely long and intensive physical activity, but by the lower estrogen levels.

The Natural Course of Development of Bone Mass During Youth

Before speculating about the possibility of influencing peak bone mass during youth to delay the age at which the loss of bone mass (due to aging) begins (especially in postmenarchal women where it reaches the borderline of osteoporotic bone), we must get insight into the development of the bone mass and at what point in time of life the maximal amount of bone mass will be reached. Therefore, in this section we will review the literature about bone development in boys and girls before puberty, estimate the importance of the pubertal period in the total development of bone mass, and try to determine the age at which maximal or peak bone mineral density occurs in males and females.

Development of Bone Density Before Puberty

Cross-sectional studies (8,25,26,28,30,31) and the longitudinal study of Theintz et al. (80), conclude that between boys and girls there is no significant difference between the bone mineral density of the radius and the lumbar spine. This indicates that the development of BMD before puberty is not dependent on steroids. Although there is a trend of a gradual increase from birth to puberty in bone mass, from the publications reviewed it is not possible to make a quantitative estimation of the proportional contribution to the total (adult) bone mass. Before puberty there is no difference in BMD between boys and girls.

Development of Bone Density During Puberty

The relatively short period of life of the pubertal stage of boys and girls (about 3 to 5 years) seems to be a very important one for the development of bone mass according to the literature. The results of cross-sectional studies of Gilsanz et al. (26), Glastre et al. (28), Geusens et al. (25), Bonjour et al. (8), Gordon et al. (30), and Grimston et al. (31) report increases of BMD that vary between 15 and 75% of total adult values in girls and between 5 and 70% of total adult values in boys (see Figure 5.3).

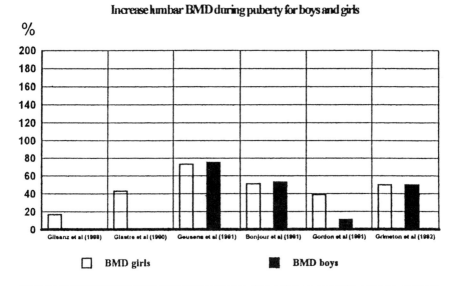

Figure 5.3.   Percentage increase in bone mineral density of boys and girls during puberty.

The high variation in the results can be attributed to several factors:

1. Differences in the classification of the pubertal stages (79)
2. Confounding factors such as nutritional and/or activity patterns that are different for the populations studied
3. The possible influence of early or late maturation: Early maturation coincides with a relatively longer exposition to sex specific hormones than late maturation. Dhuper et al. (18a) showed that estrogen levels in girls and Riis et al. (64) showed that testosterone levels in boys are related to bone mass development. This could also be confirmed in the retrospective cohort study of Finkelstein et al. (22), who found in males with a delayed puberty a lower radial BMD compared to males with advanced puberty.

The cross-sectional data of Bonjour et al. (8) indicate that in boys and girls the pubertal years add 53% and 51% respectively to total bone mass of the lumbar spine. This is 31% for the radial bone mass in boys (64).

Recently however, Bailey et al. (5) reported that the BMD changes should be interpreted with caution. Determination of BMD by projectional methods like Dual X-ray Absorptiometry (DEXA) provide areal densities (g/cm2) which are confounded by size changes accompanying growth. The calculated volumetric BMD percentage increases were substantially less than the corresponding area BMD values. This dimensional consideration explains why Gilsanz et al. (26) showed the lowest increase (15%), because they were the only ones who used the quantified computerized tomography (QCT) to measure BMD, and this method provides real volumetric BMDs.

The BMD changes during the growth period that are reported in the literature and indicate that around puberty 50% of BMD is accreted must be doubted, because the measurement of area BMD by the DEXA method overestimates due to the accompanying size changes of the growing bones. The only study with QCT method reports a 15% volume BMD increase in pubertal girls, which seems to be a more realistic value.

Age at Which Maximal Bone Mass Is Reached (Peak Bone Mineral Density, PBMD)

Most of the anatomical structures and physiological functions, such as muscle mass, cardiorespiratory functions, immune system, and central nervous system, show a typical pattern over time. This is characterized by a steep increase during the growth period till the age of 20 years, and thereafter a much slower decrease and gradual decline during aging (40). This pattern implies that there is a point or period of time when the human functions reach their maximal capacities. The question is whether there is a same pattern observable in the development of the bone mass, and if so, at what point in time of life does the peak bone mineral density (PBMD) occur.

Cross-Sectional Studies

Of the 12 studies published between 1981 and 1992, seven are performed in girls (10,11,27,42,59,65,75) and five in both boys and girls (8,25,28,30,60).

Although a cross-sectional design in principle is not adequate to indicate individual changes over time and moreover also has methodological constraints (such as cohort effects, secular trend, etc.), with certain restrictions we give the results of some of them. Only cross-sectional studies with acceptable methodology and with sufficient information from the publication are taken into account.

The five acceptable studies left (8,10,25,27,28) report an age period of reaching PBMD in females between 16 and 23 and in boys between 16 and 25 years.

Longitudinal Studies

Eight longitudinal studies investigated the development of BMD and PBMD. All of them used female subjects. From a methodological point of view, the studies of Riggs et al. (62), Moen et al. (49), and Schlechte et al. (1992) can be seriously questioned, and these studies tend to confirm the cross-sectional results that PBMD occurs before the age of 20.

However, the two most valid studies from Davies et al. (18) with a follow-up of 4 years and from Recker et al. (58) with a follow-up of 5 years show very clearly that at least in females the age of PBMD is reached much later than 20 years; lumbar, radial, and total BMD reach the highest values around the age of 30 years (Figure 5.4). Because no data are available for males, it remains unknown at what age PBMD will be reached in males.

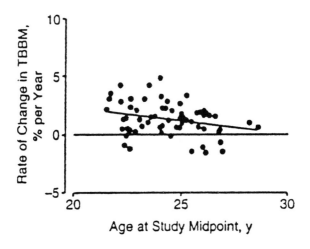

Figure 5.4.   Rate of change in total bone body mass (TBBM) as a percentage per year between the ages 20 and 30 years.
After Recker et al., 1992.

The discrepancies between the results of cross-sectional and longitudinal studies can therefore be attributed to confounding factors. In general, the valid cross-sectional studies tend to establish PBMD in females between 16 and 25 years of age and the longitudinal investigations much later, around the age of 30. Because longitudinal data are more adequate to detect age changes, it is more likely to believe that PBMD in females is occurring not in their late teens but in their late twenties.

Results of the Amsterdam Growth and Health Study About the Effects of Weight-Bearing Activities and Dietary Calcium Intake on PBMD

In the Amsterdam Growth and Health Study, 98 females and 84 males were measured longitudinally from age 13 till age 27. Since by 1991 of these subjects reached the 26-29 age range, the period when PBMD is supposed to be reached, BMD of the lumbar region was determined in this population by DEXA (41).

In the preceding 15 years measurements were taken six times of anthropometric, physiological, and psychological characteristics and also two aspects of their lifestyle by cross-check interviews of daily nutritional intake (57) and habitual physical activity (84). From the nutritional intake the calcium contribution was calculated and from the physical activity the contribution of weight-bearing activities was calculated: The dietary calcium intake was related to body height

(CAIH) and the weight-bearing activities as multiples of basal metabolic rate (WBA).

The longitudinal information of CAIH and WBA were considered over three periods: (1) the adolescent period from 13 to 18 years, (2) the period between 13 and 22 years, and (3) the total period between the ages of 13 and 28 years. In multiple linear regression analyses, we entered body weight, calcium intake, and weight-bearing activity separately for males and females in order to explain differences in lumbar bone mineral density at the age of 27 (86).

The results showed that only WBA and body weight were significant positive contributors to the final model of lumbar BMD at the age of 27. In males, the final model contained WBA in all three age periods, and in the total period body weight also was a significant predictor (Table 5.1).

In females, only body weight was in all age periods a significant predictor of BMD at the age of 27 years (Table 5.2).

These variables accounted for 16 to 17% and 9 to 14% of the total variance in males and females respectively. Calcium intake never appeared as a significant predictor of BMD in the three periods in both sexes.

It is interesting to see that WBA during the adolescent period are even more important for the BMD than WBA measured at age 21 or at age 27. The minor role for dietary calcium intake can be explained by the relatively high calcium

Table 5.1   Prediction of peak bone mineral density (PBMD) in males from weight bearing activities (WBA), calcium intake (CAI), and body weight (WT)

Age period	Variables	Regression coefficient	Explained variance
13-17 years	WBA	0.18	16%
13-21 years	WBA	0.16	17%
13-27 years	WBA WT	0.59	17%

Table 5.2   Prediction of peak bone mineral density (PBMD) in females from weight bearing activities (WBA), calcium intake (CAI), and body weight (WT)

Age period	Variables	Regression coefficient	Explained variance
13-17 years	WT	0.56	9%
13-21 years	WT	0.64	12%
13-27 years	WT	0.72	14%

intake of the Dutch subjects. Over the 15-year study, the calcium intake met in general in both sexes the recommendations of the daily allowances (DRDA). Only in teenage boys was the low calcium intake group (<P25) far below the DRDA of 900-1200 mg/day, and in teenage girls the low calcium intake group approximated the DRDA of 700-1000 mg/day.

From the results we can conclude that PBMD in the lumbar spine may be influenced by body weight and a high level of weight-bearing physical activity carried out during youth. It stresses the importance of a sufficient amount of physical activity during growth and development in order to reach a high peak bone mass at young adult age and, therefore, to delay the attainment of a critical minimal bone mass resulting in osteoporosis and fractures at older ages. These preventive effects of WBA during youth on BMD, however, have to be confirmed in a true experimental design, because the significant differences in BMD can still be explained by self-selection of activity levels during puberty.

General Conclusions

In this chapter we have provided a critical review about the natural development of bone mineral density during youth and the effects of biomechanical load from physical activity.

Bone mass increases during youth and development. The quantitative increases in terms of BMD are probably an over estimation, because these measures do not take into account differences in dimensional growth of the bones in question. Before puberty there are no differences in BMD between boys and girls. During the pubertal growth spurt, it is likely that the increases in BMD are between 10 and 20%. The longitudinal studies indicate that, in females, the BMD reaches its peak value (PBMD) in the late twenties. No data of peak BMD are available for males.

The effects of extra mechanical load on the BMD show that in almost all studies with post-menarchal women, physical activity results in a significant increase in BMD and/or a retardation of the age dependent BMD loss.

Extreme long and intensive physical activity does not decrease BMD in males; only in amenorrheic females.

In young subjects only effect studies are done in females, and they show no effects on BMD. Explanation of these negative results may be the short duration of the training programs and the relatively high habitual physical activity of young females compared to older post-menarchal females.

The only preventive effect of weight-bearing activities on the peak bone mineral density is shown in the Amsterdam Growth and Health Longitudinal Study. Both 27-year-old males and females with a relatively high habitual physical activity pattern during the foregoing 15 years had significantly higher PBMD than their inactive counterparts. The higher PBMD built up during youth can delay the age at which the osteoporotic border will be reached.

References

1. Aloia, J.F. Prevention of involutional bone loss by exercise. Ann. Int. Med. 89:356-358; 1978a.
2. Aloia, J.F.; Cohn, S.H.; Bahn, T.; Abesamis, C.; Kalici, N.; Ellis, K. Skeletal mass and body composition of marathon runners. 27:1743-1746; 1978b.
3. Andersson, S.M.; Nilsson, B.E. Changes in bone mineral content following ligamentous knee injuries. Med. Sci. Sports Exerc. 11:351-353; 1979.
4. Bailey, D.A.; Martin, A.D.; Howie, J.L.; Houston, C.S.; Simpson, C.; Harrison, E.; Lee, E. Bone density and physical activity in young women. In: Pusso, P., ed. Exercise, nutrition and performance. Sidney: Cumberland College of Health Science; 1986.
5. Bailey, D.; Drinkwater, B.; Faulkner, R.; McKay, H. Proximal femur bone mineral changes in growing children: dimensional considerations. Ped. Exerc. Science 5:388; 1993.
6. Bassett, C.A. Biophysical principles affecting bone structure. In: G. H. Bourne, ed. The biochemistry and physiology of bone. New York: Academic Press; 1976: 1-76.
7. Blimkie, C.J.; Rice, S.; Webber, J.; Martin, J.; Levy, D.; Parker, D. Bone density, physical activity, fitness, anthropometry, gynecologic, endocrine and nutrition status in adolescent girls. In: Coudert, J.; v. Praagh, E., ed. Pediatric work physiology. Masson; 1993: 201-204.
8. Bonjour, J.F.; Theintz, G.; Buchs, B.; Slosman, D.; Rizzoli, R. Critical years and stages of puberty for spinal and femoral bone mass accumulation during adolescence. J. Clin. Endocrin. Soc. 73:555-563; 1991.
9. Brewer, V.; Meyer, B.M.; Keele, M.S.; Upton, S.J.; Hagen, R.D. Role of exercise in prevention of involutional bone loss. Med. Sci. Sports Exerc. 15:445-449; 1983.
10. Buchanan, J.; Meyers, C.; Lloyd, T.; Leuenberger, P.; Demers, L. Determinants of peak trabecular bone density in women: the role of androgens, estrogen, and exercise. J. Bone Min. Res. 3:673-680; 1988a.
11. Buchanan, J.R.; Meyers, C.; Lloyd, T.; Greer, R.B. III. Early vertebral trabecular bone loss in normal premenopausal women. J. Bone Min. Res. 3:445-449; 1988b.
12. Cann, C.E.; Martin, M.C.; Genant, H.K.; Jaffe, R.B. Decreased spinal mineral content in amenorrheic women. JAMA 251:626-629; 1984.
12a. Carter, D.R. Mechanical loading histories and cortical bone remodeling. Calc. Tissue Int. (Suppl.) 36:19-24; 1984.
13. Cavanagh, D.J.; Cann, C.E. Brisk walking does not stop bone loss in postmenopausal women. Bone 9:201-204; 1988.
14. Chamay, A.; Tschantz, P. Mechanical influences in bone remodeling. Experimental research on Wolff's law. J. Biomech. 5:173-180; 1972.
15. Chow, R.; Harrison, J.E.; Notarius, C. Effect of two randomised exercise programs on bone mass of healthy post menopausal women. Brit. Med. J. 295:1441-1444; 1985.
16. Dalen, N.; Olssen, K.E. Bone mineral content and physical activity. Acta. Orthop. Scand. 45:170-174; 1974.
17. Dalsky, G.P.; Stocke, K.S.; Ehsani, A.A.; Slatopresky, E.; Lee, W.C.; Birge, S.J. Weight bearing exercise training and lumbar bone mineral content in postmenopausal women. Ann. of Int. Med. 108:824-828; 1988.
18. Davies, K.M.; Recker, R.R.; Stegman, M.R.; Heaney, R.P.; Kimmel, D.B.; Leist, J. Third decade bone gain in women. In: Cohn, D. V.; Glorieux, F.H.; Martin, T.J., ed. Calcium regulation and bone metabolism. Elsevier Science; 1990:497-50.
18a. Dhuper, S.; Warren, M.P.; Brooks-Gunn, J.; Fox, R. Effects of hormonal status on bone density in adolescent girls. J. Clin. Endocrinol. Metab. 71:1083-1088; 1990.
19. Doyle, F.; Brown, J.; Lanchance, C. Relation between bone mass and muscle weight. 1:391-393; 1970.
20. Drinkwater, B.; Wilson, K.; Chesnut, C. III; Brenner, W.; Shainholtz, S.; Southworth, M. Bone mineral content of amenorrheic and eumenorrheic athletes. N.E.J.M. 311:277-281; 1984.

21. Drinkwater, B.; Wilson, K.; Chesnut, C. III. Bone mineral density after resumption of menses in amenorrheic athletes. JAMA 256:380-382; 1986.
22. Finkelstein, J.S.; Neer, R.M.; Biller, B.M.K.; Crawford, J.D.; Klibanski, A. Osteopenia in men with a history of delayed puberty. N.E.J.M. 27:600-603; 1992.
23. Fisher, E.; Nelson, M.; Frontera, W.; Turksoy, R.; Evans, W. Bone mineral content and level of gonadotropinins and estrogens in amenorrhea of college athletes in relation to age of onset of training. J. Clin. Endocrin. Metab. 62:1232-1236; 1986.
24. Frisch, R.; Gotz-Welbergen, A.; McArthur, J.; Albright, T.; Witschi, J.; Bullen, B.; Birnholz, J.; Reed, R.; Hermann, H. Delayed menarche and amenorrhea of college athletes in relation to age of onset of training. JAMA 246:1559-1563; 1981.
25. Geusens, P.; Cantatore, F.; Nijs, J.; Proesmans, W.; Emma, F.; Dequeker, J. Heterogeneity of growth of bone in children at the spine, radius and total skeleton. 55:249-256; 1991.
26. Gilsanz, V.; Gibbons, D.T.; Roe, T.F.; Carlson, M. Vertebral bone density in children: effect of puberty. 166:847-850; 1988a.
27. Gilsanz, V.; Gibbons, D,T.; Carlson, M. Peak trabecular vertebral density: a comparison of adolescent and adult females. Calcif. Tissue Int. 43:260-262; 1988b.
28. Glastre, C.; Braillon, P.; David, L.; Cochat, P.; Meunier, P.J.; Delmas, P.D. Measurement of bone mineral content of the lumbar spine by dual energy X-ray absorptiometry in normal children: correlations with growth parameters. J. Clin. Endocrin. and Metab. 70:1330-1333; 1990.
29. Gleeson, P.B.; Protas, E.J.; LeBlanc, A.D.; Schneider, V.S.; Evans, H.J. Effects of weight lifting on bone mineral density in premenopausal women. J. Bone. Min. Res. 5:153-158; 1990.
30. Gordon, C.L.; Halton, J.M.; Atkinson, S.A.; Webber, C.E. The contributions of growth and puberty to peak bone mass. 55:257-262; 1991.
31. Grimston, S.K.; Morrison, K.; Harder, J.A.; Hanley, D.A. Bone mineral density during puberty in Western Canadian children. 19:85-96; 1992.
32. Heinonen, A.; Vuori, I; Kannus, P.; Oja, P.; Sievänen, H. Bone mineral density in competitive female athletes. Med. Sci. Sports Exerc. (Suppl.) 24:S45; 1992.
33. Heinrich, C.H.; Going, S.B.; Pamenter, R.W.; Perry, C.D.; Boyden, T.W.; Lohman, T.G. Bone mineral content of cyclically menstruating female resistance and endurance trained athletes. 22:558-563; 1990.
34. Huddleston, A.L.; Rockwell, D.; Kulund, D.N.; Harrison, R.B. Bone mass in lifetime tennis athletes. J. Appl. Physiol. 244:1013-1020; 1980.
35. Issekutz, B.; Blizzard, J.J.; Birkhead, N.C.; Rodahl, K. Effect of prolonged bed rest on urinary calcium output. J. Appl. Physiol. 21:1013-1020; 1966.
36. Jacobson, P.C.; Beaver, W.; Grubb, S.A.; Taft, T.N.; Talmage, R.V. Bone density in women: college athletes and older athletic women. J. Orthop. Res. 2:328-332; 1984.
37. Jones, H.; Priest, J.D.; Hayes, W.C.; Chinn Tichenor, C.; Nagel, D.A. Humeral hypertrophy in response to exercise. 59-A:204-208; 1977.
38. Kanders, B.; Lindsay, R.; Dempster, D.; Markhard, L.; Valignette, G. Determinants of bone mass in young healthy women. 22:337-339; 1988.
39. Kemper, H.C.G. Lichaamsbeweging en osteoporose. In: Stasse-Wolthuis, M.; W. Geerts-van der Wey, A.C., eds. Voeding en Osteoporose. Houten: Bohn Stafleu Van Loghum; 1990: 38-54.
40. Kemper, H.C.G. Binkhorst, R.A. Exercise and the physiological consequences of the aging process. In: J.J.F. Schroots, ed. Aging, health and competence. Elsevier, Amsterdam 6: 109-126, 1993.
41. Kemper, H.C.G. The Amsterdam growth and health study, health, fitness and lifestyle in longitudinal perspective; a follow-up of males and females from 13 to 27 years of age. Champaign, IL: HKP monograph, Human Kinetics; 1995.
42. Krolner, B.; Tondervald, E.; Toft, B.; Berthelsen, B.; Nielsen, S.P. Bone mass of the axial and the appendicular skeleton in women with Colles' fracture: its relation to physical activity. Clin. Physiol. 2:147-157; 1982.

43. Krolner, B.; Toft, B. Vertebral bone loss: an unheeded side effect of therapeutic bed rest. Clin. Science 64:537-540; 1983.
44. Louis, O.; Demeirleir, K.; Kalender, W.; Keizer, H.A.; Platen, P.; Hollmann, W.; Osteaux, M. Low vertebral bone density values in young non-elite female runners. Int. J. Sports Med. 12:214-217; 1991.
45. Marcus, R.; Cann, C.; Madvig, P.; Meukoff, J.; Goddard, M.; Bayer, M. Menstrual function and bone mass in elite women distance runners. Ann. Int. Med. 102:158-163; 1985.
46. Marcus, R. Exercise and the regulation of bone mass. Arch. Intern Med. 149:2170-2171; 1989.
47. Marcus, R.; Drinkwater, B.; Dalsky, G.; Dufek, J.; Raab, D.; Slemenda, C.; Snow-Harter, C. Osteoporosis and exercise in women. Med. Sci. Sports Exerc. 24:301-307; 1992.
48. Margulies, J.Y.; Simkin, A.; Leichter, I.; Bivas, A.; Steinberg, R.; Giladi, M.; Stein, M.; Kashtan, H.; Milgrom, C. Effect of intense physical activity on the bone mineral content in the lower limbs of young adults. 68a:1090-1093; 1986.
49. Moen, S.; Sanborn, C.; Bonnick, S.; Keizer, H.; Gench, B.; DiMarco, N. Longitudinal lumbar bone mineral density changes in adolescent female runners. 24:1992.
50. Montoye, H.J.; Smith, E.L.; Fardon, D.F.; Howley, E.T. Bone mineral in senior tennisplayers. Scan. J. Sports Sci. 2:26-32; 1980.
51. Nelson, M.; Fisher, E.; Catsos, P.; Meredith, C.; Turksoy, R.; Evans, W. Diet and bone status in amenorrheic runners. 43:910-916; 1986.
52. Nichols, D.; Sanborn, C.; Bonnick, S.; Dieringer, K.; Gench, B.; Sanborn, C.; DiMarco, N. Relationship of muscle mass to bone mineral density in female intercollegiate athletes. Med. Sci. Sports Exerc. (J.A.C.S.M.) 28:46; 1992.
53. Nilsson, B.E.; Westlin, N.E. Bone density in athletes. Clin. Orthopaed. 77:179-182; 1971.
54. O'Conner, J.A.; Lanyon, L.E. The influence of strain rate on adaptive bone remodelling. 15:767-781; 1982.
55. Oyster, N.; Morton, M.; Linell, S. Physical activity and osteoporosis in post-menopausal women. Med. Sci. Sports Exerc. 16:44-50; 1984.
56. Pocock, N.; Eisman, J.; Gwinn, T.; Sambrook, P.; Kelly, P.; Freund, J.; Yeates, M. Muscle strength, physical fitness and weight but not age predict femoral neck bone mass. J. Bone & Min. Res. 4:441-448; 1989.
57. Post, G.B. Nutrition in adolescence, a longitudinal study in dietary patterns from teenager to adult. Thesis, Agriculture University Wageningen, SO 16, de Vrieseborch, Haarlem 1989.
58. Recker, R.R.; Davies, K.M.; Hinders, S.M.; Heaney, R.P.; Stegman, R.P.; Kimmel, D.B. Bone gain in young adult women. JAMA 268:2403-2408; 1992.
59. Ribot, C.; Tremollieres, F.; Pouilles, J.M.; Louvet, J.P.; Guiraud, R. The influence of the menopause and aging on spinal density in French women. 5:89-97; 1988.
60. Rico, H.; Revilla, M.; Hernandez, E.R.; Villa, L.F.; Alvarez del Buergo, L. Sex differences in the acquisition of total bone mineral mass peak assessed through dual energy X-ray absorptiometry. Calcif. Tissue Int. 51:251-254; 1992.
61. Riggs, B.L.; Melton, L.J. Involutional osteoporosis. N. Engl. J. Med. 413:1676-1686; 1986a.
62. Riggs, B.L.; Wahner, H.W.; Melton, L.J.; Richelson, L.S.; Judd, H.L.; Offord, K.P. Rates of bone loss in the appendicular and axial skeletons of women. J. Clin. Invest. 77:1487-1491; 1986b.
63. Rigotti, N.A.; Nussbaum, S.R.; Herzog, D.B.; Neer, R.M. Osteoporosis in women with anorexia nervosa. N.E.J.M. 11:1601; 1984.
64. Riis, B.J.; Krabbe, S.; Christiansen, C.; Catherwood, B.D.; Deftos, L.J. Bone turnover in male puberty: a longitudinal study. Calcif. Tis. Int. 37:213-217; 1985.
65. Rodin, A.; Murby, B.; Smith, M.A.; Caleffi, M.; Fentiman, I.; Chapman, M.G.; Fogelman, I. Premenopausal bone loss in the lumbar spine and neck of femur: a study of 225 Caucasian women. Bone 11:1-5; 1990.

66. Rubin, C.T.; Lanyon, L.E. Regulation of bone mass by strain magnitude. 37:411-417; 1985.
67. Sandler, R.B.; Cauley, J.A.; Hom, D.L.; Sashin, D.; Kriska, A.M. The effects of walking on the cross-sectional dimensions of the radius in postmenopausal women. Calcif. Tissue Int. 41:65-69; 1987.
68. Sinaki, M.; Offord, K.P. Physical activity in postmenopausal women: effect on back muscle strength and bone mineral density of the spine. Arch. Phys. Med. Rehab. 69:277-280; 1988.
69. Slemenda, C.W.; Miller, J.Z.; Hui, L.S.; Reister, T.K.; Johnston, C.C. Role of physical activity in the development of skeletal mass in children. J. Bone Min. Res. 6:1227-1233; 1991.
70. Smith, E.L.; Reddan, W. Physical activity: a modality for bone accretion in the aged. Am. J. Roentgen 126:1297; 1976.
71. Smith, E.L.; Reddan, W.; Smith, P.E. Physical activity and calcium modalities for bone mineral increase in aged women. Med. Sci. Sports Exercise 13:60-64; 1981.
72. Smith, E.L.; Smith, P.E.; Ensign, C.J.; Shea, M.M. Bone involution decrease in exercising middle-aged women. Calcif. Tissue Int. 36:129-138; 1984.
73. Smith, E.L.; Raab, D.M. Osteoporosis and physical activity. Acta. Med. Scand. 711:149-156; 1986.
74. Smith, E.L.; Gilligan, C. Exercise and bone mass. In: DeLuca, H.F.; Hazess, R., eds. Osteoporosis: physiological basis, assessment and treatment. Amsterdam: Elsevier Science; 1990: 285-293.
75. Snow-Harter, C.; Marcus, R. Exercise, bone mineral density and osteoporosis. 1991.
76. Stillman, R.J.; Lohman, T.G.; Slaughter, M.H.; Massey, B.H. Physical activity and bone mineral content in women aged 30 to 85 years. Med. Sci. Sports Exerc. 18:576-580; 1986.
77. Talmage, R.V.; Anderson, J.J.B. Bone density loss in women: effects of childhood activity, exercise, calcium intake and oestrogen therapy. Calcif. Tissue Int. 36:522; 1984.
78. Talmage, R.V.; Stinnett, S.S.; Landwehr, J.T.; Vincent, L.M.; McCartney, W.H. Age related bone loss of bone mineral density in non-athletic women. 1:115-125; 1986.
79. Tanner, J.M. Growth and adolescence. Oxford: Blackwell; 1962.
80. Theintz, G.; Buchs, B.; Rizolli, R.; Slosman, D.; Clavien, H.; Sizonenko, P.C.; Bonjour, J.P.H. Longitudinal monitoring of bone mass accumulation in healthy adolescents: evidence for a marked reduction after 16 years of age at the levels of lumbar spine and femoral neck in female subjects. J.C.E & M. 75:1060-1066; 1992.
81. Todorov, T. Tennis de haut niveau: modifications osseuses et articulaires du membre superieure actif du joueur. Ann ENSEPS 8:21-26; 1975.
82. Tulloh, N.M. Relation between carcass composition and live weight of sheep. Nature 197:809-810; 1963.
83. Turner, C.H. Functional determinants of bone structure: beyond Wolff's law of bone transformation. Bone (editorial bone) 13:403-409; 1992.
84. Verschuur, R. Daily physical activity and health, longitudinal changes during the teenage period. Thesis University of Amsterdam. S.O. 12 de Vrieseborch, Haarlem, 1987.
85. Virvidakis, K.; Georgiou, E.; Korkotsidis, A.; Nitalles, K.; Proukakis, C. Bone mineral content of junior competitive weight lifters. Int. J. Sports Med. 11:244-246; 1990.
86. Welten, D.C.; Kemper, H.C.G.; Post, G.B.; Mechelen, W.v.; Twist, J.; Lips, P.; Teule, G.J. Weight bearing activity during youth is a more important factor for peak bone mass than calcium intake. J. Bone Min. Res. 9(7):1089-1096; 1993.
87. Woo, S.L.Y.; Kuei, S.C.; Amiel, D.; Gomez, M.A.; Hayes, W.C.; White, F.C.; Akeson, W.H. The effect of prolonged physical training on the properties of long bone: a study on Wolff's law. J. Bone Joint Surg. 63a:780-786; 1981.
88. Yano, K. Bone mineral measurement among middle-aged and elderly Japanese residents in Hawaii. Am. J. Epidem. 119:751-764; 1984.

Chapter 6

The Role of Mechanical Loading in the Regulation of Skeletal Development During Growth

Donald A. Bailey, PED

Introduction

It has been recognized for over 100 years that skeletal tissue has the ability to adapt to a changing mechanical environment. In 1859, Darwin, in the first edition of his classical treatise *The Origin of Species by Means of Natural Selection*, referred to this capacity of bone as "functional adaptation." He used the domestic duck to illustrate this process, in which

> the bones of the wing weigh less and bones of the leg more, in proportion to the whole skeleton, than do the same bones in the wild duck; and this change may be safely attributed to the domestic duck flying less and walking more than its wild parents (9).

An anatomist from Berlin, Julius Wolff, is generally given credit for first articulating a law to explain this phenomenon. He noted that bone tissue reorganizes when mechanical forces change (39). His seminal work in German has recently been translated into English (22) and Wolff's Law, as it has come to be known, can be restated as follows: the general form of bone being given, alterations to the internal architecture and external form occur as a consequence of primary changes in mechanical stress.

The influence of mechanical stress on bone development can best be thought of in the following terms. At conception, humans are provided with a basic skeletal template dictated by the laws of heredity. During growth and throughout life, mechanical forces can modify this basic skeletal plan, within set limits, allowing the skeleton to cope with the physical demands and needs imposed on it by different levels and types of physical activity. Thus, in many respects the skeleton becomes self-designed to meet individual needs (6), thereby allowing functional activity to proceed in situations where a less adaptable skeleton might fail.

Bone Shaping Processes

The plasticity and adaptability of bone to respond to persistently altered mechanical forces is evident in the three different processes that are involved in changing the shape and architecture of bone: *growth, modeling, and remodeling.* Of these processes, a single one may dominate at different times during the life span, or the three processes may function concurrently at other times. While each process appears to have a different function, it is clear that mechanical loading is an important factor affecting the expression of each.

Growth

Growth is the expression of the genetically programmed process of enlargement of the skeleton under the control of the endocrine system. The genetic potential for growth, however, can be affected by extraneous factors of which mechanical loading is a preeminent factor along with nutrition and disease. Figure 6.1 shows

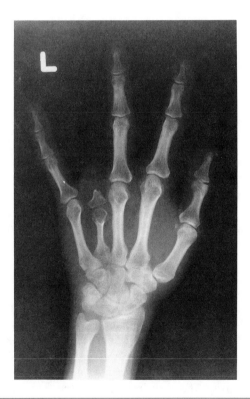

Figure 6.1.   Growth retardation of the fourth metacarpal in a 34-year-old woman following amputation of the ring finger at 21 months.

a radiograph of the hands of a 34-year-old woman who lost the ring finger on her left hand in an accident at the age of 21 months (17). In the absence of the missing phalanges there was no mechanical loading on the fourth metacarpal of the injured hand and no associated muscular forces acting on it. This resulted in a virtual cessation of growth in this bone as evidenced by a comparison with the same bone in the uninjured hand. This observation leads to interesting speculations as to the skeletal growth and integrity of children who may in the future be born in the gravitationally free environment associated with space exploration.

It should be noted that historically, from a growth perspective, there has been more concern with too much rather than too little mechanical loading. A good example of this would be the child workers of the early industrial revolution who experienced a stunting of growth. Of interest recently are two studies suggesting that some elite gymnastic training programs for growing children that involve intensive mechanical loading many hours a week may have a detrimental effect on somatic growth (37,40). Thus, there appears to be a "golden mean" in terms of mechanical loading and growth.

Modeling

Modeling is the process that alters the external form and internal architecture of specific bones in response to local factors. It occurs mainly during the growing years and is distinguished from growth by the fact that it is a regional response to specific loading factors. The modeling response to the mechanical loading involved in weight-bearing physical activity in young people may result in a reserve of bone beyond that needed for normal activity (12). Thus, it is possible that the student who finds recreation in weight lifting may be less vulnerable to fractures later in life than a comparable piano player with a smaller bone reserve (32).

An example of modeling in the young has been provided in a study of the bone density in the proximal femur of children with unilateral Legg Calvé Perthes Disease (2). This is a painful osteochondrotic condition of the hip causing a limp and compromised weight-bearing on the affected side. As indicated in Figure 6.2, the bone mineral density in specific femoral regions on the unaffected side, which has assumed an increased weight-bearing responsibility, is greater than age and sex specific baseline norms. Conversely, on the painful affected side values are generally below baseline norms. This indicates that bone mineral density can be modulated as a result of differential loading, a perfect example of modeling.

Remodeling

Remodeling, although present in young individuals, is the predominant bone process modifying shape and mass in adults. The maintenance of skeletal integrity is the goal of remodeling. Remodeling does not make a net contribution to the

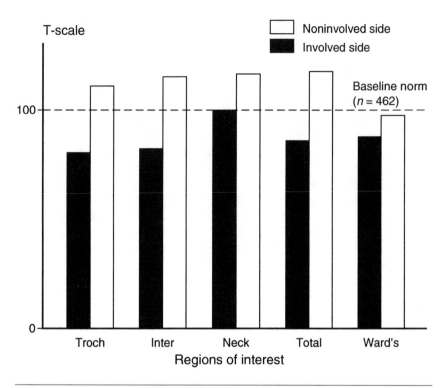

Figure 6.2.   Bone mineral density in regions of the affected and unaffected proximal femur in 18 children with unilateral Legg Calvé Perthes Disease.

"bone bank." In fact, just the opposite is true; over time unopposed remodeling results in a net bone loss.

The primary function of remodeling is to repair microfractures that occur with normal everyday living and to maintain a properly mineralized bone matrix. In normal remodeling the bone resorbing osteoclast cells and the bone forming osteoblast cells are coupled so that formation follows resorption. This process allows the skeleton to maintain its mechanical integrity through the renewal of bone and provides a mechanism for the maintenance of calcium homeostasis (11). The net bone loss that accompanies aging, when formation fails to keep up with resorption, is essentially the result of long-term remodeling.

Mechanical Strain and the Regulation of Bone Mass

The key intermediate variable between skeletal loading induced by physical activity and the adaptation of bone mass is the induced mechanical strain. Changes in internal strain in bone, defined as the minute deformation of bone in response to a mechanical load, appear to activate osteocytes which in turn alter the delicate balance between bone resorption and formation.

Repeated physical activity producing strain above an upper limit will induce modeling to increase bone mass in response to the increased load requirement. The increased bone mass has the effect of reducing the internal strain from a given load, because the same load will be distributed over a larger amount of bone. This reduced strain dampens the drive to bone formation, and a new equilibrium between resorption and formation is established, now at a higher level of bone mass. This mechanism for controlling bone mass is localized since different levels of mechanical strain exist in different parts of the skeleton, so there may be net bone loss and net bone gain occurring simultaneously in different locations.

A series of animal studies, particularly those of Lanyon (21) and his colleagues, have demonstrated that the effects of loading on bone cells are directly related to the level of strain and the loads must be cyclic in nature; static loads are not of themselves osteogenic. The most surprising finding from the research on loading and bone adaptation is that only a few repetitions seem to be necessary to produce an osteogenic effect (30). The results from animal studies suggest that the optimal type of bone promoting exercise should provide high levels of strain at high strain rates distributed throughout the skeleton.

Loading studies on humans, taken as a whole, suggest that the positive effect of physical activity on adult bone is modest in the short term, but may be quite powerful in more intense programs that overload the muscular system over a longer term (23). In children, however, our knowledge about the long-term effects of physical activity on bone accretion is incomplete, and studies on pediatric populations have only recently been undertaken.

However, because net bone mass is increased by the modeling process which is regulated by skeletal loading, and because modeling occurs mainly during the growing and early adult years, the importance of promoting load-bearing physical activity in children and young adults becomes apparent.

Relevance to Osteoporosis

The current interest in osteoporosis has resulted in considerable research aimed at identifying the factors that underlie age-related bone loss, particularly in females where the problem is pronounced. Skeletal fragility in the elderly represents a major public health problem particularly in developed countries with aging populations. Three determinants have been advanced to explain the cause of dangerously reduced bone mass in older people: failure to attain a sufficiently high level of bone mass during the growing years, failure to maintain peak bone mass for a sufficient period of time during the adult years, and unusually accelerated bone loss in later years (7). It is probable that reduced bone mass in the elderly results from some combination of these factors as depicted in Figure 6.3.

DETERMINANTS OF SKELETAL INTEGRITY
(with strategies for the prevention of osteoporosis)

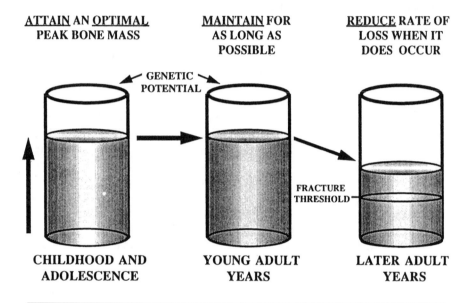

ATTAIN AN OPTIMAL PEAK BONE MASS

MAINTAIN FOR AS LONG AS POSSIBLE

REDUCE RATE OF LOSS WHEN IT DOES OCCUR

GENETIC POTENTIAL

FRACTURE THRESHOLD

CHILDHOOD AND ADOLESCENCE

YOUNG ADULT YEARS

LATER ADULT YEARS

Figure 6.3. Conditions controlling bone status over the lifespan.

Most research to date has been directed at understanding the mechanisms of, and providing strategies for, reducing the rate of bone loss in the adult and elderly populations. As a result we know much more about bone loss in adults than we do about bone accretion during the growing years when skeletal modeling can be stimulated by weight-bearing activity. Failure to attain a sufficient level of bone mass during childhood and adolescence may be a significant contributing cause of dangerously low bone status in older populations (29). Because bone loss is a normal consequence of aging, people who acquire a greater bone mass during the first two decades of life should have a reduced risk of skeletal fragility in later life. Inasmuch as 90% of the total adult bone investment has been deposited by the end of adolescence (14,24), it has been suggested that the best single predictor of bone status in later life is the level of peak bone mass attained in the early years (18). This has led to the study of factors that may enhance the attainment of an optimal level of peak bone mass.

Peak Bone Mass

The concept of peak bone mass is straightforward; however, because most current techniques measure bone mineral content (BMC) or, in an attempt to control for size, bone mineral density (BMD) at specific skeletal sites, there is some confusion in the literature. For instance, the peak bone mass of women is generally less than that of men because women's skeletons are physically smaller. But, dimorphism in BMD is not nearly as clear cut and probably varies with skeletal site (4). This issue is complicated further by the use of different types of instrumentation in different studies. For example, while a computed tomography study showed no difference between trabecular vertebral BMD of boys and girls measured in gm/cm^3 (13), other evidence, using dual energy X-ray absorptiometry, has been presented showing girls to have a greater vertebral density than boys as measured in gm/cm^2 (20).

Clearly, differences in measurement technique must be considered in interpreting BMD values, especially when these values are used to monitor bone accretion in growing children. A number of studies have demonstrated dramatic increases in bone density during adolescence in both sexes (25,36). However, methodological questions have been raised as to whether the magnitude of the observed bone density changes is an accurate reflection of change or simply a manifestation of increasing size during growth (1). Currently popular projectional methods used to measure bone density, such as the photon absorption techniques (i.e., single photon, dual photon, and dual energy X-ray absorptiometry), measure an area density. Thus, larger bones resulting from growth will yield higher BMD values than previously smaller bones even if there is no difference in true density (5). This has led to some confusion as to magnitude of change in adolescent bone density in the acquisition of a peak bone mass.

Thus, while peak bone mass is a simple concept, there are still several important issues that need clarification. For instance, the age of attaining peak bone mass is still not precisely defined and is probably site specific, and the question of sexual dimorphism remains controversial. In spite of these unanswered questions, it is clear that adolescence is a crucial time in terms of bone accretion (27), and we need more information about the determinants of bone gain in children and peak bone mass in young adults (28). The determinants of peak bone mass are graphically presented in Figure 6.4, showing that the genetically programmed skeletal template can, within limits, be positively influenced by osteogenic mechanical loading factors, which depend on a proper nutritional, hormonal, and lifestyle climate for maximum expression.

As the following quotations indicate, the possibility of maximizing bone mass during the growing years is an area of considerable current interest, especially in view of the significant relationship between adult bone density status and fracture risk in the elderly (19,38).

1. Deciphering the complex network of factors that determine peak bone mass may be the key to preventing osteoporosis (27).
2. Abundant evidence indicates that a high peak bone mass is the best single protection against osteoporosis in later life (16).
3. The ultimate target population for osteoporosis prophylaxis may indeed be the young, rather than the elderly, female (8).
4. Factors influencing the attainment of peak bone density early in life are likely to play an important role in determining the risk for fracture after the menopause and in the latter decades of life (33).

DETERMINANTS OF PEAK BONE MASS

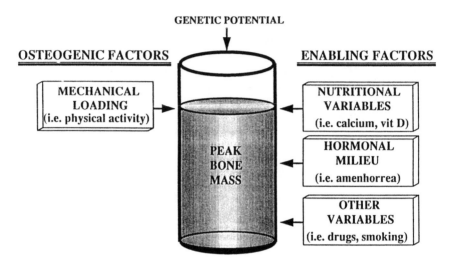

GENETIC POTENTIAL

OSTEOGENIC FACTORS   ENABLING FACTORS

MECHANICAL LOADING (i.e. physical activity)

NUTRITIONAL VARIABLES (i.e. calcium, vit D)

PEAK BONE MASS

HORMONAL MILIEU (i.e. amenhorrea)

OTHER VARIABLES (i.e. drugs, smoking)

Figure 6.4.   Conditions influencing the attainment of peak bone mass.

Physical Activity and Bone Gain in the Young

The potential of weight-bearing physical activity to reduce the rate of bone density loss in adults has been widely studied, and there are a number of excellent reviews covering this topic (10,15,35). In children, however, our knowledge about the long-term effects of physical activity on bone density accretion is incomplete, and studies on adolescent populations have only recently been undertaken. We have recently reviewed the few studies that have investigated the relationship between bone mineral density accretion and physical activity in the under 21 age group (3). Studies were categorized according to the experimental design that was followed, including

- controlled trials (randomized and non-randomized) and prospective observational studies;
- cross-sectional observational studies, which included studies using retrospective questionnaires to assess historical childhood and adolescent physical activity patterns; and
- unilateral studies in which one limb was preferentially stressed with each individual acting as his/her own control.

The results of the prospective studies suggest that physical activity must be vigorous if bone mineral density is to be enhanced in young individuals. This is consistent with the results of animal trials; however, studies of longer duration with larger sample sizes are needed to further test this. In studies that have used physical activity questionnaires to classify subjects into levels of activity, most have reported a significant but modest association between activity as a youth and bone density at certain skeletal sites. Childhood activities that preferentially stress one side of the body over the other provide the strongest evidence that physical activity can modulate bone mineral density during the growing years over and above genetic considerations.

While these studies suggest that bone mineral density can be enhanced by local mechanical factors, there remain more questions than answers when it comes to activity prescription issues such as how much, how often, how intense, and what type. There is, however, one piece of evidence over which there is no dispute. Immobility and lack of weight bearing has a detrimental effect on the skeleton. From space flight to casting after injury to bed rest, studies on children, adults, and animals all demonstrate the skeletal danger of immobilization.

Conclusions

Slemenda et al. (1991) (34) recently suggested that children who are more physically active may emerge from adolescence with a 5 to 10% greater bone mass and bone density than less active children, depending on skeletal site. Any advantage derived from optimizing the level of bone density at maturity is likely to persist through adult life and provide some protection against skeletal fragility in later years (31).

Clearly, studies of osteoporosis are needed that address not only age-related bone loss, but also the mechanisms of bone gain during the years of growth. It is possible that the attainment of an optimal level of peak bone mass in young adults may be more effective in terms of osteoporosis prevention than measures taken to preserve bone in later life. More information is needed regarding the exact relationship between levels of activity and bone density accrual during the growing years. Our knowledge is currently incomplete in this regard. To this end, a mixed longitudinal study of bone density changes during the growing years in boys and girls, with special reference to physical activity and nutritional factors, is now in progress in our laboratory at the University of Saskatchewan. More than 200 children ranging in age from 8 to 16 years are being followed on a longitudinal basis. The testing procedures include annual bone mineral density measurements of the whole body, lumbar spine and proximal femur, and whole body soft tissue analyses using dual energy X-ray absorptiometry. As well, anthropometric size and shape growth measurements are taken at 6-month intervals, and dietary intake and physical activity assessments are collected every 4 months. In addition to the children's study, which is now in its third year, bone density measurements have been collected on 75 mothers and 24 maternal grandmothers of children in the study to investigate genetic links (26). The aim of this research is to better understand the factors that influence bone density accretion during the growing years, with the goal of attaining an optimal level of bone density in young people.

There are many issues that need to be addressed related to questions of whether or not there are childhood activity antecedents for adult skeletal health problems. For instance, if the failure to attain sufficient bone mass and bone density during the growing years is related to skeletal fragility in later years, how do you relate a disease of the elderly to a teenage population that will not be at risk for 40 or 50 years? How are high risk individuals to be identified? What level of physical activity is needed for the attainment of optimal skeletal status? The list goes on.

Taking into account that there are many more questions than answers related to these and other issues, it is still possible, on the basis of the studies that have been conducted to date, to offer some sound lifestyle advice to young people in the hope of avoiding many of the problems associated with skeletal fragility in later years.

Recommendations

- Develop a lifelong enthusiasm for physical activity and exercise.
- Promote activities that increase muscular strength as these will enhance bone density. Short daily activity is better than prolonged activity done infrequently, and weight-bearing activity is better than weight-supported activity.
- Avoid immobilization and minimize periods of immobility; where this is not possible (as in bed rest during sickness) even brief daily weight-bearing movements can help to reduce bone loss.
- Eat a well-balanced diet that meets the recommended dietary allowance for calcium. The substitution of diet soft drinks for milk should be avoided. Soft drinks are highly acidic with a high phosphorus content that can lead to increased calcium excretion.
- Teenagers should avoid cigarettes as these are anti-estrogenic and may interfere with the attainment of a normal peak bone mass.
- In girls, abnormal delay of menarche and chronic irregular menstruation should be avoided, and natural means to restore an energy balance (reduced endurance activity and greater caloric intake) should be advocated to normalize menarche and regulate menstruation where possible.
- Eating disorders are destructive to the skeleton. These disorders often begin in adolescence and are frequently found in young female athletes and other adolescent children. Parents, teachers, and coaches should be alerted to the skeletal dangers of disordered eating behavior.

References

1. Bailey, D.; Drinkwater, D.; Faulkner, R.; McKay, H.; McCulloch, R.; Houston, C. Longitudinal bone mineral changes in the femoral neck in growing children: dimensional considerations. J. Bone Miner. Res. 8(S1):S266; 1993.

2. Bailey, D.; Daniels, K.; Dzus, A.; Yong-Hing, K.; Drinkwater, D.; Wilkinson, A.; Houston, S. Bone mineral density in the proximal femur of children with Legg Calve Perthes Disease. J. Bone Miner. Res. 7(S1):S287; 1992.

3. Bailey, D.A.; Martin, A.D. Physical activity and skeletal health in adolescents. Pediatric Exercise Science 6:330-347; 1994.

4. Bonjour, J.P.; Theintz, G.; Buchs, B.; Slosman, D.; Rizzoli, R. Critical years and stages of puberty for spinal and femoral bone mass accumulation during adolescence. J. Clin. Endocrinol. Metab. 73:555-563; 1991.

5. Carter, D.R.; Bouxsein, M.L.; Marcus, R. New approaches for interpreting projected bone densitometry data. J. Bone Min. Res. 7:137-145; 1992.

6. Carter, D.R.; Wong, M.: Orr, T.E. Musculoskeletal ontogeny, phylogeny, and functional adaptation. J. Biomechanics. 24S1:3-16; 1991.

7. Chesnut, C. Theoretical overview: bone development, peak bone mass, bone loss, and fracture risk. Am. J. Med. 91(5B):2S-4S; 1991.

8. Chestnut, C.H. Is osteoporosis a pediatric disease? Peak bone mass attainment in the adolescent female. Public Health Rep. Supp. 1:50-08; 1989.

9. Darwin, C. The origin of species. (6th Edition). New York: New American Library; 1872.

10. Drinkwater, B.L. Physical exercise and bone health. J. Am. Med. Women's Assoc. 45(3):91-97; 1990.

11. Eriksen, E.F.; Steiniche, T.; Mosekilde, L.; Melsen, F. Histomorphometric analysis of bone in metabolic bone disease. In: Tiegs, R.D., ed. Metabolic bone disease, part I, endocrinology and metabolism clinics of North America. Philadelphia: W.B. Saunders; 1989:919-954.

12. Frost, H. Mechanical usage, bone mass, bone fragility: a brief overview. In: Kleerekoper, M.; Krane, S., eds. Clinical disorders of bone and mineral metabolism. New York: Mary Ann Liebert; 1989:15-40.

13. Gilsanz, V.; Gibbens, D.T.; Roe, T.F.; Carlson, M.; Senac, M.O.; Boechat, M.I.; Huang, H.K.; Schulz, E.E.; Libanati, M.D.; Cann, C.C. Vertebral bone density in children: effect of puberty. Radiology. 166:847-850; 1988.

14. Glastre, C.; Braillon, P.; David, L.; Cochat, P.; Meunier, P.J.; Delmas, P.D. Measurement of bone mineral content of the lumbar spine by dual energy X-ray absorptiometry in normal children: correlations with growth parameters. J. Clin. Endocrinol. Metab. 70(5):1330-1333; 1990.

15. Gutin, B.; Kasper, M. Can vigorous exercise play a role in osteoporosis prevention? A review. Osteoporosis Int. 2:55-69; 1992.

16. Heaney, R. The effect of calcium on skeletal development, bone loss, and risk of fractures. Am. J. Med. 91(5B):23S-28S; 1991.

17. Houston, C.A. The radiologist's opportunity to teach bone mechanics. J. Can. Assoc. Radiol. 29:232-238; 1978.

18. Hui, S.L.; Slemenda, C.W.; Johnston, P.H.; Johnston, C.C. Baseline measurements of bone mass predicts fracture in white women. Ann. Intern. Med. 111:355-361; 1989.

19. Johnston, C.; Slemenda, C. Risk prediction in osteoporosis: a theoretical overview. Am. J. Med. 91(5B):47S-48S; 1991.

20. Kroger, H.; Kotaniemi, A.; Vainio, P.; Alhava, E. Bone densitometry of the spine and femur in children by dual-energy X-ray absorptiometry. Bone Mineral. 17:75-85; 1992.

21. Lanyon, L.E. Control of bone architecture by functional load bearing. J. Bone Miner. Res. 7(S2):S369-S375; 1992.

22. Maquet, P.; Furlong, R. (translators) The laws of bone remodeling. Julius Wolff, Berlin: Springer; 1986.

23. Marcus, R.; Drinkwater, B.; Dalsky, G.; Dufek, J.; Raab, D.; Slemenda, C.; Snow-Harter; C. Osteoporosis and exercise in women. Med. Sc. Sport Ex. 24(6S):S301-S307; 1992.

24. Matkovic, V.; Fonatana, D.; Tominac, C.; Goel, P.; Chesnut, C.H. Factors which influence peak bone mass formation: a study of calcium balance and the inheritance of bone mass in adolescent females. Am. J. Clin. Nut. 52:878-888; 1990.

25. McCormick, D.P.; Ponder, S.W.; Fawcett, H.D.; Palmer, J.L. Spinal bone mineral density in 335 normal and obese children and adolescents: evidence for ethnic and sex differences. J. Bone Miner. Res. 6:507-513; 1991.

26. McKay, H.; Bailey, D. Bone mineral density: a mother-daughter-grandmother comparison. J. Bone Miner. Res. 8(S1):S266; 1993.

27. Ott, S. Bone density in adolescents. N. Engl. J. Med. 325:1646-1647; 1991.

28. Raisz, L.G. Letter to the editor. N. Engl. J. Med. 795:319; 1988.

29. Recker, R. Bone mass and calcium nutrition. Nutr. Res. 11:19-21; 1987.

30. Rubin, C.T.; Lanyon, L.E. Regulation of bone formation by applied dynamic loads. J. Bone Joint Surg. 66:397-402; 1984.

31. Sandler, R.B.; Slemenda, C.W.; LaPorte, R.E.; Cauley, J.A.; Schramm, M.M.; Barrest, M.C.; Kriska, A.M. Postmenopausal bone density and milk consumption in childhood and adolescence. Am. J. Clin. Nut. 42:270-274; 1985.

32. Schultheis, L. The mechanical control system of bone in weightless space flight and in aging. Experimental Gerontology. 46:203-214; 1991.

33. Seeman, E.; Young, N.; Szmukler, G.; Tsalamandris, C.; Hopper, J. Risk factors for osteoporosis. Osteoporosis Int. 3(S1):40-43; 1993.

34. Slemenda, C.W.; Millder, J.Z.; Hui, S.L.; Reister, T.K.; Johnston, C.C. Role of physical activity in the development of skeletal mass in children. J. Bone Miner. Res. 6:1227-1233; 1991.

35. Snow-Harter, C.; Marcus, R. Exercise, bone mineral density and osteoporosis. Ex. Sport Sc. Rev. 19:351-388; 1991.

36. Southard, R.N.; Morris, J.D.; Mahan, J.D.; et al. Bone mass in healthy children: measurement with quantitative DXA. Radiology. 179:735-738; 1991.

37. Theintz, G.E.; Howald, H.; Weiss, V.; Sizonenko, P.C. Evidence for a reduction of growth potential in adolescent female gymnasts. J. Pediatr. 122:306-313; 1993.

38. Wasnich, R. Bone mass measurements in diagnosis and assessment of therapy. Am. J. Med. 91(5B):47S-48S; 1991.

39. Wolff, J. Das gesetz der transformation der knochen. A. Hirschwald, Berlin: 1892.

40. Ziemilska, A. Effect of intensive gymnastic training on growth and maturation of children. Biology of Sport. 2(4):279-294; 1985.

Chapter 7

Nutritional Factors in Bone Growth and Development

Susan I. Barr, PhD, RDN

Nutrition can have a major influence on both the growth of bone (i.e., the amount of bone tissue formed) and on its development (i.e., the nature or quality of bone formed). Nutritional factors may be an important determinant of peak bone mass during early adulthood, which in turn affects the risk of fracture in later life. This review will briefly describe the influence of nutrients on bone matrix and will then focus on the roles of energy, protein, vitamin D, and calcium on bone growth and development. To the extent possible, data obtained in young athletes will be incorporated.

Nutrition and Bone Matrix Development

Bone is described as a specialized form of connective tissue composed of a ground substance (or matrix) within which is deposited bone mineral. Collagen, a family of proteins that make up the body's major extracellular proteins, is the predominant protein of bone, and synthesis of Type I collagen by osteoblasts is the initial step in matrix formation (47). Matrix also contains a number of noncollagenous proteins, including proteoglycans, phosphoproteins, glycoproteins, and gamma-carboxyglutamic acid (gla)-proteins, which are proposed to function in regulating mineralization and the type and size of Ca-P crystal that is formed (47).

Several nutrients potentially affect matrix formation (8,47), although they are rarely limiting. Not surprisingly, protein deficiency and starvation inhibit synthesis of collagen (8) and noncollagenous proteins. Protein synthesis is closely associated with zinc, and zinc deficiency also affects bone matrix formation (47). Vitamin C's role as a cofactor in the hydroxylation of proline and lysine residues in collagen is well-known, and it also aids in synthesis of noncollagenous proteins (8). Vitamin A has major roles in cellular differentiation, including effects on collagen. Collagen synthesis has been reported to be inhibited by vitamin A as retinol in chick and murine calvarial organ culture, and by retinoic acid in murine calvaria (47). Vitamin D, while mainly known for its role in bone mineralization, also appears to increase levels of noncollagenous proteins in osteoblast cell cultures (47). The post-translational gamma-carboxylation of glutamate residues in osteocalcin is vitamin K dependent, and vitamin K deficiency affects synthesis of this protein (47). Thus, while many nutrients can influence matrix development, in cases other than severe deficiencies they rarely impact on bone growth.

Nutrition and Bone Mineralization and Growth

It appears that most of the variability in bone growth and mineral density is associated with genetic factors (25,38); however, environmental factors such as nutrition and physical activity appear to have the potential to make an important contribution to adult peak bone mass and density. Given that relatively small differences in bone density are associated with substantial differences in fracture risk (41), greater attention to the role of nutrition could be of significant health benefit. The remainder of this review will focus on the roles of energy, protein, vitamin D, and calcium in bone growth and development.

Energy

One only needs to examine the literature documenting the effects of chronic undernutrition on growth to understand the key role of energy intake on bone growth (20,62). Children whose energy intakes are marginal for prolonged periods may not appear emaciated or visibly malnourished; instead, their growth rate is reduced and they experience stunting (62). Height-for-age and weight-for-age are both reduced, but weight-for-height may fall within the normal range. Energy shortages are clearly not a problem in most of the developed world; conversely, childhood obesity has been identified as a growing concern in the United States (19). However, linear growth of some children living in a plentiful environment may still be compromised by an inadequate energy intake, either as a result of what has been termed "fear of obesity," or in association with intense athletic training in sports that place a premium on small body size.

Fear of obesity was first described as leading to short stature by Pugliese et al. in 1983 (44). Of 201 children attending a clinic for investigation of short stature or delayed puberty, 14 were identified as having no organic cause for the growth delay. All children were underweight (<5th percentile of weight-for-age) and 11 of the 14 were below the 5th percentile of height-for-age. Weight-for-height was 10% below average. Further investigation of these subjects revealed energy intakes that averaged 55% of expected for children of the same age, and interviews revealed a fear of becoming fat in almost all the affected children. Nutrition counseling and intervention resulted in increased intakes, suggesting that the children's concern about short stature and pubertal delay was sufficient to allow them to increase their food intake. Normal growth resumed in most subjects, although some whose epiphyses had already closed remained at a lower than expected height (44). These children and others like them have neither the extreme emaciation nor the psychopathology typical of patients with anorexia nervosa (49); instead, they may reflect the effects of socio-cultural or possibly physiological influences on food intake and thereby on growth (49).

Since Pugliese's initial report, additional cases of slowed growth have been reported in children counseled to follow cholesterol-lowering diets (32). Eight children of a group of 40 were found to have growth failure; 5 experienced weight loss and 3 had nutritional dwarfing. The latter group obtained less than 60% of the recommended energy intake for age and sex, and obtained only 20.5% of energy from fat. Intake of all nutrients except vitamins C and E also fell below the RDAs (32). A school-based survey has also suggested that significant proportions of children in the general population may be experiencing some degree of nutritional dwarfing (45).

Inadequate energy intake has also been suggested to affect growth and maturation of children involved in intense athletic training, and particularly close scrutiny has been received by the sport of gymnastics. This sport is unusual in terms of the early age at which intense training is initiated; the large volume of training required of elite athletes; the subjective element of judging, in which physical appearance may play a role; and the competitive advantage conferred by being small and having a prepubertal physique (e.g., greater ease in completing elements such as somersaults, due to faster rotation of a small body, and vaults, associated with the greater propulsion with a higher center of gravity).

Cross-sectional studies of gymnasts have shown that short stature and pubertal delay are common. A study of competitors with an average age of 14 at the 1984 European Junior Championships suggested that the growth rate of the gymnasts was normal, but delayed, consistent with their not having attained menarche (10). In contrast, ''non-talented'' gymnasts had growth curves which corresponded to growth standards (10). Benardot et al. (5), studying junior elite gymnasts at a training camp, obtained somewhat different results that may be explained by the younger age and slightly lower competitive level of the athletes they studied. They found that the gymnasts aged 7 to 10 years were at the 48th percentile of both weight-for-age and height-for-age, and at the 50th percentile for weight-for-height. The 11- to 14-year-old group, however, were at the 20th percentiles for weight-for-age and height-for-age, while remaining at the 50th percentile of weight-for-height. As has been reported by other authors (7), these authors also found the energy and nutrient intakes of the gymnasts to be low in comparison to standards (6). Thus, they speculated that the low energy intakes, especially when considered relative to expenditure, may have compromised the linear growth of these young athletes.

While providing grounds for further investigation, the results of cross-sectional studies must be interpreted with caution, particularly when there is a distinct competitive advantage to being small. As the authors themselves identify (5), it is possible that the gymnasts who were genetically predestined to be smaller were more successful in the sport and were therefore more likely to remain in it. In contrast, those who were destined to be taller could have been more likely to retire from competition at an early age, and therefore would not have been represented in the older group. Consistent with this hypothesis are the data of Theintz et al. (60), which indicate that expected heights of successful female gymnasts, based on weighted mid-parental heights, are below average.

Data on reported energy intakes must also be interpreted cautiously, as revealed by the results of studies using doubly-labeled water to quantitate energy expenditure (51). In this method, subjects ingest a dose of heavy water (labeled with $^2H_2$ and ^{18}O), and samples of body fluids (e.g., blood, urine, or saliva) are taken at intervals for up to two weeks. The difference between the disappearance rate of the two isotopes (^{18}O is eliminated as both water and carbon dioxide, while $^2H_2$ is eliminated only as water) can be used to calculate the rate of carbon dioxide production, which in turn is used to estimate oxygen consumption and energy expenditure (51). For individuals who are in energy balance and who are maintaining weight, average energy expenditure is by definition equal to average energy intake over the same time period. The method is advantageous in that it is non-invasive and does not interfere with the subjects' usual activity patterns.

Results of studies using the doubly-labeled water method indicate that self-reported energy intakes generally underestimate average energy expenditures, and that the degree of underestimation is not consistent, but varies with age, body weight, and the extent of weight concern (9,51). Livingstone et al. studied children aged 7 through 18 years using both weighed diet records and doubly-labeled water (33). They found that the 7- and 9-year-old children reported energy intakes that corresponded well to their energy expenditures. In the adolescents, however, the reported intakes ranged from 89 ± 12% of expenditure in 12-year-olds to 73 ± 25% of expenditure in 18-year-olds (33). It is possible that the older children were more aware of the social desirability of being thin and were thus more likely to underestimate their intakes. Bandini et al. (4), studying normal weight and obese adolescents, reported that the normal weight subjects had self-reported energy intakes averaging 81% of their energy expenditure, while the overweight subjects reported intakes averaging only 59% of their energy expenditure, indicating that underreporting may be a greater problem in adolescents with above-average weight. Finally, underestimation of intakes has also been reported in women athletes (51), who are also frequently concerned about weight. Thus, the low reported energy intakes of the gymnasts may not reflect actual intakes.

Few prospective data are available on growth of young female gymnasts. Theintz et al. (61) studied adolescent female swimmers and gymnasts, initially aged 12.3 ± 0.2 years (mean ± SEM) every 6 months for an average of 2.35 years. The gymnasts trained for an average of 22 hours per week, while the swimmers trained for 8 hours weekly. For each athlete, a target height was predicted from a weighted mid-parental height, and a predicted adult height was determined at each visit based on attained height at current bone age. As described earlier, the gymnasts were genetically destined to be short of stature: Their target height, as assessed by the height of their parents, was significantly lower than the target height of the swimmers (160.6 ± 1.0 vs. 165.1 ± 1.1 cm, P<0.01). At a bone age of 10 years, predicted heights for both groups of athletes were similar to their target heights. Over the course of the study, however, a significant drop in predicted height occurred for the gymnasts (r=−.629, P<0.001), whereas no change was observed in predicted height for the swimmers (r=0.160, NS). At a bone age of 15 or above, gymnasts' height was 95% of target, compared to 101% for the swimmers. The authors also report that the reduction in gymnasts' growth was most marked in the lower segments. Sitting height increased with age, while leg length did not change after a bone age of 12 years. This would suggest that the gymnasts, in addition to not attaining their maximum potential height, would also have altered bodily proportions. In this regard, it should be noted that elite gymnasts who were studied at the Rotterdam World Championships were reported as being short but normally proportioned (14). Theintz et al. conclude by stating that "heavy training in gymnastics (>18 hr/wk), starting before puberty and maintained through puberty can alter growth rate to such an extent that full adult height will not be reached" (61). Further work in this area is clearly warranted, and it is also important to recognize that it is unlikely that physical training per se compromised linear growth. Instead, energy intakes inadequate to meet the demands of both training and growth are likely responsible. Whether the inadequate intake results from an inability to ingest sufficient food to meet needs, a conscious or unconscious desire on part of the athlete to remain small, or some combination thereof cannot be determined at present.

It is thus clear from a number of different lines of evidence that a relative inadequacy of energy intake, whether occurring as a result of poverty-associated malnutrition, fear of obesity, or intense athletic training, can compromise growth, including growth of bone.

Protein

As the major constituent of bone matrix, protein is obviously necessary for bone growth (8). However, high protein intakes have been linked with calciuria (22,27,28,35,36,63), with lower values for bone mineral density (46), and with hip fracture (1). A discussion of protein's role in bone growth and mineralization is also of relevance for the young athlete, given that adult athletes appear to require larger protein intakes to meet requirements than do normally-active adults (30,31,42,58,59).

The higher protein requirements observed in athletes appear to exist for both strength-trained athletes (31,58) and for endurance-trained athletes (42,59). Additional protein is required to increase lean body mass during the initial stages of strength training (31) and to compensate for the oxidation of amino acids as a fuel source during activity. Although the relative contribution of protein to energy needs is generally regarded as small, it can be appreciable in those exercising for prolonged periods on a daily basis and thereby contribute to a higher requirement (30). The amounts of protein required by young, growing athletes have not been evaluated, but given the data from adults, they may well be above the requirements of normally-active children and adolescents.

In adults, increased intakes of protein, especially from purified sources, lead to increases in urinary calcium excretion and negative calcium balance (27). Although the specific mechanism is not completely clear (2), increases in endogenous acid excretion from the oxidation of excess sulfur-containing amino acids appear to have an important role in contributing to the calciuretic effect of high protein intakes (52,63). The key role of acid excretion is illustrated by the finding that ingestion of sodium bicarbonate reversed the acidification of urine and the increased urinary calcium excretion observed with increased protein intake (35). Another line of evidence implicating the role of acidification of urine by oxidation of sulfur-containing amino acids relates to the finding that protein sources lower in these amino acids, such as soy, may be associated with reduced urinary calcium loss (66).

Much of the work in this area has been conducted using purified protein sources, and of potential practical relevance are studies that indicate that the effects of high protein intakes are much less pronounced when the protein is ingested as food sources, such as meat (56,57). The additional phosphorus that accompanies food sources of protein exerts a hypocalciuric effect, by increasing the renal tubular reabsorption of calcium (21). Although high phosphorus intakes appear to be beneficial in terms of reducing calcium loss in urine, the long-term consequences of high phosphorus intakes, especially in association with low calcium intakes, have been questioned (11). Young women studied for 28 days on a high-phosphorus, low-calcium diet were found to develop mild hyperparathyroidism, which could stimulate bone resorption (12).

Unfortunately, the effects of protein and phosphorus intakes on calcium balance in growing children, and especially in young athletes, do not appear to have been studied systematically. However, given the importance of adequate protein in promoting normal growth and development and the possibility that protein requirements of young athletes are higher than those of normally-active children, restriction of dietary protein intakes as a means of promoting bone mineral accretion during growth does not appear warranted at present.

Vitamin D

The key role of vitamin D in enhancing calcium absorption and bone mineralization has been known for many years, and rickets has been largely eradicated through the fortification of fluid milk and infant formulas with vitamin D (23). In recent years, however, the condition has again been diagnosed in young children living in Connecticut, Chicago, and Philadelphia (3,17,48), confirming the importance of receiving either a dietary source of the vitamin or exposure to enough ultraviolet irradiation to permit endogenous synthesis. Risk factors for development of rickets identified in these children included prematurity, reduced exposure to sunlight either in absolute terms or in association with pigmented skin, prolonged unsupplemented breast feeding, and vegetarian diets (48).

Calcium

The amount of calcium necessary to allow bone to be mineralized is quite low, and only very inadequate calcium intakes lead to rickets and delayed growth (15,29). In recent years, the effect of calcium intakes beyond this minimal requirement has been receiving much attention, and data exist to both support and refute a beneficial effect of calcium in promoting and maintaining bone density and in protecting against fracture risk.

Matkovic et al. were among the first to suggest that calcium intake during growth influenced values for peak bone mass and thereby was associated with decreased fracture rates in later life (41). The original study was based on a cross-sectional survey of adults, aged 30 to 90, living in two regions of the former Yugoslavia (41). In the "high calcium" district, calcium intakes approached 1,000 mg per day, while in the "low calcium" district, the average intake was about 500 mg per day. Bone mineral density, assessed as metacarpal cortical area/ metacarpal total area (MCA/MTA), was found to be at maximal levels at age 30 and to decline thereafter. Residents of the high calcium district had higher values for MCA/MTA at 30 years of age, and the differences were maintained throughout life. Corresponding to the higher values for MCA/MTA were differences in the rates of hip fracture: Among those aged 70 and above, women living in the high calcium district experienced fractures at only 31% of the rate of those living in the low calcium district; among men, the rate in the high calcium district was 49% of that in the low calcium district. This study has been criticized insofar as variables other than calcium also differed between the two regions. For example, diets differed in protein and other nutrients as well as in calcium, and women in the high calcium district had higher energy intakes than women in the low calcium district. Because body weights were similar, it is possible that physical activity differed between the two groups and may have contributed to the differences in fracture rate. Nevertheless, the study had great significance in terms of shifting research attention toward factors that influence peak bone mass. Subsequently, much work has been done in this area and evidence has accumulated to indicate that achieving maximal values for peak bone mass during growth may be important in reducing the risk of osteoporosis in later life (24,37,40).

Evidence for a role of calcium in contributing to higher values for bone mineral density during growth may be obtained from retrospective, cross-sectional, longitudinal, and experimental studies. In addition to the study of Matkovic (41), retrospective data suggesting the importance of calcium intake during childhood and adolescence was reported by Sandler et al. (50). They studied bone density in postmenopausal women in relationship to milk intake during childhood, during adolescence, and during adulthood. Women who "always" drank milk during their early years had higher values for bone density than those who "rarely" drank milk, while current milk use was not associated with bone density (50).

The results of cross-sectional studies of bone density and calcium intake in children have been inconsistent (13,16,18,26,53,55,64,65). For example, Chan evaluated the association between calcium intake and bone mineral content of the radius in 164 children aged 2 to 16 years (13). Each child's bone mineral content was expressed in terms of the number of standard deviation units it was from the mean for all children of that age (i.e., as z-scores), thus avoiding confounding of the results by the expected changes in bone mineral content with age. Calcium intake was positively associated with z-scores for bone mineral content, and children ingesting over 1,000 mg calcium per day had higher values than those consuming less than 1,000 mg per day (13). Calcium intake was also significantly associated with bone density at the hip for 15- to 17-year-old girls (64) and in the lumbar spine in girls aged 8 to 18 (53). In contrast, no associations between dietary calcium and bone density were detected in other studies (16,18,26,55,65). Several factors may contribute to the lack of consistency of these results. First, calcium intakes are difficult to quantitate accurately. Miller et al. (43) reported that at least 9 days of intake in girls and 18 days in boys were needed to obtain reasonably reliable estimates of calcium intake. Many studies assessed intakes using only one or two days of records (16,65) or did not provide details on how calcium intake was assessed (18,26,55). Small sample sizes and a wide range of subject age in some studies could also make detection of a small effect difficult.

Another factor which may contribute to discrepant findings among studies is the relative adequacy of the subjects' calcium intakes. Calcium has been suggested to behave as a "threshold" nutrient, where the threshold represents the level of nutrient intake below which some aspect of nutrient status is influenced by intake of the nutrient, and above which is independent of intake. Matkovic and Heaney analyzed the results of over 500 calcium balance studies from 34 reports in the literature (39). They found evidence of thresholds for calcium in all four age groups they assessed (infancy, childhood, adolescence, and young adulthood) (39). Two-component split linear regression models were used to identify the thresholds, below which calcium intake was positively associated with calcium balance and above which no association was detected. In each case these models predicted more of the variability in calcium balance than did simple linear regression (39). Thus, it is possible that some subjects in studies that did not detect a relationship between calcium and bone density may have had intakes that met or exceeded the threshold, again making detection of an association difficult. Whether or not physical activity influences the threshold for calcium intakes has not been systematically studied. Data obtained in young adult women, however, suggest that the positive effects of physical activity and calcium intake on bone mineral density are independent (46).

Several experimental studies have been conducted to directly evaluate the effect of calcium supplementation on bone accretion during growth. Initially, Matkovic et al. reported the results of a trial in 28 adolescent girls, initially 14 years of age (38). Although balance studies conducted in the subjects showed a clear positive relationship between calcium intake and calcium balance, after 2 years of supplementation, no difference in bone density existed between girls in the control group (n=8) and girls in the groups receiving 500 mg additional calcium per day. However, the increments in bone density between ages 14 and 16 were small, and the sample size was likely inadequate to detect a difference between the supplemented and unsupplemented subjects. Johnston et al. (25) conducted a 3-year study of supplementation with 1,000 mg calcium versus placebo in 45 pairs of identical twins whose initial ages ranged from 6 to 14 years and whose dietary calcium intake averaged over 900 mg/day. Among the 22 pairs of twins who were prepubertal throughout the study, the supplemented twins experienced significantly greater gains in bone density than their unsupplemented partners at the midshaft of the radius (5.1%), the distal radius (3.5%), and the lumbar spine (2.8%). No effects of supplementation were detected in the twin pairs who were pubertal at the start of the study or who became pubertal during the study, although the numbers of pairs in these groups were smaller. Finally, Lloyd et al. conducted an 18-month supplementation trial of 500 mg calcium versus placebo in 94 girls initially 11.9 years old, with calcium intakes averaging 960 mg/day (34). They detected significantly greater increases in lumbar spine bone mineral density (18.7% vs. 15.8%) and in whole body bone mineral density (9.6% vs. 8.3%) in the supplemented group than in the placebo group.

An important question is whether the beneficial effects of calcium supplementation on bone density are maintained when supplementation is stopped, or whether they are associated with slowed remodeling and are transient. Preliminary data from a 1-year post-supplementation follow-up study of the prepubertal twins who gained more bone with calcium supplementation, suggest that the latter may be true (54). During the 1 year off supplements, dietary calcium intake of the twins averaged 1,020 mg/day, and at the end of the year, the significant differences between the formerly supplemented and unsupplemented twins disappeared. The twins formerly on placebo gained more bone than those formerly on calcium at all sites evaluated, and the differences were significant at the spine and nearly so at the distal radius (54). It is possible that the high calcium intakes would need to be maintained indefinitely for the difference in bone density to persist. Additional work in this area will be important in providing a clear answer to the question of whether current dietary recommendations are adequate for maximizing peak bone mass and thereby reducing the risk of osteoporosis.

In conclusion, there is clear evidence that calcium intakes during growth influence bone mineral density. Debate still exists as to the levels of calcium intake that are sufficient to maximize the beneficial influence.

References

1. Abelow, B.J.; Holford, T.R.; Insogna, K.L. Cross-cultural association between dietary animal protein and hip fracture: a hypothesis. Calcif. Tissue Int. 50:14-18; 1992.
2. Anderson, J. Nutritional biochemistry of calcium and phosphorus. J. Nutr. Biochem. 2:300-307; 1991.
3. Bachrach, S.; Fisher, J.; Parks, J.S. An outbreak of vitamin D deficiency rickets in a susceptible population. Pediatrics 64:871-877; 1979.

4. Bandini, L.G.; Schoeller, D.A.; Cyr, H.; Dietz, W.H. A validation of reported energy intake in obese and non-obese adolescents. Am. J. Clin. Nutr. 52:421-425; 1990.
5. Benardot, D.; Czerwinski, C. Selected body composition and growth measures of junior elite gymnasts. J. Am. Diet. Assoc. 91:29-33; 1991.
6. Benardot, D.; Schwarz, M.; Heller, D.W. Nutrient intake in young, highly competitive gymnasts. J. Am. Diet. Assoc. 89:401-403; 1989.
7. Benson, J.E.; Allemann, Y.; Theintz, G.E.; Howald, H. Eating problems and calorie intake levels in Swiss adolescent athletes. Int. J. Sports Med. 11:249-252; 1990.
8. Berg, R.A.; Kerr, J.S. Nutritional aspects of collagen metabolism. Annu. Rev. Nutr. 12:369-390; 1992.
9. Black, A.E.; Prentice, A.M.; Goldberg, G.R.; et al. Measurements of total energy expenditure provide insights into the validity of dietary measurements of energy intake. J. Am. Diet. Assoc. 93:572-579; 1993.
10. Caldarone, G.; Leglise, M.; Giampietro, M.; Berlutti, G. Anthropometric measurements, body composition, biological maturation and growth predictions in young female gymnasts of high agonistic level. J. Sports Med. 26:263-273; 1986.
11. Calvo, M.S. Dietary phosphorus, calcium metabolism and bone. J. Nutr. 123:1627-1633; 1993.
12. Calvo, M.S.; Kumar, R.; Heath, H. III. Persistently elevated parathyroid hormone secretion and action in young women after four weeks of ingesting high phosphorus, low calcium diets. J. Clin. Endocrinol. Metab. 70:1334-1340; 1990.
13. Chan, G.M. Dietary calcium and bone mineral status of children and adolescents. Am. J. Dis. Child. 145:631-634; 1991.
14. Claessens, A.L.; Veer, F.M.; Stijnen, V.; et al. Anthropometric characteristics of outstanding male and female gymnasts. J. Sports Sci. 9:53-74; 1991.
15. Davidovits, M.; Levy, Y.; Avramovitz, T.; Eisenstein, B. Calcium-deficiency rickets in a four-year-old boy with milk allergy. J. Pediatr. 122:249-251; 1993.
16. Dhuper, S.; Warren, M.P.; Brooks-Gun, J.; Fox, R. Effects of hormonal status on bone density in adolescent girls. J. Clin. Endocrinol. Metab. 71:1083-1088; 1990.
17. Edidin, D.V.; Levitsky, L.L.; Schey, W.; Dumbovic, N.; Campos, A. Resurgence of nutritional rickets associated with breast-feeding and special dietary practices. Pediatrics 65:232-235; 1980.
18. Glastre, C.; Braillon, P.; David, L.; Cochat, P.; Meunier, P.H.; Delmas, P.D. Measurement of bone mineral content of the lumbar spine by dual energy X-ray absorptiometry in normal children: correlations with growth parameters. J. Clin. Endocrinol. Metab. 70:1330-1333; 1990.
19. Gortmaker, S.L.; Dietz, W.H.; Sobol, A.M.; Wehler, C.A. Increasing pediatric obesity in the United States. Am. J. Dis. Child. 141:535-540; 1987.
20. Habicht, J-P.; Martorell, R.; Yarborough, C.; Malina, R.M.; Klein, R.E. Height and weight standards for preschool children. How relevant are ethnic differences in growth potential? Lancet 1:611-615; 1974.
21. Heaney, R.P.; Recker, R.R. Effects of nitrogen, phosphorus, and caffeine on calcium balance in women. J. Lab. Clin. Med. 99:46-55; 1982.
22. Hegsted, M.; Linkswiler, H.M. Long-term effects of level of protein intake on calcium metabolism in young adult women. J. Nutr. 111:244-251; 1981.
23. Holick, M.F. Vitamin D. In: Shils, M.E.; Olson, J.A.; Shike, M., eds. Modern nutrition in health and disease, 8th edition. Philadelphia: Lea & Febiger; 1994: 308-325.
24. Hui, S.L.; Slemenda, C.W.; Johnston, C.C. Jr. The contribution of bone loss to postmenopausal osteoporosis. Osteoporosis Int. 1:30-34; 1990.
25. Johnston, C.C.; Miller, J.Z.; Slemenda, C.W.; et al. Calcium supplementation and increases in bone mineral density in children. N. Engl. J. Med. 327:82-87; 1992.
26. Katzman, D.K.; Bachrach, L.K.; Carter, D.R.; Marcus, R. Clinical and anthropometric correlates of bone mineral acquisition in healthy adolescent girls. J. Clin. Endocrinol. Metab. 73:1332-1339; 1991.

27. Kerstetter, J.E.; Allen, L.H. Dietary protein increases urinary calcium. J. Nutr. 120:134-136; 1990.

28. Lakshmanan, F.L.; Rao, R.B.; Church, J.P. Calcium and phosphorus intakes, balances, and blood levels of adults consuming self-selected diets. Am. J. Clin. Nutr. 40:1368-1379; 1984.

29. Legius, E.; Proesmans, W.; Eggermont, E.; Vandamme-Lombaerts, R.; Bouillon, R.; Smet, M. Rickets due to dietary calcium deficiency. Eur. J. Pediatr. 148:784-785; 1989.

30. Lemon, P.W.R.; Proctor, D.N. Protein intake and athletic performance. Sports Med. 12:313-325; 1991.

31. Lemon, P.W.R.; Tarnopolsky, M.A.; MacDougall, J.D.; Atkinson, S.A. Protein requirements and muscle mass/strength changes during intensive training in novice bodybuilders. J. Appl. Physiol. 73:767-775; 1992.

32. Lifshitz, F.; Moses, N. Growth failure. A complication of dietary treatment of hypercholesterolemia. Am. J. Dis. Child. 143:537-542; 1989.

33. Livingstone, M.B.E.; Prentice, A.M.; Coward, W.A.; et al. Validation of estimates of energy intake by weighed dietary record and diet history in children and adolescents. Am. J. Clin. Nutr. 56:29-35; 1992.

34. Lloyd, T.; Andon, M.B.; Rollings, N.; et al. Calcium supplementation and bone mineral density in adolescent girls. J. Am. Med. Assoc. 270:841-844; 1993.

35. Lutz, J. Calcium balance and acid-base status of women as affected by increased protein intake and by sodium bicarbonate ingestion. Am. J. Clin. Nutr. 39:281-288; 1984.

36. Margen, S.; Chu, J.Y.; Kaufmann, N.A.; Calloway, D.H. Studies in calcium metabolism. 1. The calciuretic effect of dietary protein. Am. J. Clin. Nutr. 27:584-589; 1974.

37. Matkovic, V. Calcium and peak bone mass. J. Int. Med. 231:151-160; 1992.

38. Matkovic, V.; Fontana, D.; Tominac, C.; Goel, P.; Chestnut, C.H. Factors which influence peak bone mass formation: study of calcium balance and the inheritance of bone mass in adolescent females. Am. J. Clin. Nutr. 52:878-888; 1990.

39. Matkovic, V.; Heaney, R.P. Calcium balance during human growth: evidence for threshold behavior. Am. J. Clin. Nutr. 55:992-996; 1992.

40. Matkovic, V.; Ilich, J.Z. Calcium requirements for growth: are current recommendations adequate? Nutr. Rev. 51:171-180; 1993.

41. Matkovic, V.; Kostial, K.; Simonovic, I.; Buzina, R.; Brodarec, A.; Nordin, B.E.C. Bone status and fracture rates in two regions of Yugoslavia. Am. J. Clin. Nutr. 32:540-549; 1979.

42. Meredith, C.N.; Zackin, M.J.; Frontera, W.R.; Evans, W.J. Dietary protein requirements and body protein metabolism in endurance-trained men. J. Appl. Physiol. 66:2850-2856; 1989.

43. Miller, J.; Kimes, T.; Hui, S.; Andon, M.B.; Johnston, C.C. Nutrient intake variability in a pediatric population: implications for study design. J. Nutr. 121:265-274; 1991.

44. Pugliese, M.T.; Lifshitz, F.; Grad, G.; Marks-Katz, M. Fear of obesity: a cause of short stature and delayed puberty. N. Engl. J. Med. 309:513-518; 1983.

45. Pugliese, M.; Recker, B.; Lifshitz, F. A survey to determine the prevalence of abnormal growth patterns in adolescence. J. Adolesc. Health Care. 9:181-187; 1988.

46. Recker, R.R.; Davies, K.M.; Hinders, S.M.; Heaney, R.P.; Stegman, M.R.; Kimmel, D.B. Bone gain in young adult women. J. Am. Med. Assoc. 268:2403-2408; 1992.

47. Roughead, Z.K.; Kunkel, M.E. Effect of diet on bone matrix constituents. J. Am. Coll. Nutr. 10:242-246; 1991.

48. Rudolf, M.; Arulanantham, K.; Greenstein, R.M. Unsuspected nutritional rickets. Pediatrics 66:72-76; 1980.

49. Sandberg, D.E.; Smith, M.M.; Fornari, V.; Goldstein, M.; Lifshitz, F. Nutritional dwarfing: is it a consequence of disturbed psychosocial functioning? Pediatrics 88:926-933; 1981.

50. Sandler, R.B.; Slemenda, C.W.; LaPorte, R.E.; et al. Postmenopausal bone density and milk consumption in childhood and adolescence. Am. J. Clin. Nutr. 42:270-274; 1985.

51. Schoeller, D.A.; Bandini, L.G.; Dietz, W.H. Inaccuracies in self-reported intake identified by comparison with the doubly-labeled water method. Can. J. Physiol. Pharmacol. 68:941-949; 1990.

52. Schuette, S.A.; Zemel, M.B.; Linkswiler, H.M. Studies on the mechanism of protein-induced hypercalciuria in older men and women. J. Nutr. 110:305-325; 1980.

53. Sentipal, J.M.; Wardlaw, G.M.; Mahan, J.; Matkovic, V. Influence of calcium intake and growth indexes on vertebral bone mineral density in young females. Am. J. Clin. Nutr. 54:425-428; 1991.

54. Slemenda, C.W.; Reister, T.K.; Peacock, M.; Johnston, C.C. Bone growth in children following the cessation of calcium supplementation. J. Bone Min. Res. 8(suppl 1):S154; 1993.

55. Southard, R.N.; Morris, J.D.; Magan, J.D.; et al. Bone mass in healthy children: measurement with quantitative DXA. Radiology 179:735-738; 1991.

56. Spencer, H.; Kramer, L. The calcium requirement and factors causing calcium loss. Federation Proc. 45:2758-2762; 1986.

57. Spencer, H.; Kramer, L. Does dietary protein increase urinary calcium? J. Nutr. 121:151; 1990.

58. Tarnopolsky, M.A.; Atkinson, S.A.; MacDougall, J.D.; Chesley, A.; Phillips, S.; Schwarcz, H.P. Evaluation of protein requirements for trained strength athletes. J. Appl. Physiol. 73:1986-1995; 1992.

59. Tarnopolsky, M.A.; MacDougall, J.D.; Atkinson, S.A. Influence of protein intake and training status on nitrogen balance and lean body mass. J. Appl. Physiol. 64:187-193; 1988.

60. Theintz, G.E.; Howald, H.; Allemann, Y.; Sizonenko, P.C. Growth and pubertal development of young female gymnasts and swimmers: a correlation with parental data. Int. J. Sports Med. 10:87-91; 1989.

61. Theintz, G.E.; Howald, H.; Weiss, U.; Sizonenko, P.C. Evidence for a reduction of growth potential in adolescent female gymnasts. J. Pediatr. 122:306-313; 1993.

62. Torun, B.; Chew, F. Protein-energy malnutrition. In: Shils, M.E.; Olson, J.A.; Shike, M., eds. Modern nutrition in health and disease, 8th edition. Philadelphia: Lea & Febiger; 1994: 950-976.

63. Trilok, G.; Draper, H.H. Sources of protein-induced endogenous acid production and excretion by human adults. Calcif. Tissue Int. 44:335-338; 1989.

64. Turner, J.G.; Gilchrist, N.L.; Ayling, E.M.; Hassall, A.J.; Hooke, E.A.; Sadler, W.A. Factors affecting bone mineral density in high school girls. N. Zeal. Med. J. 105:95-96; 1992.

65. White, C.M.; Hergenroeder, A.C.; Klish, W.J. Bone mineral density in 15- to 21-year old eumenorrheic and amenorrheic subjects. Am. J. Dis. Child. 146:31-35; 1992.

66. Zemel, M.B. Calcium utilization: effect of varying level and source of dietary protein. Am. J. Clin. Nutr. 48:880-883; 1988.

Part III

Training and Congenital Heart Disease

Chapter 8

Benefits of Exercise Training After Surgical Repair of Congenital Heart Disease: A Theoretical Perspective

Hélène Perrault, PhD

Individuals who undertake exercise training generally do so in hope of gaining benefits. Benefits may be improving athletic performance or preventing or rehabilitating from disease. Most of our knowledge regarding the physiological effects of exercise training comes from the adult population. In this chapter, I will use adult responses as the basis for reflections and speculations concerning their application to children who have had surgery for a congenital heart defect.

Training for Athletic Performance

Training for athletic performance implies stressing or overloading the physiological characteristics that are the major determinants of performance for a given event. Maximal aerobic power ($\dot{V}O_2$max) and aerobic endurance are important determinants of athletic performance in all "endurance classified" sports. It is therefore not surprising that one of the criteria for successful endurance training is an increase in maximal oxygen uptake. With appropriate intensity, duration, and frequency of exercise training, an increase in $\dot{V}O_2$max of up to 20% is generally observed after several months of training, reflecting synchronized histological and systemic adaptations of the components of the oxygen transport system (48).

The increase in maximal oxygen uptake results from both peripheral adaptations dictating the oxygen extraction capabilities and central adaptations reflecting the "pumping" capacity of the system. Oxygen utilization is dependent upon morphological and biochemical characteristics of skeletal muscles (48). Muscular adaptations to endurance training will include changes in slow twitch muscle fibers at both the cellular and subcellular levels, including fiber hypertrophy, increased intermyofibrilar mitochondrial protein volume, and myofibrilar protein turnover rate (29). These adaptations in turn will influence substrate utilization and energy production. On the other hand, oxygen availability is dictated by the arterial oxygen content, which, in the absence of any impairment in alveolar-arterial oxygen diffusion or right-to-left shunting, is directly related to alveolar oxygen tension.

Finally, an increase in maximal cardiac output could also contribute to enhance the capabilities of the oxygen transport system. The extent to which each of these components contributes, if at all, to the increase in maximal aerobic power most likely varies from one individual to another, as well as from one type of individual to another, accounting for a number of limiting factors rather than a ''single'' common limitation to maximal oxygen uptake.

Because an in-depth review of these adaptations is beyond the scope of this presentation, I have chosen to restrict the focus of this chapter to selected adaptations that could ''theoretically'' benefit patients who have had surgery for a congenital heart defect, be it in terms of athletic performance, disease prevention, or rehabilitation. I refer the reader to selected reviews for a complete overview of the specific effects of exercise training.

Metabolic Adaptations

The most obvious metabolic adaptation to endurance training is the shift in muscle substrate utilization during exercise, which leads to greater free fatty acid utilization and thus delays the occurrence of muscle glycogen depletion (4,5). The shift to fatty acid metabolism may result from changes in lipid mobilization due to an increase in hormone-sensitive triglyceride lipase or to an enhancement of beta-adrenergic binding affinity of adipocytes (5). Enhancement of lipid utilization could result from a decrease in circulating insulin, which has been reported after endurance training. An increase in capillarization, resulting in a 5 to 10% increase in the capillary:fiber ratio, as well as up to twofold increases in the oxidative enzyme activities and mitochondrial volume density may also contribute to facilitate lipid utilization (4,5,46).

Could such adaptations be of specific benefit to individuals who have undergone surgery for a congenital heart defect? Results from Ericksson and Hanson (15), obtained from a progressive cycling exercise study in 16 men, who as children had undergone surgery for coarctation of the aorta, and their age-matched controls indicate systematically higher muscle lactate concentrations in patients for any level of blood lactate. Because the glycogen depletion pattern and blood lactate concentrations in relation to relative exercise intensities were not different between groups, it was concluded that an impairment in leg blood flow must persist in these patients thereby reducing metabolic clearance and favoring muscle lactate accumulation. Peripheral circulatory adaptations could of course contribute to increased circulating substrate utilization and favor lactate clearance. In the absence of increased capillarization, a shift in substrate utilization favoring fatty acid oxidation and glycogen sparing could probably also improve exercise tolerance in patients with peripheral flow limitations by delaying intramuscular lactate accumulation, which has been associated with inhibition of glycolysis and the onset of fatigue (46,47).

Cardiovascular Adaptations

Cardiovascular adaptations and, more specifically, those affecting pump function, are perhaps more directly related to patients who have had surgery for a congenital heart defect. It is well known that endurance exercise training induces adaptations in exercise stroke volume and heart rate, which may or may not be reflected in maximal cardiac output (45). Although the kinetics of the exercise-induced increase in stroke volume with exercise intensity is independent of training state, absolute values of stroke volume are higher in fit individuals and athletes for any absolute exercise intensity (60). Since stroke volume is the difference between end-diastolic and end-systolic volumes, the higher stroke volume of athletes can result from a decrease in end-systolic volume, an increase in end-diastolic volume, or a combination of these two factors (28,45).

Effects of Training on End-Diastolic Volume
Two factors may account for an increase in end-diastolic volume following endurance training: training bradycardia and training-induced hypervolemia.

A decrease in resting and submaximal exercise heart rates is probably the most anticipated and recognized effect of endurance training. The occurrence of training bradycardia may be due to any combination of three factors: a reduction in the intrinsic rate of depolarization of the cardiocytes of the sinus node; a decrease in the sympathetic stimulation of the sinoatrial node; or an increase in the parasympathetic stimulation to the sinus node. Traditionally, training bradycardia has been attributed to an increase in the parasympathetic influence on the sinoatrial node (45). The experimental evidence on this topic is, however, far from convincing. In rats, atropine administration, which blocks the parasympathetic influence on the sinus node, was found to cause a smaller rather than a larger rise in heart rate in trained animals, suggesting a lower vagal tone in trained animals (50). More recent studies using combined parasympathetic and sympathetic blockade in rats suggest a decrease in the intrinsic heart rate following endurance training rather than a decrease in sympathetic or an increase in vagal influence (37,49,51).

In humans, results appear to be more controversial. Results obtained in trained and untrained subjects following B-blockade administration showed a greater decrease in heart rate of sedentary subjects, which suggests a lower sympathetic drive to the sinus node in athletes (45). Results from dual blockade experiments used in cross-sectional comparisons of athletes and non-athletes or following an endurance training program, indicate a lower intrinsic rate in athletes (31) or following training (33,52), which could also be associated with an enhanced vagal influence (52). Investigations of heart rate variability in athletes or following endurance training indicate an increase in both the high frequency (parasympathetic) (13,21) and the low frequency (sympathetic) (21) components of the power spectrum. In addition to the traditional view of an increase in vagal tone, adaptations in cellular metabolism of sinoatrial cardiocytes could partially explain the observed decrease in resting heart rate.

Would endurance training also induce bradycardia following surgical correction of a congenital heart disease? It is widely recognized that, despite excellent surgical outcome, patients who have had surgery for a congenital heart defect exhibit a chronotropic limitation to maximal exercise (10). At present, there is no clear explanation for this finding. Results from electrophysiological investigations of patients who have undergone surgery for tetralogy of Fallot, however, indicate sinoatrial as well as atrioventricular conduction abnormalities, (23,55) which could contribute to the observed limitation. It has also been associated with the anatomical disruption of the sympathetic innervation following transventricular surgical procedures. However, findings of a study of similar chronotropic limitation to exercise following long-term successful repair of isolated ASD (39) suggest that the etiology may not be restricted to the transventricular surgical approach, but could be associated to a common denominator of all open-heart surgical procedures. Results from a comparative study of the response to exercise of patients in whom a VSD had either closed spontaneously or was surgically repaired, patients who had undergone surgery for patent ductus arteriosus, and healthy controls showed the maximal heart rate to be abnormal only in those who had had open-heart surgical repair for the VSD. Because this procedure involves placement of cannulae in the superior vena cava for cardiopulmonary bypass, it could lead to injury of the sinoatrial node area, disturbing its physiological integrity and altering the control of heart rate during exercise. Surgical fibroelastosis, possibly resulting from transient hypoxia, interstitial edema, and poor lymph drainage, has been reported following the cardiopulmonary bypass procedure (3). This could account for an irreversible impairment to the sinoatrial node.

In light of these observations, it is reasonable to ask whether the potential of sinoatrial cardiocytes to adapt to training is altered after open-heart surgery. Disturbances in the autonomic control of heart rate have been reported in children with congenital heart defects. Whether this is inherent to the heart malformation or results from the surgical correction of the defect remains to be clarified.

Using spectral analysis of heart rate variability, Finley et al. (17) described the amplitude of the low and the high frequency component of the R-R variability. When patients were in the supine position, both before and after surgery a lower HF component was found in ASD, suggesting either a change in coupling between respiration and the heart or an alteration in the parasympathetic control of heart rate. Much information on the autonomic control of heart rate in these patients remains to be provided. Is training-induced bradycardia a common observation in these patients, and if it is, what are the factors responsible for its occurrence?

Training-Induced Hypervolemia. Cross-sectional comparisons of endurance athletes and non-athletes clearly demonstrate a 20 to 25% larger blood volume in both male and female trained subjects, independent of age (8). A general observation associated with endurance training is that plasma volume expansion is a rapid adaptation phenomenon occurring after a single exercise session. The extent of the expansion is directly proportional to the intensity and duration of the exercise. Increases in plasma volume ranging between 12 and 15% are generally reported following endurance training of 1 day to 4 months in duration, the effects being more pronounced with running than cycling exercise (8). Although the precise mechanism has not been completely elucidated, the hypervolemia has been associated with the regular training-induced increases in plasma renin activity and arginine vasopressin concentration (9). In humans, the net increase in body fluids with exercise training has been associated with increased water intake and decreased urine output, probably through increased renal tubular reabsorption of sodium due to a more sensitive aldosterone action.

A teleological explanation for this phenomenon is that hypervolemia may provide an advantage for heat dissipation and thermoregulatory stability in addition to providing a larger vascular volume and filling pressure for greater cardiac stroke volume and lower heart rates during exercise. How would patients exhibiting chamber volume overload or an altered hydro-mineral hormonal status respond to exercise training? In previous investigations of patients who have a good clinical status after undergoing successful Fontan correction, we have found abnormal ANP, AVP, and PRA responses to dynamic exercise, which suggest alterations in the control of fluid-regulating hormonal responses (41). A similar response was observed in patients following cardiac transplantation due to the effects of cardiac denervation and the immunosuppresive therapy (40). Would the conditions for training-induced hypervolemia still be fulfilled in these patients? And assuming that training induced a similar hypervolemia in these patients, would the teleological advantages still stand in view of the chronic cardiac overload already sustained in these patients? The observation of a decrease rather than an increase in plasma hematocrit following exercise in these patients suggests an increase in lymphatic drainage following exercise, which could provide beneficial effects.

Training Effects on the End-Systolic Volume

Generally, little improvement in myocardial contractility in healthy sedentary adults is reported following training when using resting echocardiographic indices of contractility. It has been argued that such changes might be observed only under conditions soliciting an enhanced contractile function such as maximal exercise. Echocardiographic measurements of contractility indices have been obtained during steady-state exercise in subjects with high, moderate, and low levels of fitness. Although the PEP/LVET ratio appeared to be enhanced in highly fit individuals, presumably because of the effects of training, no significant differences between groups could be observed (60). These observations are in accordance with others reported following endurance training (45) and may reflect an absence of adaptation or adaptations that remain below the practical resolution of the echocardiographic technique.

Results from animal studies are conflicting. Examinations of mechanical properties of isolated papillary muscles in trained and untrained animals have not provided evidence that training has a clear effect on ventricular performance. While swimming almost always induces myocardial adaptations in rats, this model has been criticized because it may more closely resemble a "hypoxic" stress. Some improvement in indices of contractility have been reported in rats subjected to treadmill running; however, the reports were not made in a systematic fashion (50).

Such adaptations could be related to intrinsic biochemical/functional properties of the contractile machinery and other cellular components, by impacting on either the proteins involved in ATP degradation/energy transformation or subcellular components involved in calcium transport to and from the contractile material (1,56). Trained animals have been shown to exhibit higher peak tension of the papillary muscle for any given external concentration of calcium, which could be caused by an increase in sarcolemnal calcium binding sites (56). Similarly, three myosin isosymes designated as V1, V2, and V3 have been identified in mammalian hearts. In rats subjected to 8 and 12 weeks of swim training a 20% increase in myosin Ca-ATPase activity of myofibrils was observed (38), which was in proportion to an increase in the relative amount of V1, the myosin isosyme with the highest Ca-dependent ATPase activity. Whether such adaptations take place in healthy human hearts or in hearts subjected to chronic volume or pressure overload has yet to be determined.

Thus, independent of changes in ventricular systolic function, an increase in $\dot{V}O_2$max may take place following endurance training because of peripheral adaptations favoring oxygen extraction and/or changes in cardiac output resulting from an increase in end-diastolic volume. Whether patients who have undergone surgery for a congenital heart defect exhibit potential similar to that of their healthy counterparts for improving aerobic power, and the extent to which each of the aforementioned mechanisms can contribute to this improvement, remain to be determined.

Training for the Prevention of Coronary Artery Disease

The association between physical activity level and atherosclerosis is based on a substantial body of evidence that suggests that habitual activity leads to a blood lipoprotein profile that is favorable with respect to preventing or delaying the atherosclerotic process (62). In the literature there is ample evidence that plasma total cholesterol is positively associated with incidence of coronary artery disease; that the principal carrier of cholesterol in the plasma, LDL lipoprotein, is positively associated with CAD; and that plasma concentration of HDL cholesterol is inversely related to the relative risk of CAD (30,35,61). Moreover, endurance training can positively affect the patient with diabetes mellitus, a primary risk factor for coronary artery disease. Although much remains to be clarified regarding the definite effects of regular physical activity on the prevention of atherosclerosis or the mechanisms responsible for this effect, there is general agreement on a number of issues. I briefly summarize these in the next sections.

Lipoprotein Metabolism

Cross-sectional comparisons of untrained and endurance-trained individuals indicate that total plasma cholesterol is not much different or only slightly greater in trained subjects. Highly trained endurance athletes may exhibit somewhat lower LDL-cholesterol (10-12%) values than non-athletes, but differences between active and inactive individuals in the general population are generally not found. In male endurance-trained subjects, HDL-cholesterol appears to be consistently higher (20-25%) than in untrained subjects, although the influence of diet may be a confounding factor in these studies (54). Results from longitudinal studies generally show an increase of 10 to 15% in HDL cholesterol, provided the endurance training program exceeds 10 weeks in duration (27,54,62). The precise mechanism for these adaptations are still not completely understood. Several lipoproteins and their apoproteins play an active part in lipid metabolism. Chylomicrons, very low density lipoproteins (VLDL), low density lipoproteins (LDL), intermediate density lipoproteins (IDL), and high density lipoproteins (HDL) act as transporters of triglyceride, phospholipids, and cholesterol, the proportion of these determining the density of the lipoprotein. Similarly, several enzymes regulate the lipid exchanges between circulating lipoproteins or between lipoproteins and tissues. Lipoprotein lipase (LPL), the heparin-releasable hepatic lipase (HRHL), and lecithin cholesterol acyl transferase (LCAT) are important modulators of lipoprotein metabolism, and all appear to be involved in the exercise-training effect on circulating lipoproteins (27).

Although still only fragmentary, results from cross-sectional studies have provided evidence of differences in enzymatic activities which could help explain the elevation of circulating HDL-cholesterol associated with endurance training. First, an increase in skeletal and cardiac muscle LPL activity has been reported that could enhance fatty acid fluxes and the apoprotein C and E transfer to HDL. Second, an increase in LCAT activity has been found favoring cholesteryl ester formation and making cholesterol less accessible to tissues. High circulating levels of apoprotein AI, which has the capacity to activate LCAT activity, has also been associated with a protective effect for the development of coronary artery disease. Finally, lower HRHL, which could delay the transformation of HDL_2 to HDL_3 and promote their uptake by the liver, has also been reported. Again, a higher circulating HDL_2 concentration is associated with a reduced risk of CAD (62).

Diabetes Mellitus

Diabetes mellitus is another known risk factor for the development of CAD. Cross-sectional investigations have shown lower fasting and glucose-stimulated insulin levels and an increase in glucose tolerance or hepatic and peripheral insulin sensitivity in endurance-trained athletes and trained subjects when compared to sedentary individuals (58,59). Using the hyperinsulinemic euglycemic clamp technique, researchers found in trained distance runners an insulin sensitivity 25 to 40% higher than in controls

(58). Similarly, endurance training may also result in an increased glucose uptake in diabetic Type I patients. Studies in rats suggest several contributing factors including an increase in skeletal muscle insulin binding receptor density, capillary density, or oxidative mitochondrial enzymes, as well as insulin-stimulated glucose uptake, oxidation, and incorporation into fatty acids in adipocytes (59). Moreover, recent evidence of a twofold increase in glucose transporter (GLUT 4) protein turnover rate of skeletal muscles following endurance training in rats suggests that the increase in insulin sensitivity could be related to the enhancement of the facilitated diffusion of glucose across the plasma membrane. According to these recent observations, the relative insulin resistance observed in diabetic or obese individuals could be related to defects in the signal recognition or intracellular behavior of the glucose transporter protein (32).

Although there are many reasons to suggest the adoption of an active lifestyle for the general population, there might be even more reasons to do so for children who have undergone surgery for a congenital heart defect or for heart transplantation. Because there is not much information yet on the long-term natural history of such patients, it remains to be seen whether these patients are more prone to adopt a sedentary lifestyle in their adult life. Also, while coronary atherosclerosis is a recognized complication after heart transplantation, there is still little information as to the likelihood of suffering Type II diabetes or the susceptibility to coronary artery disease in patients who have had surgery for a congenital heart defect, in light of or independent of their activity level.

Hypertension

It is generally accepted that endurance training can reduce arterial blood pressure in individuals with essential hypertension. The reductions reported average roughly 5 to 25 mmHg in systolic pressure and 3 to 15 mmHg in diastolic blood pressure (24). When the endurance training is combined with a significant weight reduction, even greater decreases are reported. Again, a precise mechanism for the observed effect of endurance training has not been identified. It is possible, however, that the training effect reflects the cumulative influence of regularly repeated dynamic exercise (24). Using ambulatory blood-pressure monitoring in hypertensive adult patients, Pescatello et al. (43) observed a significant drop in systolic and diastolic blood pressures persisting for up to 13 hours following a single 30-minute moderate cycling exercise. This, however, was not observed in normotensive controls. Because acute dynamic exercise is characterized by disturbances in sympatho-adrenal and hydro-mineral hormonal status as well as cortical and medullary activity, the reported decreases in blood pressure cannot be ascribed to a single factor but instead to a combination of factors. A detailed account of all possible explanations is beyond the scope of this article, but I refer the reader to a recent review article by Tipton (57).

However, in the last 5 years, much attention has been devoted to the role of baroreflex function for the control of peripheral vascular resistance in hypertensive individuals (7,19). Cardiopulmonary baroreflexes have been shown to be involved in the control of peripheral vascular resistance through tonic inhibition of the sympathetic outflow to systemic arterioles (26,34). In hypertensive subjects, an acute cycling exercise induced a significant decrease in arterial blood pressure, which was associated with an increase in forearm blood flow. This resulted in a downward shift in the relationship between central venous pressure and peripheral vascular resistance, suggesting that the anti-hypertensive effect of exercise could be related to a modulation of cardiopulmonary baroreflex control (7).

Little information is available regarding baroreflex functions following corrective surgery for a congenital heart defect. Using phenylephrine and nitroprusside injections to increase or decrease heart rate, Beekman et al. (1983) reported an alteration in the arterial baroreceptor function curve after repair of coarctation of the aorta (2). While carotid and aortic baroreceptors primarily operate via changes in the heart rate, cardiopulmonary baroreflexes act to regulate skeletal muscle vascular resistance (34). In patients who underwent surgery for coarctation of the aorta showing exercise-induced hypertension, a normal cardiac output response to exercise was reported, suggesting that a potential disturbance in the control of peripheral resistance could be involved in the etiology of the hypertensive response (36). Cardiopulmonary baroreflex function has not been widely investigated in patients who have undergone surgery for a congenital heart defect. However, considering that surgical repair of congenital heart defects is often associated with impaired chamber diastolic function (10), it is highly probable that the sensitivity of the cardiopulmonary receptors to volume loading and unloading could be affected. Whether exercise training could positively affect children who have had surgery for a congenital heart defect by delaying or preventing hypertension remains to be determined.

Training for Cardiac Rehabilitation

Finally, exercise training has been used for rehabilitation after myocardial infarction or coronary artery disease. Cardiac rehabilitation generally results in a significant increase in maximal exercise tolerance or maximal aerobic power for a given anginal threshold, determined by the double product of heart rate and systolic blood pressure (18,20,44). The increase in exercise tolerance has generally been attributed to peripheral adaptations favoring skeletal muscle oxygen extraction (6,12) and reducing coronary flow requirements for any given absolute work load rather than an increase in myocardial oxygen delivery (16). Present knowledge does not support the development of coronary collateral circulation as a result of exercise conditioning in humans, although evidence of increased myocardial capillary growth and/or enhanced myocardial flow in response to an ischemic challenge has been reported in animals (20). More recently, it has been suggested that the traditional absence of ventricular adaptations to exercise training could be the result of insufficient training stimuli. Evidence has now been provided for improvements in left ventricular function during isometric exercise leading to an increase in left ventricular stroke work following 1 year of endurance training in patients having sustained myocardial infarction (14,25).

Similarly, improvements in myocardial performance have been reported in patients with severe left ventricular dysfunction who have been subjected to endurance training (53). It has not been established whether this is the result of true myocardial adaptations, or whether this reflects the natural healing process of the myocardium following the initial insult.

The effects of endurance training following corrective surgery for a congenital heart defect have been described predominantly in terms of maximal exercise capacity and aerobic power (22). In addition, most of these controlled studies are restricted in duration to several weeks or months. Myocardial infarction is not a major concern in most patients with a congenital heart defect. Nonetheless, an increase in myocardial performance in the years following surgery could be of potential value for the long-term prognosis of the child who has undergone surgery for a congenital heart defect. Moreover, while the surgical repair can restore the heart's proper physiological function, there are situations where this is achieved at the expense of anatomical and histological integrity. Would exercise-training following transposition of the great arteries benefit the patient?

Conclusion

Surgical correction of congenital heart defects has become common practice. However, the information regarding the long-term natural history of these patients into adulthood is limited. Similarly, the short-term and long-term effects of exercise training on their natural history, on their clinical status, or on their quality of life remains to be fully documented. Chapter 9 covers some of the available information that suggests children who have had surgery for congenital heart defects indeed can benefit from exercise training. From a physiologist's perspective, I believe that not only the patient will benefit from exercise training after surgical repair of a congenital heart defect, but the researcher will benefit as well.

References

1. Baldwin, K.M. Effects of chronic exercise on biochemical and functional properties of the heart. Med. Sci. Sports Exerc. 17:522-528; 1985.
2. Beekman, R.H.; Katz, B.P.; Moorehead-Steffens, C.; Rocchini, A.P. Altered baroreceptor function in children with systolic hypertension after coarctation repair. Am. J. Cardiol. 52:112-117; 1983.
3. Bharati, S.; Lev, M. The myocardium, the conduction system and general sequelae after surgery for congenital heart disease. In: Engle, J.A.; Perloff, K.F. Congenital heart disease after surgery: benefits, residua, sequelae. New York: Yorke Medical Books; 1983: 240-260.
4. Bjorntorp, P. Adipose tissue adaptation to exercise. In: Exercise fitness and health. Bouchard, C.; Shephard, R.J.; Stephens, T.; Sutton, J.R.; McPherson B.D. A consensus of current knowledge. Champaign, IL: Human Kinetics; 1990: 315-323.
5. Brooks, G.A.; Fahey, T.D. Exercise physiology. Human bioenergetics and its applications. New York: Wiley & Sons; 1984.

6. Clausen, J.P. Circulatory adjustments to dynamic exercise and effect of physical training in normal subjects and in patients with coronary artery disease. Prog. Cardiovasc. Dis. 18:459-470; 1976.

7. Cleroux, J.; Kouame, N.; Nadeau, A.; Coulombe, D.; Lacourciere, Y. Baroreflex regulation of forearm vascular resistance after exercise in hypertensive and normotensive humans. Am. J. Physiol. 263:H1523-1531; 1992.

8. Convertino, V.A. Blood volume: its adaptation to endurance training. Med. Sci. Sports Exerc. 23:1338-1348; 1991.

9. Convertino, V.A.; Keil, L.C.; Greenleaf, J.E. Plasma volume, renin and vasopressin responses to graded exercise after training. J. Appl. Physiol. 54:508-514; 1983.

10. Cumming, G.R. Children with heart disease. In: Skinner, J.S. Exercise testing and exercise prescription for special cases. Theoretical basis and clinical application. Philadelphia: Lea and Febiger; 1987: 241-260.

11. Davies, K.J.A.; Packer, L.; Brooks, G.A. Biochemical adaptation of mitochondria, muscle, and whole-animal respiration to endurance training. Arch. Biochem. Biophys. 209:538-553; 1981.

12. Detry, J.M.; Rousseau, M.; Vandenbroucke, G.; Kusumi, F.; Brasseur, L.A.; Bruce R.A. Increased arteriovenous oxygen differences after physical training in coronary heart disease. Circulation 44:109-118; 1971.

13. Dixon, E.M.; Kamath, M.V.; et al. Neural regulation of heart rate variability in endurance athletes and sedentary controls. Cardiovasc. Res. 26:713-719; 1992.

14. Ehsani, A.A.; Martin, W.H. III; Heath, G.W.; Coyle, E.F. Cardiac effects of prolonged and intense exercise training in patients with coronary artery disease. Am. J. Cardiol. 50:236-253; 1982.

15. Eriksson, B.O.; Hanson, E. Muscle metabolism during exercise in men operated upon coarctation of the aorta in childhood. Scand. J. Clin. Invest. 41:135-141; 1981.

16. Ferguson, R.J.; Cote, P.; Gauthier, P.; Bourassa, M.G. Changes in exercise coronary sinus blood flow with training in patients with angina pectoris. Circulation 58:41-47; 1978.

17. Finley, J.P.; Nugent, S.; Hellenbrand, W.; Craig, M.; Gillis, D.A. Sinus arrhythmia in children with atrial septal defect: an analysis of heart rate variability before and after surgical repair. Br. Heart J. 61:280-284; 1989.

18. Fletcher, G.F.; Froelicher, V.F.; Hartley, H.; Haskell, W.L.; Pollock, M.L. Exercise standards: a statement for health professionals from the American Heart Association. Circulation 82:2286-2322; 1990.

19. Floras, J.S.; Sinkey, C.A.; Aylward, P.E.; Seals, D.R.; Thoren, P.; Mark, A.L. Postexercise hypotension and sympathoinhibition in borderline hypertensive men. Hypertension 14:28-35; 1989.

20. Froelicher, V.F. Exercise, fitness and coronary heart disease. In: Bouchard, C.; Shephard, R.J.; Stephens, T.; Sutton, J.R.; McPherson, B.D. Exercise fitness and health. A consensus of current knowledge. Champaign, IL: Human Kinetics; 1990: 429-450.

21. Furlan, R.; Piazza, S.; Dell'Orto, S.; Gentile, E.; Cerutti, S.; Pagani, M.; Malliani, A. Early and late effects of exercise and athletic training on neural mechanisms controlling heart rate. Cardiovascular Res. 27:483-488; 1993.

22. Galioto, F.M.; Tomassoni, T.L. Exercise rehabilitation in congenital cardiac disease. Prog. Ped. Cardiol.: pediatric cardiovascular exercise responses part II. 2:50-66; 1993.

23. Gillette, P.C.; Yeoman, M.A.; Mullins, C.E.; McNamara, D.G. Sudden death after repair of tetralogy of Fallot. Electrocardiographic and electrophysiological abnormalities. Circulation 56:566-571; 1977.

24. Hagberg, J.M. Exercise, fitness and hypertension. In: Bouchard, C.; Shephard, R.J.; Stephens, T.; Sutton, J.R.; McPherson, B.D. Exercise fitness and health. A consensus of current knowledge. Champaign, IL: Human Kinetics; 1990: 455-466.

25. Hagberg, J.M.; Ehsani, A.A.; Holloszy, J.O. Effect of 12 months of intense exercise training on stroke volume in patients with coronary artery disease. Circulation 67:1194-1199; 1983.

26. Hainsworth, R. Reflexes from the heart. Physiol. Rev. 71:617-658; 1991.
27. Haskell, W.L. The influence of exercise on the concentrations of triglyceride and cholesterol in human plasma. In: Ex. Sport Sciences Reviews 12:205-244; 1984.
28. Higginbotham, M.B.; Morris, K.G.; Williams, R.S.; McHale, P.A.; Coleman, R.E.; Cobb, F.R. Regulation of stroke volume during submaximal and maximal upright exercise in normal man. Circ. Res. 58:281-291; 1986.
29. Holloszy, J.O.; Booth, F.W. Biochemical adaptations to endurance exercise in muscle. Ann. Rev. Physiol. 38:273-291; 1976.
30. Kannel, W.B.; Belanger, A.; D'Agostino, R.; Israel, I. Physical activity and physical demand on the job and risk of cardiovascular disease and death: the Framingham study. Am. Heart J. 112:820-825; 1986.
31. Katona, P.G.; McClean, M.; Dighton, D.H.; Guz, A. Sympathetic and parasympathetic cardiac control in athletes and nonathletes at rest. J. Appl. Physiol. Respirat. Environ. Exercise Physiol. 52:1652-1657; 1982.
32. Khan, B.B. Facilitative glucose transporters: regulatory mechanisms and dysregulation in diabetes. J. Clin. Invest. 89:1367-1374; 1992.
33. Lewis, S.F.; Nylander, E.; Gad, P.; Areskog, N.H. Non-autonomic component in bradycardia of endurance trained men at rest and during exercise. Acta Physiol. Scand. 109:297-305; 1980.
34. Mancia, G.; Donald, D.; Shepherd, J.T. Inhibition of adrenergic outflow to peripheral blood vessels by vagal afferents from the cardiopulmonary region in the dog. Circ. Res. 33:713-721; 1973.
35. Morris, J.N.; Everitt, M.G.; Pollard, R.; Chave, S.P.W. Vigorous exercise in leisure-time: protection against coronary heart disease. LANCET ii:1207-1210; 1980.
36. Murphy, A.M.; Blades, M.; Daniels, S.; James, F.W. Blood pressure and cardiac output during exercise: a longitudinal study of children undergoing repair of coarctation. Am. Heart J. 117:1327-1332; 1989.
37. Negrao, C.E.; Moreira, E.D.; Santos, M.C.L.M.; Farah, V.M.A.; Krieger, E.M. Vagal function impairment after exercise training. J. Appl. Physiol. 72:1749-1753; 1992.
38. Pagani, E.D.; Solaro, J.J. Swimming exercise, thyroid state and the distribution of myosin isosymes in rat heart. Am. J. Physiol. 245:H713-7120; 1983.
39. Perrault, H.; Drblik, S.P.; Montigny, M.; Davignon, A.; Lamarre, A.; Chartrand, C.; Stanley, P. Comparison of cardiovascular adjustments to exercise in adolescents 8 to 15 years of age after correction of tetralogy of Fallot, ventricular septal defect or atrial septal defect. Am. J. Cardiol. 64:213-217; 1989.
40. Perrault, H.; Melin, B.; Jimenez, C.; Dureau, G.; Dureau, E.; Allevard, A.M.; Cottet-Emard, J.M.; Gharib, C. The response of fluid-regulating and sympathoadrenal hormones to exercise following orthotopic heart transplantation. J. Appl. Physiol. 76(1):230-235; 1994.
41. Perrault, H.; Miro, J.; Davignon, A.; Beland, M.; Armstrong, B.; Thibault, G.; Cantin, M.; Chartrand, C. Decreased plasma atriopeptin response to volume-overloading maneuvers and exercise after atriopulmonary anastomosis of Fontan. Am. J. Cardiol. 69:1325-1328; 1992.
42. Perrault, H; Drblik, S.P. Exercise after surgical repair of congenital cardiac lesions. Sports Medicine 7:18-31; 1989.
43. Pescatello, L.S.; Fargo, A.E.; Leach, C.N.; Scherzer, H.H. Short-term effect of dynamic exercise on arterial blood pressure. Circulation 83:1557-1561; 1991.
44. Redwood, D.R.; Rosing, D.R.; Epstein, S.E. Circulatory and symptomatic effects of physical training in patients with coronary-artery disease and angina pectoris. N. Engl. J. Med. 286:959-965; 1972.
45. Rowell, L.B. Human circulation during physical stress. New York: Oxford University Press; 1986: 257-287.
46. Sahlin, K. Discussion: Effects of exercise on aspects of carbohydrate, fat and amino acid metabolism. In: Bouchard, C.; Shephard, R.J.; Stephens, T.; Sutton, J.R.; McPherson. B.D. Exercise fitness and health. A consensus of current knowledge. Champaign, IL: Human Kinetics; 1990: 309-314.

47. Sahlin, K.; Katz, A.; Henricksson, J. Redox state and lactate accumulation in human skeletal muscle during dynamic exercise. Biochem. J. 245:551-556; 1987.

48. Saltin, B. Cardiovascular and pulmonary adaptation to physical activity. In: Bouchard, C.; Shephard, R.J.; Stephens, T.; Sutton, J.R.; McPherson, B.D. Exercise fitness and health. A consensus of current knowledge. Champaign, IL: Human Kinetics; 1990: 187-205.

49. Schaefer, M.E.; Allert, A.; Adams, H.R.; Laughlin, M.H. Adrenergic responsiveness and intrinsic sinoatrial automaticity of exercise trained rats. Med. Sci. Sports Exerc. 24:887-894; 1992.

50. Scheuer, J.; Tipton, C.M. Cardiovascular adaptations to physical training. Annu. Rev. Physiol. 39:221-251; 1977.

51. Sigvardsson, K.; Svanfeldt, E.; Kilbom, A. Role of the adrenergic nervous system in development of training-induced bradycardia. Acta Physiol. Scand. 101:481-488; 1977.

52. Smith, M.L.; Hudson, D.L.; Graitzer, H.M.; Raven, P.B. Exercise training bradycardia: the role of autonomic balance. Med. Sci. Sports Exerc. 21:40-44; 1989.

53. Sullivan, M.J.; Higginbotham, M.B.; Cobb, F.R. Exercise training in patients with severe left ventricular dysfunction. Hemodynamic and metabolic effects. Circulation 78:506-515; 1988.

54. Superko, H.R.; Haskell, W.H. The role of exercise training in the therapy of hyperlipoproteinemia. Cardiology Clinics 5:285-310; 1987.

55. Tamer, D.; Wolff, G.C.; Ferrer, P.; Pickoff, A.S.; Casta, A.; Ashok, V.M.; Gracia, O.; Gelband, H. Haemodynamic and intracardiac conduction after operative repair of tetralogy of Fallot. Am. J. Cardiol. 51:552-556; 1983.

56. Tibbits, G.F. Regulation of myocardial contractility in exhaustive exercise. Med. Sci. Sports Exerc. 17:527-529; 1985.

57. Tipton, C.M. Exercise training and hypertension. Ex. Sport Sciences Reviews 19:447-505; 1991.

58. Vranic, M.; Wasserman, D. Exercise, fitness and diabetes. In: Bouchard, C.; Shephard, R.J.; Stephens, T.; Sutton, J.R.; McPherson, B.D. Exercise fitness and health. A consensus of current knowledge. Champaign, IL: Human Kinetics; 1990: 467-490.

59. Wallberg-Henriksson, H. Exercise and diabetes mellitus. Ex. Sport Sciences Reviews 20:339-368; 1992.

60. Wolfe, L.A.; Cunningham, D.A.; Davis, G.M.; Rosenfeld, H. Relationship between maximal oxygen uptake and left ventricular function in exercise. J. Appl. Physiol. 44:44-49; 1978.

61. Wood, P.D.; Terry, R.B.; Haskell, W.L. Metabolism of substrates: diet, lipoprotein metabolism and exercise. Fed. Proc. 44:358-363; 1985.

62. Wood, P.D.; Stefanick, M.L. Exercise, fitness and atherosclerosis. In: Bouchard, C.; Shephard, R.J.; Stephens, T.; Sutton, J.R.; McPherson, B.D. Exercise fitness and health. A consensus of current knowledge. Champaign, IL: Human Kinetics; 1990: 409-424.

Chapter 9

Training and the Pediatric Patient: A Cardiologist's Perspective

Gerald Barber, MD

Introduction

The physiologic responses of normal adults to training or of adults with various diseases to exercise rehabilitation have been well studied. While training or rehabilitation may be even more significant in the life of a child, data are much more limited. These studies have frequently attempted only non-invasive measurements of physiologic changes. Only a limited number of patients have been involved secondary to difficulty in recruiting volunteers and in obtaining compliance throughout the course of the program. For these reasons, not only have individual studies not been helpful, they have sometimes been contradictory in their conclusions.

In an attempt to increase the power of these studies and to clarify the response to training in pediatric patients, I will briefly review the results of 28 pediatric training studies (1-28) conducted over the past 31 years using weighted averaging of the data when possible. To be included in this review, the training sessions had to last longer than a month with the patient's physiologic status assessed prior to and immediately following the training program. Excluded from this review are training programs for individuals with neuromuscular or musculoskeletal abnormalities, cross-sectional studies comparing athletes to controls, and studies of athletes before and after their primary season.

Patients

Of the training programs reviewed, 427 patients successfully completed their training programs. Since the number of individuals starting but not finishing a training program was not consistently available, it is impossible to assess the dropout rate. Trainee ages ranged from 5 to 30 years with the majority of patients being teenagers. Trainees were divided into six groups based on diagnosis. Eleven studies (7-9,13,14,18,19,22,24,27,28), accounting for 170 trainees, involved normal individuals or normal controls for one of the other groups. Twelve studies (1-3,6,10,16,17,19,22,23,25,26) were performed in children with cardiac abnormalities. These studies accounted for 124 trainees. Hypertension was the indication for training in four studies (5,11-13) involving 68 trainees. Diabetes was the diagnosis in three studies (4,14,15) totaling 34 patients. One study each was performed in 21 patients with cystic fibrosis (21) and 10 patients with Down's syndrome (20).

Protocols

One of the difficulties in summarizing pediatric training data is the lack of a consistent protocol. The duration of training ranged from 1.5 to 14 months with a mean duration of 4 months. Thirty-six percent of the training programs lasted less than 3 months, 36% lasted 3 months, and 28% lasted more than 3 months. Frequency of training sessions was also very variable with a range of 1 to 5 sessions per week and a mean frequency of 3 sessions per week. Twenty-two percent of the training programs involved less than 3 sessions per week, 57% involved 3 sessions per week, and 22% involved more than 3 sessions per week. A target intensity for the training sessions was documented in only 60% of the programs. The heart rate at 70 to 80% of the peak oxygen consumption on the pre-training exercise test was used in 13% of the programs. Seventy-three percent of the programs used a target heart rate of between 60 and 80% of the maximum heart rate, with 7% each using a target heart rate of less than 60% or more than 80% of the maximum heart rate.

Results

There are several reasons why individuals might undergo a training program: improved performance by altering physiologic responses, decreased risk of coronary artery disease, increased working capacity or rehabilitation after an illness or operation, or improved psychologic well-being.

Physiologic Responses to Training

Very little is known about the physiologic responses to training in children. None of the articles reviewed address the issue of glycogen storage or other metabolic adaptations, flow redistribution, or hydromineral changes with training. Peak oxygen consumption is the only area in which any information is available.

Table 9.1 summarizes the acute changes in peak oxygen consumption over the course of the training program. There is a wide variation in responses between the various groups from −5% in the patients with Down's syndrome to +13% in the patients with cystic fibrosis. The explanation for this probably relates to two

Table 9.1   Percent change in peak oxygen consumption from beginning to end of the training program

Category	% Change	Number of patients
Normal	+4%	170
Cardiac	+11%	67
Hypertensive	+7%	57
Diabetic	+2%	20
Cystic fibrosis	+13%	20
Down's syndrome	−5%	10
Total	**+6%**	**344**

factors: how well-trained the individuals were at the start of the training program and how cooperative the individuals were throughout the training program. The relatively minor change in the normal children and in children with diabetes mellitus probably represents the effect of training in an already well-trained population. In both groups, mean values of peak oxygen consumption frequently exceeded 50 ml/kg/min prior to training (4,7,13). When the pre-training oxygen consumptions were lower, more substantial increases were seen (8,14). Lack of consistent effort during the training session probably explains the negative result in the children with Down's syndrome. In this study (20), while the mean peak oxygen consumption prior to training was low (26 ml/kg/min), the authors report that "if left to themselves, they would stop immediately, especially if there were diversions of any type." The remaining three groups probably represent the true effects of training in individuals who are not well-trained at the start of the program and who are cooperative within the program.

The 6% overall increase in peak oxygen consumption raises two additional questions: How persistent is this effect once the training program stops? and What physiologic changes cause the increase in oxygen consumption? Very little data are available to answer either of these questions.

Mathews (19) evaluated 8 individuals (4 normals and 4 cardiac patients) 6 months following his training program. On long-term follow-up the normal individuals demonstrated a 1% increase and the cardiac patients a 16% increase in peak oxygen consumption when compared to the pre-training values. These represented a fall from 7% and 34% increases respectively, immediately following the training program. Hagberg (11) evaluated 25 hypertensive children 9 months following training. Although these patients demonstrated a 10% increase in peak oxygen consumption immediately following training, on long-term follow-up peak oxygen consumption was not significantly different from the pre-training value.

There is a little more data available to explain the causes of the, at least initial, increase in peak oxygen consumption. Four studies have attempted to determine changes in peak cardiac index following a training program. Peak cardiac index increased 12% in 21 normal individuals (8,27) and 11% in 18 cardiac patients (23,25). In the cardiac patients this is presumably secondary to changes in both heart rate and stroke volume index. Peak heart rate increased 5% in 52 cardiac patients (2,3,19,22,23,25) and stroke volume increased 3% in 10 cardiac patients (2) immediately following the training program. Stroke volume data are not available for any of the other groups. Peak heart rate fell 1% in 105 normal individuals (7-9,18,19,22,27,28) and 3% in 10 children with Down's syndrome (20). Peripheral changes that might explain an increase in peak oxygen consumption have not been addressed in children.

Prevention of Coronary Artery Disease

The prevention of coronary disease with an exercise program consists of three components: the changes in lipoprotein metabolism, the antihypertensive effects of exercise, and the insulin-like effect of exercise.

Percent body fat is the most frequently made but crudest measure of lipoprotein metabolism. In 159 individuals no change in percent body fat could be detected over the course of the training program. There also does not seem to be a significant difference in this parameter between the normal individuals (9,13,19, 22,27), the cardiac patients (19,22,23,26), or hypertensive children (11,13). It was not assessed in the other groups. Serum cholesterol was measured in 33 patients. There was a 4% rise in 14 children with diabetes mellitus (15) and a 4% fall in 15 normal individuals (9,19). Although the numbers are very limited, the greatest change occurred in 4 cardiac patients (19). In this group the mean serum cholesterol fell from 204 mg/dl to 151 mg/dl over the course of the training. Furthermore, it remained low (149 mg/dl 6 months after the completion of the training program). High density lipoprotein concentration was assessed in only 8 trainees (4 normal individuals and 4 cardiac patients). In the normal individuals there was a 1% increase in serum HDL, and this persisted on retesting at 6 months. In the cardiac patients the immediate post-training HDL fell 4%, but it was 5% higher than pre-training at the 6-month follow-up evaluation. Serum triglycerides have been studied in 19 individuals. There was a 19% fall in 15 normal individuals (9,19) and a 33% fall in 4 cardiac patients (19) at the conclusion of the training program. While long-term response was not addressed in the majority of the normal individuals, the fall in the 4 cardiac patients was maintained with a 29% fall in serum triglycerides on 6 month follow-up when compared to pre-training.

The effect of training on blood pressure has been assessed in 126 trainees. In 48 normal individuals (8,13,19) training resulted in a 2% fall in systolic blood pressure. Diastolic blood pressure was reported in 44 of these individuals with no significant change. Ten cardiac patients (1,19) demonstrated a 6% fall in systolic blood pressure. While a smaller percentage changed, the biggest absolute change occurred in 68 hypertensive individuals (5,11,13). In this group, systolic blood pressure fell 5% and diastolic blood pressure fell 4%. Unfortunately this change was not sustained in long-term follow-up in a subgroup of 25 individuals. At 9 months the systolic blood pressure had risen to 2% greater than the pre-training value (11). Diastolic blood pressure also rose in these 25 individuals when compared to the immediate post-training value, but it remained 2% below the pre-training value. Epinephrine and norepinephrine levels were assessed prior to and following the training program in only one study (12). In the 12 patients studied, no differences could be detected in either the resting or peak exercise levels.

The insulin-like effect of exercise has been studied only in the diabetic patients. Even in this group, most of the data are from short duration sports camps, not true training programs. Sports camps are not an ideal time to look at the insulin-like effect because of the confounders of education and dietary changes that occur during these camps. Two of the three training studies of diabetic patients reviewed here used sports camps in addition to a longer training program. In these two studies, glucosuria decreased 44% (15) and 77% (14) during the 1 week sports camp. During the longer training programs, hemoglobin A_1 fell 9% in the one study in which it was measured (4). No change in insulin requirements was detected, but caloric intake increased by as much as 60% (14). Thus, training produced a net positive shift in relationship between insulin requirement and caloric intake.

Work Capacity/Rehabilitation

Some measure of performance or work capacity was performed in 14 of the training studies involving four of the subgroups (Table 9.2). While this represents the second most frequently assessed variable, it is also one of the hardest to

Table 9.2   Percent change in an index of work capacity from beginning to end of the training program

Category	% Change	Number of patients
Normal	+30%	74
Cardiac	+21%	104
Hypertensive		
Diabetic	+16%	20
Cystic fibrosis		
Down's syndrome	+8%	10
Total	**+23%**	**208**

analyze because work capacity was determined in a wide variety of ways including maximum work in kpm/min (8,10), work in kpm/min at a heart rate of 170 beats/min (14,15), duration of exercise (1-3,19,20,22,23,25), time to complete a 150 meter run (28), and an index combining measures of cardiovascular endurance, strength, flexibility, and coordination (17). Regardless of the index of work capacity used, the percent change was calculated by dividing the difference between the post and pre-training values by the pre-training value.

Work capacity increased significantly in all four of the groups assessed. While an increase in cardiac output and peak oxygen consumption probably accounts for some of this increase, the magnitude of increase is too great to be explained by this alone. Two other factors probably play a significant role. Training probably improves work efficiency such that at equivalent levels of oxygen consumption more work can be done. Several studies have demonstrated either a lower heart rate (7,8,10,24) or a lower oxygen consumption at submaximal workloads (10). Another possible explanation, not well addressed by any of the studies, is an improvement in anaerobic tolerance or performance. In such a case, increases in exercise time might be the result of increased performance beyond the anaerobic threshold with a subsequent increase in oxygen debt. Anaerobic threshold was assessed in only two of the studies reviewed here (18,23). A mean increase of 16% was detected in these 18 patients. While this is greater than the mean 6% increase in peak oxygen consumption, it is still probably not adequate to explain the total increase in work capacity.

Longmuir (16) has reported the 5-year follow-up of work capacity in 40 children following surgical repair of congenital heart disease. Most of her patients had simple lesions including a patent ductus arteriosus, coarctation of the aorta, an atrial septal defect, a ventricular septal defect, or aortic stenosis. Her study demonstrates that even with these simple lesions, without a postoperative training program work capacity remains significantly below that of healthy peers. The children who completed a simple home exercise program during the first 3 postoperative months achieved normal levels of physical fitness and maintained these levels for at least 5 years without any additional intervention.

Psychological Well-Being

Very little data are available on the psychological benefits of training. Of the studies reviewed here, psychological benefits are commented upon in only three studies, all involving cardiac patients.

Ruttenberg (22) studied nine patients with a variety of lesions including tetralogy of Fallot, aortic stenosis, transposition of the great arteries, and atrioventricular canal. Anecdotally, he reports that "some parents told us that, as a result of the training, their children became more outgoing, and better able to participate socially, as well as athletically, in peer activities."

Calzolari (3) reports on nine children who underwent training following total correction for tetralogy of Fallot. He reports that "at the end of the programme, the children all showed increased independence and initiative and more self-confidence in establishing social relations.'' While the basis for this statement is not clearly explained in the paper, at least two of the coauthors on this paper are psychologists.

Donovan (6) evaluated four children and their mothers prior to and following a training program using an open-ended questionnaire and a series of self tree drawings. Three of the children had undergone surgical repair of aortic stenosis, coarctation of the aorta, and tetralogy of Fallot, respectively. The fourth child had pulmonic stenosis that had not been previously operated upon. Prior to training, the mothers reported a fear that their child would die suddenly during physical activity. For this reason all the mothers tried to restrict their child's activity and were subsequently afraid of adolescent rebellion because of these restrictions. They had no clear understanding of the true limitations or safety of exercise for their child. Similarly, prior to the training program, three of the four children admitted a fear of dying. All of the children felt inadequate in pursuing physical activities. They were unable to talk spontaneously about their own body, but they openly responded to questions about weakness, ugliness, and lazy behaviors. The psychological status of both mothers and children improved after training. The mothers lost their fear of sudden death and stopped restricting their child's physical activities. They developed a better understanding of their child's strengths and limits and became less focused on the ''heart problem'' and more focused on the potential for physical normalcy. The children felt adequate and in control of their bodies during exercise. They developed a better self-image with improved school performance and were better able to communicate their concerns and fears.

Discussion

Averaging the data from multiple studies utilizing different protocols, while increasing numbers, has the potential for minimizing any true change. The results of effective protocols and training sessions with compliant patients are diluted by the lack of results from protocols in which the training program was of insufficient length, frequency, or intensity or in which the patients were non-compliant with the program. Thus, it is extremely encouraging that, at least for some children, these studies indicate that training can increase psychological well-being, work performance, oxygen consumption, and cardiac index while decreasing blood pressure, cholesterol, and triglyceride levels.

The studies, however, leave many questions unanswered. Future research is essential to utilize training to its fullest. The physiologic and psychologic responses to training need to be better understood. Almost nothing is known about the peripheral adaptations to training. How does training affect mitochondrial concentrations or glycogen storage? How does it affect the distribution of blood flow during exercise? What happens to hydromineral balance? Central adaptations also need further investigation. Almost nothing is known about the pulmonary adaptations to training. While a little more is known about the cardiac adaptations, these studies are only the beginning. Interesting questions concerning cardiac adaptations ask: what changes occur in cardiac chamber dimensions and geometric configuration, what changes occur in wall stress and cardiac work, what changes occur in heart rate and stroke volume, and what is the true cause of an increase in stroke volume. Finally, even the overall effects of training need to be clarified. What percentage of the change in work capacity is secondary to improved aerobic performance, and what percentage is secondary to greater anaerobic performance? For the improvement in aerobic performance, what percentage is due to an increased aerobic capability, and what percentage is due to an increased efficiency at the same aerobic level? Finally, what percentage of these changes are secondary to central adaptations, and what percentage is secondary to peripheral adaptations?

Protocols are another essential area of investigation. What are the optimal duration, frequency, and intensity of a training program? Is this the same for all individuals or diagnoses, or must different schemes be worked out for different individuals? How does one best monitor intensity to assure that the training is effective? Should the training be home based, school based or hospital based?

Selection of individuals is another major question. As some of the studies of normal individuals demonstrated, it is not effective to attempt to train someone who is already well-trained. Yet some of the normal individuals had diminished performance prior to training and improved following training. Lack of a medical diagnosis, therefore, does not necessarily mean that the individual will not benefit from training. Minor cardiac lesions are generally thought not to affect physical activity and, thus, patients with these lesions are generally not placed in training programs. Longmuir's 5-year follow-up data, however, suggest that this is not correct. Finally, how does one convince children or their parents that they really need and would benefit from a training program, and how does one keep their compliance once enrolled? Many of the studies reviewed here had problems with patient recruitment or compliance. Even in cases of gross abnormalities, parents believe that their child is normal and thus see no need for training. Thus, they either refuse to enroll their child in a training program or stop attending the sessions before completion of the program.

It is hoped that the apparent benefits of training in some children will motivate researchers to undertake further studies to address these questions.

Conclusion

Discrepant protocols and limited patient numbers make definitive conclusions impossible. I believe, however, that the data I have reviewed suggest the following. Normal children show an improvement in exercise efficiency with an increase in work performance with only minor changes in peak oxygen consumption, heart rate, blood pressure, or estimated body fat following a training program. Children with cardiac abnormalities, on the other hand, demonstrate an improvement in both work performance and peak oxygen consumption. Their peak heart rate increases and their blood pressure decreases. They also appear to benefit significantly psychologically following the training program. Hypertensive children demonstrate an improvement in oxygen consumption with a decrease in blood pressure. Children with diabetes mellitus demonstrate an improvement in exercise efficiency with an increase in work performance and only minor changes in peak oxygen consumption. They develop an improved caloric-insulin relationship. Inadequate data are available to even begin to assess the effects of training on children with cystic fibrosis or Down's syndrome. Finally, large, well-planned, multi-institutional studies will probably be necessary before sufficient data is collected to fully understand all the effects of pediatric training programs.

References

1. Balfour, I.C., A.M. Drimmer, S. Nouri, D.G. Pennington, C.L. Hemkens, and L.L. Harvey. Pediatric cardiac rehabilitation. Am. J. Dis. Child 145:627-630; 1992.
2. Bradley, L.M., F.M. Galioto, P. Vaccaro, D.A. Hansen, and J. Vaccaro. Effect of intense aerobic training on exercise performance in children after surgical repair of tetralogy of Fallot or complete transposition of the great arteries. Am. J. Cardiol. 56:816-818; 1985.
3. Calzolari, A., A. Turchetta, G. Biondi, F. Drago, C. De Ranieri, G. Gagliardi, I. Giambini, S. Giannico, A.M. Kofler, F. Perrotta, et al. Rehabilitation of children after total correction of tetralogy of Fallot. Int. J. Cardiol. 28:151-158; 1990.
4. Dahl-Jorgensen, K., H.D. Meen, K.F. Hanssen, and O. Aagenaes. The effect of exercise on diabetic control and hemoglobin A1 (HbA1) in children. Acta Paediatr. Scand. Suppl. 283:53-56; 1980.
5. Danforth, J.S., K.D. Allen, J.M. Fitterling, J.A. Danforth, D. Farrar, M. Brown, and R.S. Drabman. Exercise as a treatment for hypertension in low-socioeconomic-status black children. J. Consult. Clin. Psychol. 58:237-239; 1990.
6. Donovan, E.F., R.A. Mathews, P.A. Nixon, R.J. Stephenson, R.J. Robertson, F. Dean, F.J. Fricker, L.B. Beerman, and D.R. Fischer. An exercise program for pediatric patients with congenital heart disease: psychosocial aspects. J. Cardiac. Rehabil. 3:476-480; 1983.
7. Ekblom, B. Effect of physical training in adolescent boys. J. Appl. Physiol. 27:350-355; 1969.
8. Eriksson, B.O. and G. Koch. Effect of physical training on hemodynamic response during submaximal and maximal exercise in 11-13-year old boys. Acta Physiol. Scand. 89:27-39; 1972.
9. Gilliam, T.B. and P.S. Freedson. Effects of a 12-week school physical fitness program on peak VO_2, body composition and blood lipids in 7 to 9 year old children. Int. J. Sports Medicine 1:73-78; 1980.
10. Goldberg, B., R.R. Fripp, G. Lister, J. Loke, J.A. Nicholas, and N.S. Talner. Effect of physical training on exercise performance of children following surgical repair of congenital heart disease. Pediatrics 68:691-699; 1981.
11. Hagberg, J.M., D. Goldring, A.A. Ehsani, G.W. Heath, A. Hernandez, K. Schechtman, and J.O. Holloszy. Effect of exercise training on the blood pressure and hemodynamic features of hypertensive adolescents. Am. J. Cardiol. 52:763-768; 1983.
12. Hagberg, J.M., D. Goldring, G.W. Heath, A.A. Ehsani, A. Hernandez, and J.O. Holloszy. Effect of exercise training on plasma catecholamines and haemodynamics of adolescent hypertensives during rest, submaximal exercise and orthostatic stress. Clin. Physiol. 4:117-124; 1984.

13. Hansen, H.S., K. Froberg, N. Hyldebrandt, and J.R. Nielsen. A controlled study of eight months of physical training and reduction of blood pressure in children: the Odense schoolchild study. BMJ. 303:682-685; 1991.

14. Larsson, Y.A.A., B. Persson, G.C.G. Sterky, and C. Thoren. Functional adaptation to rigorous training and exercise in diabetic and nondiabetic adolescents. J. Appl. Physiol. 19:629-635; 1964.

15. Larsson, Y.A.A., G.C.G. Sterky, K.E.K. Ekengren, and T.G.H.O. Möller. Physical fitness and the influence of training in diabetic adolescent girls. Diabetes 11:109-117; 1962.

16. Longmuir, P.E., M.S. Tremblay, and R.C. Goode. Postoperative exercise training develops normal levels of physical activity in a group of children following cardiac surgery. Pediatr. Cardiol. 11:126-130; 1990.

17. Longmuir, P.E., J.A.P. Turner, R.D. Rowe, and P.M. Olley. Postoperative exercise rehabilitation benefits children with congenital heart disease. Clinical and Investigative Medicine 8:232-238; 1985.

18. Mahon, A.D. and P. Vaccaro. Ventilatory threshold and $\dot{V}O_2$max changes in children following endurance training. Med. Sci. Sports Exerc. 21:425-431; 1989.

19. Mathews, R.A., P.A. Nixon, R.J. Stephenson, R.J. Robertson, E.F. Donovan, F. Dean, F.J. Fricker, L.B. Beerman, and D.R. Fischer. An exercise program for pediatric patients with congenital heart disease: organizational and physiologic aspects. J. Cardiac. Rehabil. 3:467-475; 1983.

20. Millar, A.L., B. Fernhall, and L.N. Burkett. Effects of aerobic training in adolescents with Down syndrome. Med. Sci. Sports Exerc. 25:270-274; 1993.

21. Orenstein, D.M., B.A. Franklin, C.F. Doershuk, H.K. Hellerstein, K.J. Germann, J.G. Horowitz, and R.C. Stern. Exercise conditioning and cardiopulmonary fitness in cystic fibrosis. The effects of a three-month supervised running program. Chest 80:392-398; 1981.

22. Ruttenberg, H.D., T.D. Adams, G.S. Orsmond, R.K. Conlee, and A.G. Fisher. Effects of exercise training on aerobic fitness in children after open heart surgery. Pediatr. Cardiol. 4:19-24; 1983.

23. Sharkey, A.M., A.B. Carey, C.T. Heise, and G. Barber. Cardiac rehabilitation after cancer therapy in children and young adults. Am. J. Cardiol. 71:1488-1490; 1993.

24. Stewart, K.J. and B. Gutin. Effects of physical training on cardiorespiratory fitness in children. Res. Q. 47:110-120; 1976.

25. Tomassoni, T.L., F.M. Galioto, P. Vaccaro, and J. Vaccaro. Effect of exercise training on exercise tolerance and cardiac output in children after repair of congenital heart disease. Sports Training, Med. and Rehab. 2:57-62; 1990.

26. Vaccaro, P., F.M. Galioto, L.M. Bradley, and J. Vaccaro. Effect of physical training on exercise tolerance of children following surgical repair of D-transposition of the great arteries. J. Sports Med. Phys. Fitness 27:443-448; 1987.

27. Weber, G., W. Kartodihardjo, and V. Klissouras. Growth and physical training with reference to heredity. J. Appl. Physiol. 40:211-215; 1976.

28. Yoshida, T., I. Ishiko, and I. Muraoka. Effects of endurance training on cardiorespiratory functions of 5-year-old children. Int. J. Sports Medicine 1:91-94; 1980.

Part IV

Nutrition and Exercise in Children and Adolescents

Chapter 10

Undernutrition, Physical Activity, and Performance of Children

G.B. Spurr, PhD, and Julio C. Reina, MD

Recent media focus on episodes of famine and interventions to bring help to starving people have reminded us of the delicate balance in many populations between food availability and demand. Many people in the developed countries have returned to their daily lives relieved to know that humanitarian efforts have been successful. Unfortunately, the ongoing problem of marginal or mild-to-moderate malnutrition in the developing world goes largely unrecognized in the popular mind. The most recent estimates of malnutrition in developing countries in children under 5 years of age were 34% in 1990, down from 42% in 1975 (42). However, the absolute numbers increased from 168 to 184 million in the same period. The incidence of malnutrition, based on the stunting of children as evidenced by height less than -2 SD of a reference population (U.S. National Center for Health Statistics) tends to increase with the age of children (16), so the figures given are only a fraction of those affected. The conclusion is inescapable that chronic undernutrition of a moderate nature is a widespread problem in tropical regions of the world, although not confined to them (16,42).

The present discussion will be concerned with the limitations placed on the growth and development of children by chronic malnutrition. The daily struggle to obtain food occurs under socioeconomic circumstances which, because of poor hygiene, are conducive to a high incidence of infection in both adults and children. In the context of physical activity and performance, the limitations are related to body size and function. The discussion will be restricted to daily activity and energy expenditure and to performance in the athletic events that have been commonly measured in children. Both activity and performance are based on the physical fitness of individuals as measured by the maximal oxygen consumption ($\dot{V}O_2max$), which is affected by nutritional status (29); consequently, some discussion of this basic physiological measurement will be presented.

Anthropometry

The most visible effect of chronic marginal malnutrition is on the growth of the individual (i.e., the body size of both children and adults of affected populations).

149

This has been assumed to be an adaptive mechanism in situations of chronic shortage of nutrients; smaller bodies require less and so survive better. Yet, Martorell (20) makes a convincing case for an improved survival of bigger (taller) children and adults and a better reproductive performance of taller women. He has also demonstrated that the cause(s) of small stature is more likely to be environmental (nutrition, infectious diseases) than genetic in nature (20).

Studies of Colombian children 6 to 16 years of age have shown that both upper and lower socioeconomic children who are classified as nutritionally normal follow growth curves that are close to the 50th percentile of U.S. NCHS data until older ages when they tend to deviate toward the 25th percentile (30,33,36). Marginally malnourished children are common in lower socioeconomic groups and follow growth for weight and height that are near or below the 5th percentile of NCHS data (30,33,36). These children also show deficits of lean body mass (LBM) and body fat as well as other indicators of body composition (e.g., mid-arm circumference) (36). Other indicators are delayed sexual maturation (30,33,36) and growth spurt (30), and in small subgroups of boys, undernourished subjects had significantly higher fasting levels of circulating growth hormones (Spurr and Reina, unpublished). All of these are features of an ongoing process of undernutrition.

The picture one sees from these data is of children who, at any age, have smaller bodies and less skeletal muscle mass, because it is one of the largest components of the LBM. The question then arises about the functional consequences of smaller size in these children.

Maximal Oxygen Consumption

The maximal oxygen consumption ($\dot{V}O_2$max) is the best measure currently available of the overall physical fitness and capacity for work of human subjects. A number of factors contribute to the $\dot{V}O_2$max of an individual, among them natural endowment (genes), physical condition (training), sex, and age. Barac-Nieto et al. (3,4) demonstrated the effect of nutritional status and of dietary repletion on the body composition and $\dot{V}O_2$max of adult males living in Colombia. They showed that the major contributor to the decreased $\dot{V}O_2$max of severely malnourished men was the reduced muscle mass resulting from the nutritional deprivation (29).

In subsequent studies (5,31,36), we described the effect of chronic, marginal malnutrition on the growth of $\dot{V}O_2$max in school-aged Colombian children. Marginally undernourished children have significantly reduced $\dot{V}O_2$max (L/min) when compared to their nutritionally normal counterparts (31,36). The relationship between $\dot{V}O_2$max and body weight and LBM in both boys and girls is seen in Figure 10.1 in which age group means of $\dot{V}O_2$max (L/min) are plotted on means of body weight and LBM. The relationship is a linear one in both cases, with the girls having a significantly smaller slope in each indicating poorer physical condition (36) not related to the differences in body composition (Figure 10.1, left panel).

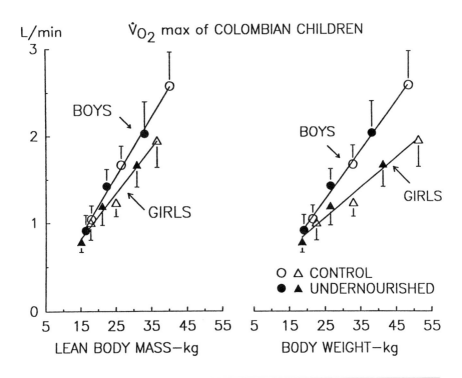

Figure 10.1. $\dot{V}O_2$max of 6-8, 10-12, 14-16-year old control and marginally undernourished children as a function of lean body mass and body weight.

When the $\dot{V}O_2$max is expressed in terms of body weight (ml/kg/min), the values of Colombian children are somewhat lower than the values of Swedish children (2) and more in line with those reported for Dutch (25) and British children (1), all of whom were measured with a treadmill protocol. The statistical difference between nutritional groups disappears when $\dot{V}O_2$max is divided by body weight or LBM as suggested in Figure 10.1. It should be emphasized, however, that the undernourished Colombian children have lower absolute values of $\dot{V}O_2$max (L/min) than their nutritionally normal counterparts, and this will have negative implications for their ability to endure heavy physical work when they are adults because the ability to perform work is related to the total $\dot{V}O_2$max (29).

The INCAP Longitudinal Study (14) recently made important contributions to our knowledge of the effects of early dietary intervention on subsequent functional abilities of Guatemalan children and young adults. Haas et al. (13) found that intervention in early life (prenatal to 3 y and 3-7 y) with a high-protein energy drink (6.4 g protein and 91 kcal/100 ml) resulted in higher $\dot{V}O_2$max values in male subjects when they were older (11-26 y) than in those subjects who had received only a low-calorie drink (0 g protein and 33 kcal/100 ml) early in life. Consequently, early interventions, if only for a restricted period, can have long-term effects on functional competence.

Physical Activity and Energy Expenditure

The methodology of measuring energy expenditure has been reviewed (37) and will not be repeated here. In free-living subjects, the doubly-labeled water (DLW) method is the most accurate although the minute-by-minute heart rate method is useful in estimating energy expenditure of groups (37) and has the additional advantage of providing data on the pattern of expenditure (37).

Preschool Children

A number of observers have reported that undernutrition reduces the activity levels of very young children in a period of their lives before they are strongly influenced by the peer pressure of their playmates. These include studies on Ugandan (23), Mexican (7), Guatemalan (43), and Jamaican children (11), although in the latter the difference from non-stunted children, while statistically significant, was small (3.4%), suggesting that the reduced activity would be unlikely to provide a large conservation of energy (11). A further cautionary note about undernutrition and physical activity of preschool children has been made by Lawrence et al. (17). They used an activity diary technique to demonstrate major differences between the activity patterns of Gambian and U.K. children. The former were much less active than the latter. However, when they compared only Gambian children above and below 80% of weight-for-age, the differences were much smaller and not statistically significant. This suggests that sociocultural differences or the absence of toys may explain the lower activity of Gambian compared to U.K. children (17). This may also be a partial explanation of the earlier results obtained by Rutishauser and Whitehead (23) in Ugandan children.

A classic study by Torún and Viteri (41) on five Guatemalan boys 30 months of age showed that when dietary energy intake was reduced from 90 to 82 kcal/kg/day, there was no significant change in growth rate (g/day), but daily energy expenditure was significantly decreased. When intake was further reduced to 71 kcal/kg/day, daily energy expenditure was not significantly altered, but growth rate was decreased significantly. These results indicate that the first line of defense against lowered energy intake in very young and growing children is concomitant reduction in energy expenditure, and only beyond some critical level of decreased intake is the growth of the child affected (41).

School-Aged Children

The BMR is a significant part of the total daily energy expenditure. Consequently, measurement of BMR in marginally undernourished children is of interest. We have reported on the BMR of Colombian children 2 to 16 years of age (38). The LBM explained more than 65% of the variation in BMR so that the differences in LBM resulting from the effects of marginal malnutrition on growth of the child affect the BMR because of body size. Ethnicity of the child (black, mestizo, or white) did not contribute significantly to the variation of BMR (38).

Satyanarayana (26) studied the habitual physical activity of undernourished school-aged children by using a questionnaire but analyzed the data from the standpoint of their effect on the physical work capacity of the subjects. It is not possible to separate the influence of nutritional status on habitual physical activity in their studies, although there was a statistically significant direct relationship between the latter and body weight.

Other studies on this topic are from our own laboratory and were carried out on children 6 to 16 years of age (33,34,35). TDEE was estimated by the minute-by-minute heart rate method. The validation of the heart rate method by whole body indirect calorimetry and doubly-labeled water has been reviewed (37). The subjects in our studies were individually calibrated Colombian school children classified as nutritionally normal (control) or marginally undernourished. The details of the methodology have been presented (33).

The boys and girls were divided into three age groups, 6 to 8, 10 to 12, and 14 to 16 years of age, and into two nutritional groups, control and marginally undernourished. The TDEE and energy expended in activity (EAC) are shown in Figure 10.2 together with the results of a two- and three-way ANOVA. There are statistically significant increases with age and lower values in girls than

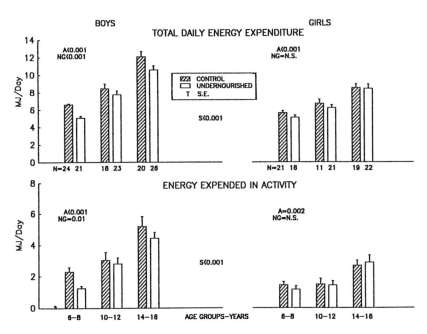

Figure 10.2.   Total daily energy expenditure and energy expended in activity (above maintenance energy requirements) of 6-8, 10-12, and 14-16-year-old control and marginally undernourished children with results of 2- and 3-way ANOVA.
With permission from Spurr (37).

boys (33). The differences between the two nutritional groups are statistically significant in the boys but are not different in the girls. We have suggested (33) that the lower values in girls are the result of cultural constraints on the activity of young girls. The results shown in Figure 10.2 are precisely what would be expected if this were the case (i.e., reduced activity to some level acceptable to the community). This would tend to reduce any differences which might exist due to nutritional status.

Because a mild stress (marginal malnutrition) might not be sufficient to produce differences in activity from non-stressed controls, we took advantage of the well-known physiological principle of superimposed stresses in an attempt to reveal an underlying effect of the marginal malnutrition on the activity pattern (34). The activity patterns of two groups of 10- to 12-year-old boys classified as control (n=14) or marginally malnourished (n=19) were studied during regular school days during 5 hours of school and 5 hours of free time (Figure 10.3). The boys were then invited to join a summer day camp, which was instituted for 8 weeks, 5 days a week, during July and August 1985. Four groups of eight to

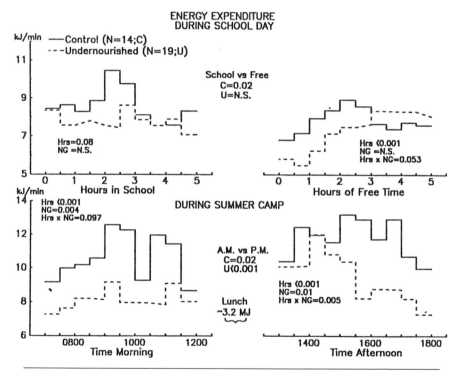

Figure 10.3. Average energy expenditure for 30 minute periods during a school day (upper) and in a summer day camp (lower) where an opportunity for increased activity was presented. Also shown is the effect of a hot lunch at mid-day on the energy expenditure in the afternoon of day camp. Where appropriate, the 2-way ANOVA is with repeated measures.
With permission from Spurr (37).

nine randomly assigned subjects were formed. Each group spent a 2-week period under the supervision of a university physical education student in various athletic activities designed to increase the level of energy expenditure. These consisted of soccer games, foot races, calisthenics, basketball, etc., which were conducted in a spirit of friendly competition, but without specific pressure being placed on any individual boy. The athletic director had no knowledge of the nutritional status of any of the subjects.

We also used the study to investigate the effect of a short-term dietary intervention on the results obtained. The subjects were picked up at 7 a.m. and taken to an athletic complex in Cali with extensive facilities for the activities described. At noon they were driven to a location where they were served a hot meal consisting of 760 kcal (3.2 MJ). At 1 p.m. they went back to their athletic activities and were returned home at 6 p.m. The data are summarized in Figure 10.3 with the results of two-way ANOVA with repeat measures in one or two directions, as appropriate. There were no significant nutritional group (NG) differences in school or free-time measurements, and there was a tendency toward lower values in free time than in school, which was statistically significant only in the control boys (P=0.02). The most striking features of the data in Figure 10.3 are found during the summer day camp measurements of EE. In the morning session, the undernourished boys were unable to keep up with their control counterparts. It has been our experience during the last 15 years in studies on Colombian children classified as nutritionally normal or undernourished that the latter generally receive only a minimal breakfast consisting usually of sweetened coffee with a little milk, while the former receive a more adequate meal. This is not documented in the present study, but our previous experience can be used as a partial explanation. Following the noon meal there was a beneficial effect on both groups of subjects. Their EE patterns were significantly higher than in the morning, and for about 2 hours the undernourished boys were able to keep up with the controls (Figure 10.3). However, following this period they were again unable to keep up and their EE values decreased to levels similar to those seen in the morning. There are no other studies with which to compare these results. The noon meal consisted of about 70% carbohydrate, and it has been found that ingestion of 100 g of glucose immediately before exercise results in a shift of work metabolism toward carbohydrate and away from free fatty acid metabolism (15). But one cannot rule out the possibility of a psychological effect from eating a well-cooked, hot meal, and what might be called the "full-tummy syndrome." In any event, the results make it clear that the undernourished boys are different in their response to superimposed exercise. Because differences in their EE on ordinary school days are due largely to differences in body size in comparison to controls (37), and because levels of activity contribute to motor (18) and cognitive and social development (24), it would seem that our marginally undernourished Colombian school children are at no real disadvantage in this regard. Whether their apparent inability to keep up in situations of increased activity above the usual has an effect on their development remains to be seen.

Strength and Motor Skill Performance

Earlier theories about the adaptive significance of small body size in chronic undernutrition supported the concept that it was advantageous (39) or that the reduced size was a costless adaptation and affected individuals were ''small but healthy'' (27). Although these views have mostly been rejected (21), they continue to surface (9).

A number of investigators have looked at performances in grip strength, running, jumping, and throwing in a spectrum of children from developing countries who showed noticeable growth deficits (6,12,19). The results are summarized in Table 10.1. For the most part, the moderately undernourished children exhibited poorer performances than the nutritionally better off children of their own culture (6,12) or when compared to children in the U.S. (19). The lack of difference in running and jumping of children in Papua, New Guinea, and of better throwing performance of boys there may be the result of cultural influences (19), although these seem not to have been studied to any extent.

Expression of these results in terms of body weight or height frequently show a proportional reduction or even an improved performance of the moderately undernourished children (12,19). However, such comparisons tend to obscure the fact that the deficit is an absolute one. If a small, undernourished boy runs a 33 meter race in 8 seconds, and his larger, nutritionally normal school mate runs it in 6 seconds, who will be chosen to represent the team at the next athletic event? The answer is obvious.

Summary

Marginal or mild-to-moderate undernutrition is largely the result of poverty,

Table 10.1   Strength and motor skills performance of undernourished (U) compared with better nourished (N) children[a]

Investigator	Country	Grip	Run	Jump	Throw
Ghesquiere & Eeckels (12)	Zaire[b]	(−)	(−)	(−)	(−)
Malina et al. (19)	Mexico[c]	(−)	(−)	(−)	(−)
Malina et al. (19)	Papau, New Guinea[c]	(−)	(0)	(0)	(+)♀
					(−)♂
Bénéfice (6)	Senegal[b]	(−)	(−)	(−)	(−)

[a](−) = U < N; + = U > N; 0 = No difference
[b]Compared with nutritionally better off national children.
[c]Compared with well-nourished Philadelphia, USA, school children.

resulting in smaller children and adults. The reduced $\dot{V}O_2$max (L/min) observed in children will one day be a detriment in the ability to produce during heavy physical work. There is also a negative effect of undernutrition in the performance of children in activities such as running, throwing, jumping, and in their grip strength. The reductions are proportional to the reduced body size so that expression in terms of body weight tend to hide the defects, which are absolute in nature. Daily activity levels are similar in nutritionally normal and undernourished children, although the latter are unable to keep up with the former in situations of artificially increased activity levels such as sustained participation in sports.

There is no "costless adaptation" to chronic undernutrition. The small size of affected populations is detrimental to survival and to the development of the full physical potential of affected individuals.

References

1. Armstrong, N.; Williams, J.; Balding, J.; Gentle, P.; Kirby, B. The peak oxygen uptake of British children with reference to age, sex and sexual maturity. Eur. J. Appl. Physiol. 62:369-375; 1991.
2. Åstrand, P.O. Experimental studies of physical working capacity in relation to age and sex. Copenhagen: Ejnar Munksgaard; 1952.
3. Barac-Nieto, M.; Spurr, G.B.; Maksud, M.G.; Lotero, H. Aerobic work capacity in chronically undernourished adult males. J. Appl. Physiol. 44:209-215; 1978.
4. Barac-Nieto, M.; Spurr, G.B.; Dahners, H.W.; Maksud, M.G. Aerobic work capacity and endurance during nutritional repletion of severely undernourished men. Am. J. Clin. Nutr. 33:2268-2275; 1980.
5. Barac-Nieto, M.; Spurr, G.B.; Reina, J.C. Marginal malnutrition in school-aged Colombian boys: body composition and maximal O_2 consumption. Am. J. Clin. Nutr. 39:830-839; 1984.
6. Bénéfice, E. Physical activity and anthropometric and functional characteristics of mildly malnourished Senegalese children. Ann. Trop. Paediat. 12:55-66; 1992.
7. Chávez, A.; Martínez, C.; Bourges, H. Nutrition and development in infants from poor rural areas. II. Nutritional level and physical activity. Nutr. Rep. Intl. 5:139-144; 1972.
8. Barac-Nieto, M.; Spurr, G.B.; Lotero, H.; Maksud, M.G.; Dahners, H.W. Body composition during nutritional repletion of severely undernourished men. Am. J. Clin. Nutr. 32:981-991; 1979.
9. Edmundson, W.D.; Sukhatme, P.V.; Edmundson, S.A. Diet, disease and development. New Delhi: Macmillan India; 1992.
10. FAO/WHO/UNU. Energy and protein requirements. Tech. Report 724. Geneva: WHO; 1985.
11. Gardner, J.M.; Grantham-McGregor, S.M.; Chang, S.M.; Powell, C.A. Dietary intake and observed activity of stunted and non-stunted children in Kingston, Jamaica. Part II: Observed activity. Eur. J. Clin. Nutr. 44(8):585-593; 1980.
12. Ghesquiere, J.; Eeckels, R. Health, physical development and fitness of primary school children in Kinshasa. In: Ilmarinen, J.; Välimäki, I., eds. Children and sport. Berlin: Springer-Verlag; 1984: 18-30.
13. Haas, J.D.; Martinez, E.I.; Murdoch, S.; Conlisk, E.; Rivera, J.; Martorell, R. Nutritional supplementation during pre-school years and physical work capacity in adolescents and young adult Guatemalans. J. Nutr. (In press, 1993).
14. Habicht, J.P.; Martorell, R. Objectives, research design and implementation of the INCAP longitudinal study. Food Nutr. Bull. (In Press, 1993).

15. Issekutz, B.; Birkhead, N.C.; Rodahl, K. Effect of diet on work metabolism. J. Nutr. 79:109-115; 1963.
16. Keller, W. The epidemiology of stunting. In: Waterlow, J.C., ed. Linear growth retardation in less developed countries. New York: Raven Press; 1988: 17-39.
17. Lawrence, M.; Lawrence, F.; Durnin, J.V.G.A.; Whitehead, R.G. A comparison of physical activity in Gambian and U.K. children aged 6-18 months. Eur. J. Clin. Nutr. 45:243-252; 1991.
18. Malina, R.M. Physical activity and motor development performance in populations at nutritional risk. In: Pollitt, E.; Amante, P., eds. Energy intake and activity. New York: Liss; 1984: 285-302.
19. Malina, R.M.; Little, B.B.; Schoup, R.F.; Buschang, P.H. Adaptive significance of small body size: strength and motor performance of school children in Mexico and Papua, New Guinea. Am. J. Phys. Anthropol. 73:489-499; 1987.
20. Martorell, R. Child growth retardation: a discussion of its causes and its relationship to health. In: Blaxter, K.; Waterlow, J.C., eds. Nutritional adaptation in man. London: Libbey, 1985: 13-30.
21. Martorell, R. Body size, adaptation and function. Hum. Organ. 48:15-20; 1989.
22. Rueda-Williamson, R.; Luna-Jaspe, H.; Ariza, J.; Pardo, F.; Mora, J.O. Estudio seccional de crecimiento, desarrollo y nutrición en 12,139 niños de Bogotá, Colombia. Pediatría 10:337-349; 1969.
23. Rutishauser, I.H.E.; Whitehead, R.G. Energy intake and expenditure in 1-3-year-old Ugandan children living in a rural environment. Br. J. Nutr. 28:145-152; 1972.
24. Sameroff, A.J.; McDonough, S.C. The role of motor activity in human cognitive and social development. In: Pollitt, E.; Amante, P., eds. Energy intake and activity. New York: Liss, 1984: 331-353.
25. Saris, W.H.M. Aerobic power and daily physical activity in children. The Netherlands: Meppel, Kripps Repro; 1982.
26. Satyanarayana, K.; Nadamuni Naidu, N.; Narasinga Rao, B.S. Nutritional deprivation in childhood and the body size, activity, and physical work capacity of young boys. Am. J. Clin. Nutr. 32:1769-1775; 1979.
27. Seckler, D. "Small but healthy": A basic hypothesis in the theory, measurement and policy of malnutrition. In: Sukhatme, P.V., ed. Newer concepts in nutrition and their implications for policy. Pune, India: Maharashtra Association for the Cultivation of Science Research Institute; 1982: 127-137.
28. Spurr, G.B.; Barac-Nieto, M.; Maksud, M.G. Childhood undernutrition: implications for adult work capacity and productivity. In: Folinsbee, L.J.; Wagner, J.A.; Borgia, J.F.; Drinkwater, B.L.; Gliner, J.A.; Bedi, J.F., eds. Environmental stress: individual human adaptations. New York: Academic Press; 1978: 165-181.
29. Spurr, G.B. Nutritional status and physical work capacity. Yrbk. Phys. Anthropol. 26:1-35; 1983.
30. Spurr, G.B.; Reina, J.C.; Barac-Nieto, M. Marginal malnutrition in school-aged Colombian boys: anthropometry and maturation. Am. J. Clin. Nutr. 37:119-132; 1983.
31. Spurr, G.B.; Reina, J.C.; Barac-Nieto, M. Marginal malnutrition in school-aged Colombian boys: functional consequences in maximum exercise. Am. J. Clin. Nutr. 37:834-847; 1983.
32. Spurr, G.B.; Prentice, A.M.; Murgatroyd, P.R.; Goldberg, G.R.; Reina, J.C.; Christman, N.T. Energy expenditure from minute-by-minute heart rate recording: comparison with indirect calorimetry. Am. J. Clin. Nutr. 48:552-559; 1988.
33. Spurr, G.B.; Reina, J.C. Patterns of daily energy expenditure in normal and marginally undernourished school-aged Colombian children. Eur. J. Clin. Nutr. 42:819-834; 1988.
34. Spurr, G.B.; Reina, J.C. Influence of dietary intervention on artificially increased activity in marginally undernourished Colombian boys. Eur. J. Clin. Nutr. 42:835-846; 1988.

35. Spurr, G.B.; Reina, J.C. Energy expenditure/basal metabolic rate ratios in normal and marginally undernourished Colombian children 6-16 years of age. Eur. J. Clin. Nutr. 43:515-527; 1989.

36. Spurr, G.B.; Reina, J.C. Maximum oxygen consumption in marginally malnourished Colombian boys and girls 6-16 years of age. Am. J. Hum. Biol. 1:11-19; 1989.

37. Spurr, G.B. Physical activity and energy expenditure in undernutrition. Prog. Food Nutr. Sci. 14:139-192; 1990.

38. Spurr, G.B.; Reina, J.C.; Hoffmann, R.G. Basal metabolic rate of Colombian children 2-16 years of age: ethnicity and nutritional status. Am. J. Clin. Nutr. 56:623-629; 1992.

39. Stini, W.A. Adaptive strategies of human populations under nutritional stress. In: Watts, E.S.; Johnston, F.E.; Lasker, G.W., eds. Biosocial interrelations in population adaptation. The Hague: Mouton; 1975: 19-41.

40. Torún, B. Short- and long-term effects of low or restricted energy intakes on the activity of infants and children. In: Schurch, B.; Scrimshaw, N.S., eds. Activity, energy expenditure and energy requirements of infants and children. Lausanne, Switzerland: Nestlé Foundation; 1990: 335-359.

41. Torún, B.; Viteri, F.E. Energy requirements of pre-school children and effects of varying energy intakes on protein metabolism. In: Torún, B.; Young, V.R.; Rands, W.M., eds. Protein-energy requirements of developing countries: evaluation of new data (Supplement 5). Tokyo: United Nations University World Hunger Program, Food and Nutrition Bulletin; 1981: 229-241.

42. United Nations—ACC/SCN. Highlights of the world nutrition situation. SCN News No. 8; 1992: 1-3.

43. Viteri, F.E.; Torún, B. Nutrition, physical activity and growth. In: Ritzen, M.; Aperia, A.; Hall, K.; Larsson, A.; Zetterberg, A.; Zetterström, R., eds. The biology of normal human growth. New York: Raven Press; 1981: 265-273.

Chapter 11

Disordered Eating
in the Young Athlete

Jack H. Wilmore, PhD

Introduction and Overview

Eating and weight disorders became a major focus in clinical medicine during
the 1980s and continue to be during the 1990s. Of the two primary eating
disorders, anorexia nervosa has been considered a clinical syndrome since the
late nineteenth century, at which time the term was coined and described (45).
Bulimia nervosa was not introduced as a distinct psychiatric illness until 1979
(32). The term bulimarexia was used initially to distinguish it from bulimia, a
term which describes only binge eating (5). The term bulimia nervosa is now
the accepted term to describe the binge-purge syndrome. Eating disorders are
found predominantly in late adolescent and early adult females. Males typically
represent less than 10% of all cases (1,2).

Why has there been such an increased focus on and concern for these two
eating disorders over the past 10 to 15 years? Rodin and Larson (38) have made
a strong case implicating sociocultural influences as major forces leading to what
appears to be an increasing prevalence in disordered eating. Physical attractiveness
and appearance are major concerns among late adolescents and young adults. With
an increasing emphasis on "thinness" or "leanness," females are hormonally at
a distinct disadvantage. At the onset of puberty, estrogen levels increase leading
to, among other alterations, an increased deposition of body fat. The adolescent
female is thus faced with a paradox, a hormonally induced increase in body fat
and a sociocultural-driven desire to be thin.

The potential for eating and weight disorders in certain sub-populations of
female athletes, and male athletes to a lesser extent, is slowly being acknowledged,
although recognition of this potential has occurred only during the past 15 years.
The athlete faces the same sociocultural factors impacting on the non-athlete,

This chapter is reproduced, in part, from: Wilmore, J.H. Eating and weight disorders in the female
athlete. Int. J. Sport Nutr. 1:104-117; 1991, with permission of the publisher.

but the athlete also must contend with the need to be thin to optimize performance. This demand to be thin can come from the appearance sports such as gymnastics, figure skating, and diving, where the athlete is scored on the basis of appearance during the performance; from the endurance sports where low body weight is equated with a more efficient performance, and thus a faster time for a given distance; or from weight-class sports, such as boxing, weight or power lifting, and wrestling, where goal weight must be met before competition is allowed. Jockeys also fall into this latter category.

The vulnerability of athletes for eating disorders is compounded by the psychological makeup of the elite athlete who is often perfectionistic, goal-oriented, and under the tight control of a strong parent or coach. It is also possible that individuals who are more prone to eating disorders are drawn to sports competition.

Eating Disorders: Definitions and Criteria

To better understand eating disorders and their etiology, it is necessary to provide a precise definition as to what constitutes an eating disorder. Many individuals, particularly athletes, have unusual eating patterns, so it is important to understand that a clinical eating disorder must meet established diagnostic criteria. These diagnostic criteria are published periodically in the American Psychiatric Association's Diagnostic and Statistical Manual (DSM) of Mental Disorders, the most recent being the third edition, revised (DSM-III-R), published in 1987 (1). According to the DSM-III-R, eating disorders are characterized by gross disturbances in eating behavior.

Anorexia nervosa is characterized by a refusal to maintain body weight over a minimal level considered normal for age and height; a distorted body image; an intense fear of fatness or gaining weight while, in fact, underweight; and amenorrhea (1). Table 11.1 lists the diagnostic criteria for anorexia nervosa. Anorectics "feel fat" even though they are underweight. The anorectic restricts eating to lose weight and is typically obsessed with exercise. Purging through self-induced vomiting and/or the use of laxatives and diuretics can also be a part of this syndrome, which may indicate the coexistence of bulimia nervosa.

Anorexia nervosa occurs predominantly in females (~95%). Its onset is usually during adolescence, but it can occur up to the early 30s (1). Mortality rates vary between 5% and 18% (1). There appears to be a familial pattern to the disorder, and its onset is often associated with a stressful life situation. Perfectionistic or "model children" and those who are slightly overweight are considered high risk populations.

The DSM-III-R diagnostic criteria for bulimia nervosa are presented in Table 11.1. Bulimics are characterized by recurrent episodes of rapid consumption of a large amount of food in a discrete period of time (binge eating); a feeling of lack of control over eating during these feeding binges; purging behavior including self-induced vomiting and/or the use of laxatives or diuretics; strict dieting or fasting, or vigorous exercise to prevent weight gain; and persistent overconcern with body shape and weight (1). The eating binge typically includes high caloric density foods (sweets), usually eaten inconspicuously or secretly. By using vomiting to relieve

Table 11.1   Diagnostic criteria for anorexia nervosa and bulimia nervosa (DSM-III-R)

Anorexia nervosa:

1. Refusal to maintain body weight over a minimal normal weight for age and height, e.g., weight loss leading to maintenance of body weight 15% below that expected: or failure to make expected weight gain during period of growth, leading to body weight 15% below that expected.
2. Intense fear of gaining weight or becoming fat, even though underweight.
3. Disturbance in the way in which one's body weight, size, or shape is experienced, e.g., the person claims to "feel fat" even when emaciated, believes that one area of the body is "too fat" even when obviously underweight.
4. In females, absence of at least three consecutive menstrual cycles when otherwise expected to occur (primary or secondary amenorrhea). (A woman is considered to have amenorrhea if her periods occur only following hormone, e.g., estrogen, administration.)

Bulimia nervosa:

1. Recurrent episodes of binge eating (rapid consumption of a large amount of food in a discrete period of time).
2. A feeling of lack of control over eating behavior during the eating binges.
3. The person regularly engages in either self-induced vomiting, use of laxatives or diuretics, strict dieting or fasting, or vigorous exercise in order to prevent weight gain.
4. A minimum average of two binge eating episodes a week for at least three months.
5. Persistent overconcern with body shape and weight.

Note. From American Psychiatric Association. *Diagnostic and Statistical Manual of Mental Disorders, Third Edition–Revised* (DSM-III-R). Washington, D.C., 1987, pp. 65-69.

abdominal discomfort, the individual can continue the binge. As with anorexia nervosa, bulimia nervosa begins in adolescence or in early adulthood (mean age of onset: 18 years) and is predominant in females (>90%) (1,32). Parents of bulimics are frequently obese, and bulimics have often been obese during adolescence.

Vomiting can become a pleasurable and addictive behavior. Bulimics have referred to their vomiting episodes as "a rush" or "a real high." Vomiting episodes can occur as frequently as 20 or more times a day, and it is not unusual for bulimics to have excessive disruption of tooth enamel from the acid in the vomitus, requiring extensive dental repair (35). Bulimia seldom results in death; however, severe electrolyte disturbances from purging behaviors, particularly hypokalemia, can lead to lethal cardiac arrhythmia (35).

Prevalence of Eating Disorders

Obtaining information on the prevalence of eating disorders has become of major concern in order to document what some have considered to be a major epidemic during the past 5 to 10 years. Prevalence data are generally lacking, but what data are available for the United States as a whole and for female and male athletic populations will be presented.

Prevalence in the United States Population

In the general U.S. population, the prevalence of anorexia nervosa is estimated to be from as low as 1 in 800 to as high as 1 in 100 females between 12 and 18 years of age (1). For bulimia nervosa, early studies of college students estimated the prevalence at between 8 and 19% of college women and up to 5% of college men (12). More recent studies have provided estimates that are substantially lower. Schotte and Stunkard (42), in their study of University of Pennsylvania undergraduate and graduate students, estimated a rate of only 1.3% for women and 0.1% for men using the strict DSM-III-R diagnostic criteria for bulimia nervosa.

Drewnowski et al. (12), using a telephone survey of a national probability sample of 1,007 college students, reported prevalence rates of 1.0% for women and 0.2% for men. Kurtzman et al. (30) assessed the prevalence of eating disorders among 716 females from selected student populations at a major west coast university. Overall prevalence across the total sample was 2.1% at the time of the survey, and 4.8% at any time during the student's life. The difference between these three recent studies with relatively low prevalence rates and the earlier studies with relatively high prevalence rates is more than likely due to the lack of application of the strict DSM-III-R criteria for determination of anorexia nervosa or bulimia nervosa. It is important to note that a number of individuals have bulimic-type behavior, but they do not meet the stringent criteria of a minimum average of two binge episodes a week for at least three months. They do have disordered eating.

Female Athletes

Prevalence figures in athletic populations are limited. First, very few studies have addressed the issue of eating disorder prevalence in athletes. Second, of those studies that have attempted to get at this issue, most have had very small and restricted sample sizes. Finally, most of these studies have failed to use the strict DSM-III-R criteria. This final point is an important one, for there may be many athletes who have disordered eating but do not meet the standard criteria for bulimia nervosa. Sundgot-Borgen (46) has defined a new category of disordered eating in athletes which includes athletes who do not meet the DSM-III-R criteria. She terms this category "anorexia athletica."

Most of the studies on athletes have used surveys or inventories to establish prevalence data in various athletic populations. The two measures used most frequently are the Eating Attitudes Test (EAT) established by Garner and Garfinkel (22), and the Eating Disorders Inventory (EDI) by Garner et al. (24). The most recent version of EAT contains 26 items, and the person taking the test responds to a series of statements (e.g., "I am terrified about being overweight,"

"I vomit after I have eaten," and "I give too much time and thought to food").
Each item is rated on a six point scale with descriptors ranging from "always"
to "never." The EDI is a 64-item questionnaire with eight subscales addressing
the following areas: drive for thinness, bulimia, body dissatisfaction, ineffec-
tiveness, perfectionism, interpersonal distrust, interceptive awareness, and maturity fears.

A summary of these studies conducted on female athletes to date are presented
in Table 11.2. These studies have been grouped by sport where possible. It is
impressive to note the very high prevalence of suspected or confirmed eating
disorders in these athletic populations. Even with the limitations noted earlier in
this section, it seems obvious that certain segments of the athletic population are at
high risk for disordered eating. The actual prevalence may be, in fact, considerably
higher than that which has been noted in Table 11.2. This is illustrated by two
examples from data collected in our laboratory.

In the first study (Wilmore, Brownell, and Rodin, unpublished, 1987), a large
questionnaire on training history, menstrual history, and eating disorders, which
contained the EAT, was administered to a group of 110 elite women athletes
representing seven different sports. The questionnaires were administered by a
physician and graduate student, and total anonymity was assured. Completed
questionnaires were returned by 87 of the athletes (79.1% return). Not a single
athlete scored in the disordered eating range of the EAT, and there were few
indications of serious disorders in other parts of the questionnaire. During the
subsequent 2-year period, 18 of these athletes received either inpatient or outpatient treatment for eating disorders. The results of the survey indicated that eating
disorders were not a serious problem in this group of athletes, yet 16.4% met
the DSM-III-R criteria for clinically disordered eating.

In a second study (52), 14 nationally ranked women distance runners were
administered the EDI. Of the total, 9 runners were amenorrheic and 5 were
eumenorrheic. The EDI identified 3 of these athletes as having "possible"
problems, but not clear eating disorders. Of the 9 amenorrheic runners, 7 were
subsequently diagnosed as having an eating disorder that required either or both
inpatient and outpatient treatment: 4 were subsequently diagnosed as having
anorexia nervosa, 2 as having bulimia nervosa, and 1 as having both. None of
the eumenorrheic group were subsequently diagnosed as having an eating disorder. Two of the three identified by the EDI as "possible" later received
treatment for an eating disorder.

These examples illustrate that at least for populations of female athletes, the
use of questionnaires, inventories, surveys, or self-reports may not be valid.
Considering the very nature of eating disorders, it is not surprising that a certain
subset of athletes with disordered eating would attempt to hide or mask their
problem. Furthermore, even though anonymity was assured, many of these athletes may have feared that their coaches would somehow discern individual
responses, even though the coaches were not allowed to look at the resulting
questionnaires. Sundgot-Borgen (46) has had much better success in the use of
questionnaires in elite Norwegian women athletes.

Table 11.2   A summary of studies surveying the prevalence of eating disorders in female athletes*

Study (first author)	Subjects	Measure of eating disorder	Outcome of the study
Dancers			
Brooks-Gunn (6)	55 female ballet dancers in regional and national companies	EAT, self-report	33.0% self-reported anorexia or bulimia.
Evers (19)	21 female university dancers	EAT	33.0% of the dancers and 13.8% of the controls scored in the range symptomatic for anorexia.
Frusztajer (20)	female ballet dancers, 10 with stress fractures, 10 without, and 10 controls	EAT, structured interview using DSM-III criteria for eating disorders	Trend (NS) for stress fractured dancers to have higher EAT scores; greater incidence of eating disorders in stress fracture group.
Garner (23)	35 female ballet students, ages 11-14, followed for 2-4 years	EDI	At follow-up, 16% of subjects had anorexia nervosa and 14% had bulimia nervosa or a ''partial syndrome.''
Hamilton (26)	55 white and 11 black female dancers in national and regional companies	EAT, self-report	15% of white dancers reported anorexia nervosa and 19% reported bulimia nervosa, while no blacks reported either.
Hamilton (27)	49 female ballet dancers, 19 from highly select and 13 from lower select American companies, and 17 Chinese highly select	EAT, self-report	11% of highly selected and 46% of less selected American dancers, and 24% of Chinese highly selected dancers experienced anorexia, bulimia, and purging behavior.

Figure skaters

Rucinski (41)	17 male and 23 female figure skaters	EAT	48% of the females and none of the males had EAT scores in the range of anorexia nervosa (>30).

Gymnasts

Rosen (39)	42 female college gymnasts, 17-22 years of age	Michigan State University Weight Control Survey	62% were using at least one pathogenic form of weight control (self-induced vomiting-25%; diet pills-24%; fasting-24%; diuretics-12%; laxatives-7%).

Runners

Brownell (7)	1,908 female and 2,634 male runners responding to a survey in *Runner's World* magazine	EAT questions on eating and diet concerns	38% of females and 23% of males indicated they ate excessively and out of control at least once a month, while 6% of females and 3% of males did this at least three times/week. 26% of females and 4% of males had purged at least once, and 4% of the females and 0.7% of the males purged at least three times/week.
Clark (10)	93 elite female runners, 75 eumenorrheic and 18 amenorrheic	Nutrition and Menstrual Patterns Questionnaire	13% reported a history of anorexia; 25% reported undesired binge eating; and 9% stated that they binged and purged. A total of 34% reported atypical eating behaviors.
Gadpaille (21)	13 amenorrheic and 19 eumenorrheic runners	Interview by a psychiatrist to establish DSM-III criteria	62% of the amenorrheic runners and none of the eumenorrheic runners reported eating disorders.

(continued)

Table 11.2 (continued)

Study (first author)	Subjects	Measure of eating disorder	Outcome of the study
Weight (50)	125 female distance runners, white and black (% distribution not indicated)	EAT, EDI	14% (18 runners) were symptomatic for anorexia nervosa, no mention was made of percentage symptomatic for bulimia.
Swimmers			
Dummer (16)	487 girls and 468 boys, 9-18 years of age	Michigan State University Weight Control Survey	15.4% of the girls and 3.6% of the boys used pathogenic weight-loss techniques. In a subgroup trying to lose weight, 12.7% of the girls and 2.7% of the boys used vomiting; 10.7% and 6.8% respectively used diet pills; 2.5% and 4.1% respectively used laxatives; and 1.5% and 2.8% respectively used diuretics.
Mixed sports			
Benson (3)	12 female gymnasts on the Swiss National Team; 18 highly trained female swimmers; 34 non-athletic school girls	EDI	Preoccupation with weight: swimmers (11%), gymnasts (1%), controls (6%) (ns); body dissatisfaction: swimmers (38%), gymnasts (1%), controls (9%) (p<0.01); more swimmers scored high on 3 EDI subscales compared to the other two groups (p<0.05).

Black (4)	695 college athletes, 55% women from 8 sports and 45% men from 7 sports	Questionnaire developed using DSM-III-R criteria	21.4% of the males and 25.1% of the females were eating <600 kcal/day; 8.6% and 14.7% respectively used fasting; 7.3% and 13.4% respectively used fad diets; 3.5% and 7.3% respectively used self-induced vomiting; 2.9% and 4.5% respectively used laxatives; 1.9% and 4.2% respectively used diuretics; and 1.9% and 1.0% respectively used enemas.
Davis (11)	Females: 64 college athletes in "thin" build sports, 62 athletes in "normal" build sports, and 64 college student controls	EDI	Athletes in "thin" build sports had greater weight concerns, more body dissatisfactions and more dieting than "normal" build athletes and controls, even though body weights were lower. Overall EDI scores were not different between groups.
Gustafson (25)	224 college female athletes in 6 sports	EAT	18.5% of the female athletes surveyed exhibited behavior characteristics of an eating disorder.
Kurtzman (30)	126 athletes from unspecified sports	EDI, eating disorder attitudes and behaviors using DSM-III diagnostic criteria	Athletes had lower scores on all eating disorders' measures than other groups surveyed.
Mallick (31)	Junior and senior high school female students: 87 athletes from track, swimming, gymnastics, and ballet; 41 with eating disorders; and 120 controls	Self-reports of dieting, vomiting, or eating disorders	Frequent dieting, vomiting, and claimed anorexia nervosa were more common in athletes than in normal controls, but less common than in eating disordered subjects.
Pasman (34)	15 males and 15 females in each of 3 groups: obligatory runners, obligatory weight lifters, sedentary controls	3 subscales of EDI	Runners and weight lifters had greater eating disturbances than controls; females had greater pathology than males.

(continued)

Table 11.2 *(continued)*

Study (first author)	Subjects	Measure of eating disorder	Outcome of the study
Rosen (40)	182 female college athletes in 9 sports from two major midwestern universities	Questionnaire on dieting and weight control practices	32% practiced at least one pathogenic weight-control behavior, including self-induced vomiting-14%; laxatives-16%; diet pills-25%; and diuretics-5%.
Sundgot-Borgen (46)	522 elite Norwegian female athletes in various sports and 448 nonathletic controls	EDI, questionnaire, interview, and clinical examination	18% of athletes vs. 5% of controls had disordered eating; 34% of those in appearance, 32% of those in weight dependent, 20% of those in endurance sports.
Sundgot-Borgen (47)	Females: 35 athletes in sports stressing leanness, 32 in sports not stressing leanness, and 101 nonathletes	EDI	5.0% of athletes in sports stressing leanness and 3.0% nonathletes demonstrated a tendency toward eating disorders, and 6.0% and 3.0% respectively showed preoccupation with weight. Athletes in sports not stressing leanness had no problems.
Walberg (48)	103 female weight lifters and body builders (12 competitive, 89 noncompetitive, and 2 unknown) and 92 female controls	EDI	Weight lifters and body builders scored significantly higher on the Drive for Thinness subscale of the EDI; were more preoccupied with weight; were more terrified of becoming fat; were more obsessed with food; and had a higher use of laxatives. Of the competitive weight lifters, 42% used to be anorexic, 67% were terrified of becoming fat, and 50% experienced uncontrollable urges to eat.

*In those studies in which both males and females were studied, the results for both are reported.

Adapted from Brownell, K.D. and J. Rodin. Prevalence of eating disorders in athletes. In *Eating, Body Weight and Performance in Athletes: Disorders of Modern Society.* K.D. Brownell, J. Rodin, and J.H. Wilmore (Eds.), Philadelphia: Lea & Febiger, 1992.

To summarize this section, it is reasonable to assume that female athletes are at higher risk than the normal population for eating disorders, and prevalence data may be underestimating the actual risk. Furthermore, athletes in sports where additional body weight may hinder optimal performance and where athletic performance is judged, at least in part, by the appearance of the athlete, comprise a subset of the female athletic population that would be considered at high risk for disordered eating.

Male Athletes

Because males account for less than 5% of all diagnosed anorexia and less than 10% of all diagnosed bulimia (2), it would be predicted that male athletes would also represent a small percentage of eating disordered athletes. While the data for women are few and incomplete, even less data are available for male athletes. The few studies that have been published are summarized in Table 11.3. As suspected, while there are symptoms of pathogenic eating behaviors in some of these athletes, the percentages are low compared to female athletes. Wrestling appears to be the one sport for males that has the highest potential for disordered eating (44).

Related Disorders—The Triad

In the example at the conclusion of the section on the prevalence of eating disorders in female athletes (52), it was noted that of 14 elite women distance runners, 7 were later diagnosed with eating disorders. These 7 athletes represented 7 of the 9 athletes who were amenorrheic. Again, none of the eumenorrheic athletes had been treated for disordered eating. Gadpaille et al. (21), using the DSM-III criteria, conducted psychiatric interviews of 13 amenorrheic and 19 eumenorrheic distance runners. Within the amenorrheic group, 11 of the 13 reported major affective disorders in themselves or in first- and second-degree relatives, and 8 of the 13 reported eating disorders. No eating disorders or major affective disorders were noted in the eumenorrheic runners, and only one from this group had first-degree relatives with major affective disorders. They also reported that 12 of the 13 amenorrheic runners were vegetarians, compared with only 3 vegetarians among the 19 eumenorrheic runners.

Brooks-Gunn et al. (6) reported similar results in a group of 55 women ballet dancers from national and regional classical ballet companies. Using EAT and self-report of anorexia nervosa or bulimia nervosa, one third of the dancers reported having had an eating problem. Analysis of the eating disorders by menstrual status revealed that 50% of these dancers who were amenorrheic had self-reported eating disorders, compared to only 13% for the eumenorrheic and 13% for the oligomenorrheic groups. Rippon et al. (37) studied the relationship between elevated scores for the EAT and EDI and menstrual dysfunction in 88 predominantly lean female marathon runners, ballet dancers, and fashion models.

Table 11.3   A summary of studies surveying the prevalence of eating disorders in male athletes*

Study (first author)	Subjects	Measure of eating disorder	Outcome of the study
		Figure skaters	
Rucinski (41) see Table 11.2			
		Runners	
Brownell (7) See Table 11.2			
		Swimmers	
Dummer (16) See Table 11.2			

Wrestlers

Study	Sample	Method	Findings
Steen (43)	42 wrestlers from two college teams	Open-ended interview	In addition to using food deprivation (21%), sauna (51%), fluid restriction (58%), and rubber or plastic suits (42%), wrestlers on one team used laxatives (5%), diuretics (5%), and vomiting (11%) to lose weight.
Steen (44)	63 college and 368 high school wrestlers	Questionnaire was developed to assess weight control and nutrition practices	Fasting at least once/week: 44% of high school (HS) and 63% of college (C) wrestlers; vomiting at least once/week: 5% of HS and 2% of C; laxatives at least once/week: 5% of HS and 3% of C; diuretics at least once/week: 4% of HS and 3% of C.
Weissinger (51)	125 high school wrestlers	32-item wrestler survey (many items taken from Michigan State University Weight Control Survey)	Wrestlers had tried or regularly used the following: fasting (51%), exercise in rubber suit (34%), diet pills (14%), diuretics (10%), laxatives (8%), vomiting (15%).
Woods (53)	49 high school wrestlers compared with competitive squash players and noncompetitive joggers	Questionnaire to determine weight control techniques	The wrestlers used dieting (73%), bingeing (27%), vomiting (8%), sweating (64%), fluid restriction (17%), fasting (10%), and exercise (76%) as methods of weight control.

(continued)

Table 11.3 *(continued)*

Study (first author)	Subjects	Measure of eating disorder	Outcome of the study
		Mixed sports	
Black (4) See Table 11.2			
Enns (17)	26 male wrestlers, 21 male swimmers and cross country skiers	EAT, Restraint Questionnaire, Body Image Assessment	Higher EAT scores in wrestlers due to higher scores on weight fluctuation and dieting. No overall differences in estimates of body size.
King (29)	10 male jockeys	EAT	The majority reported food avoidance, saunas, and laxative abuse. Diuretics and appetite suppressants were used. Bingeing was common, but vomiting was unusual.
Pasman (34) See Table 11.2			

*In those studies in which both males and females were studied, the results for both are reported in table 11.2.

Adapted from Brownell, K.D. and J. Rodin. Prevalence of eating disorders in athletes. In *Eating, Body Weight and Performance in Athletes: Disorders of Modern Society.* K.D. Brownell, J. Rodin, and J.H. Wilmore (Eds.), Philadelphia: Lea & Febiger, 1992.

Menstrual dysfunction was equally common in all groups, as was the incidence of elevated EAT and EDI scores. Menstrual dysfunction was most closely associated with elevated EAT test scores.

Weight and Noakes (50), however, were not able to substantiate this link between disordered eating and menstrual status. Of 125 women runners, only 18 (14%) were reported to have anorexia nervosa on the basis of both the EDI and EAT measures. Of these 18 runners, only 5 also had a low body mass and a past history of amenorrhea. The issue of bulimia was not addressed in this study.

Brownell et al. (8) made an important observation in their review of the literature on athletic amenorrhea. In three separate studies, amenorrheic runners consumed substantially fewer total calories/day than equally trained eumenorrheic runners. These differences generally ranged from 300 to 500 kcal/day, and the differences were independent of either total or fat-free body weight. Additional studies have been published since the publication of this review. With the exception of the Wilmore et al. (52) study, the amenorrheic runners either eat less than eumenorrheic runners, or they under-report what they eat.

It is tempting to conclude that amenorrhea secondary to exercise training is linked to disordered eating and malnutrition. However, just as eating disorder surveys are suspect in a population with a high prevalence of eating disordered athletes, nutritional surveys must be equally suspect. The linkage is certainly sufficiently strong to suggest that this would be an important area for further study.

The third member of this triad is bone mineral disturbances. Cann et al. (9) and Drinkwater et al. (14) were the first to report the disturbing finding that athletes who are training and are amenorrheic have a reduction in bone density and bone mineral content. In the Drinkwater et al. (14) study, women amenorrheic runners with a chronological age of 24.9 years had an average bone mineral density equivalent to that of women 51.2 years of age. In a follow-up study, Drinkwater et al. (15) reported that bone mineral density increased with the resumption of menses. However, further follow-up of these women indicated that bone mineral density remained well below the average for their age group 4 years after resumption of normal menses (13).

Two related points need to be addressed. First, Prior et al. (36) measured the density of spinal bone on two occasions 1 year apart in ovulatory women runners with regular menstrual cycles. These women were training intensely and they were compared to women with regular cycles who were sedentary. Bone loss over 1 year was strongly associated with ovulatory disturbances (anovulatory cycles and cycles with short luteal phases), but was unrelated to level of physical activity. Thus, it appears that menstrual dysfunction, not intense endurance training, is the primary factor for the bone loss observed in amenorrheic athletes.

Second, athletes must be aware of the potential for fracture when they are amenorrheic. Warren et al. (49) reported a strong relationship between both the age at menarche and the presence of secondary amenorrhea with fractures, where 69% of observed fractures were stress fractures, mostly in the metatarsals. Myburgh et al. (33) have also reported an increased risk of stress fracture in athletes with low bone density. The presence of amenorrhea was identified as a major contributing factor.

Thus, there is increasing evidence that disordered eating, menstrual dysfunction, and bone mineral disorders form a triad of disorders. It is possible that disordered eating, including undereating or malnutrition, is the initiating factor or triggering mechanism. Certainly, additional study is essential to determine more clearly the interrelationships between these three variables.

Summary

In summary, athletes are at an increased risk for eating disorders, particularly female athletes in endurance sports or appearance sports. Disordered eating can lead to menstrual dysfunction and disorders of bone. It is important to do everything possible to prevent the onset of a serious eating disorder. Realistic weight limits must be established for athletes, and athletes must be encouraged to eat balanced diets, not limiting protein, fat, carbohydrate, micronutrients, and total calories to the point where normal physiologic function is compromised. Several studies have demonstrated physiologic and performance decrements with anorexia (18) and significant weight reduction (28). Because weight loss to enhance performance is a probable triggering mechanism for disordered eating in athletes, future research should be focused on the potential detrimental effects of disordered eating and extreme weight loss on physiologic function and performance.

References

1. American Psychiatric Association. Diagnostic and Statistical Manual of Mental Disorders, Third Edition - Revised (DSM-III-R). Washington, D.C.; 1987: 65-69.
2. Anderson, A. Eating disorders in males: a special case? In: Brownell, K.D.; Rodin, J.; Wilmore, J.H., eds. Eating, body weight and performance in athletes: disorders of modern society. Philadelphia: Lea & Febiger; 1992: 172-188.
3. Benson, J.E.; Allemann, Y.; Theintz, G.E.; Howald, H. Eating problems and calorie intake levels in Swiss adolescent athletes. Int. J. Sports Med. 11:249-252; 1990.
4. Black, D.R.; Burckes-Miller, M.E. Male and female college athletes: use of anorexia nervosa and bulimia nervosa weight loss methods. Res. Quart. Exerc. Sport. 59:252-256; 1988.
5. Boskind-White, M.; White, W.C. Bulimarexia: historical-sociocultural perspective. In: Brownell, K.D.; Foreyt, J.P., eds. Handbook of eating disorders: physiology, psychology, and treatment of obesity, anorexia, and bulimia. New York: Basic Books; 1986: 353-366.
6. Brooks-Gunn, J.; Warren, M.P.; Hamilton, L.H. The relation of eating problems and amenorrhea in ballet dancers. Med. Sci. Sports Exerc. 19:41-44; 1987.
7. Brownell, K.D.; Rodin, J.; Wilmore, J.H. Eat, drink, and be worried? Runner's World, August 28, 1988.
8. Brownell, K.D.; Steen, S.N.; Wilmore, J.H. Weight regulation practices in athletes: analysis of metabolic and health effects. Med. Sci. Sports Exerc. 19:546-556; 1987.
9. Cann, C.E.; Martin, M.C.; Genant, H.K.; Jaffe, R.B. Decreased spinal mineral content in amenorrheic women. JAMA 251:626-629; 1984.
10. Clark, N.; Nelson, M.; Evans, W. Nutrition education for elite female runners. Phys. Sportsmed. 16 (#2):124-136; 1988.

11. Davis, C.; Cowles, M. A comparison of weight and diet concerns and personality factors among female athletes and non-athletes. J. Psychosom. Res. 33:527-536; 1989.

12. Drewnowski, A.; Hopkins, S.A.; Kessler, R.C. The prevalence of bulimia nervosa in the US college student population. Am. J. Publ. Health. 78:1322-1325; 1988.

13. Drinkwater, B.L.; Bruemner, B.; Chesnut, C.H. III. Menstrual history as a determinant of current bone density in young athletes. JAMA 263:545-548; 1990.

14. Drinkwater, B.L.; Nilson, K.; Chestnut, C.H. III; Bremner, W.J.; Shainholtz, S.; Southworth, M.B. Bone mineral content of amenorrheic and eumenorrheic athletes. NEJM 311:277-281; 1984.

15. Drinkwater, B.L; Nilson, K.; Ott, S.; Chesnut, C.H. III. Bone mineral density after resumption of menses in amenorrheic athletes. JAMA 256:380-382; 1986.

16. Dummer, G.M.; Rosen, L.W.; Heusner, W.W.; Roberts P.J.; Counsilman, J.E. Pathogenic weight-control behaviors of young competitive swimmers. Phys. Sportsmed. 15(#5):75-86; 1987.

17. Enns, M.P.; Drewnowski, A.; Grinker, J.A. Body composition, body size estimation, and attitudes toward eating in male college athletes. Psychosomat. Med. 49:56-64; 1987.

18. Essén, B; Fohlin, L.; Thorén, C; Saltin, B. Skeletal muscle fibre types and sizes in anorexia nervosa patients. Clin. Physiol. 1:395-403; 1981.

19. Evers, C.L. Dietary intake and symptoms of anorexia nervosa in female university dancers. J. Am. Dietet. Assoc. 87:66-68; 1987.

20. Frusztajer, N.T.; Dhuper, S.; Warren, M.P.; Brooks-Gunn, J.; Fox, R.P. Nutrition and the incidence of stress fractures in ballet dancers. Am. J. Clin. Nutr. 51:779-783; 1990.

21. Gadpaille, W.J.; Sanborn, C.F.; Wagner, W.W. Athletic amenorrhea, major affective disorders, and eating disorders. Am. J. Psychiat. 144:939-942; 1987.

22. Garner, D.M.; Garfinkel, P.E. The Eating Attitudes Test: an index of the symptoms of anorexia. Psychol. Med. 9:273-279; 1979.

23. Garner, D.M.; Garfinkel, P.E.; Rockert, W.; Olmsted, M.P. A prospective study of eating disturbances in the ballet. Psychother. Psychosom. 48:170, 1987.

24. Garner, D.M.; Olmsted, M.P.; Polivy, J. The eating disorder inventory: a measure of cognitive-behavioral dimensions of anorexia nervosa and bulimia. In: Anorexia nervosa: recent developments in research. New York: Alan R. Liss, Inc.; 1983: 173-184.

25. Gustafson, D. Eating behaviors of women college athletes. Melpomene J. 8:11-12; 1989.

26. Hamilton, L.H.; Brooks-Gunn, J.; Warren, M.P. Sociocultural influences on eating disorders in professional female ballet dancers. Int. J. Eating Disord. 4:465-477; 1985.

27. Hamilton, L.H.; Brooks-Gunn, J.; Warren, M.P.; Hamilton, W.G. The role of selectivity in the pathogenesis of eating problems in ballet dancers. Med. Sci. Sports Exerc. 20:560-565; 1988.

28. Ingjer, F.; Sundgot-Borgen, J. Influence of body weight reduction on maximal oxygen uptake in female elite athletes. Scand. J. Med. Sci. Sports. 1:141-146; 1991.

29. King, M.B.; Mezey, G. Eating behaviour of male racing jockeys. Psycholog. Med. 17:249-253; 1987.

30. Kurtzman, F.D.; Yager, J.; Landsverk J.; Wiesmeier, E.; Bodurka, D.C. Eating disorders among selected female student populations at UCLA. J. Am. Dietet. Assoc. 89:45-53; 1989.

31. Mallick, M.J.; Whipple, T.W.; Huerta, E. Behavioral and psychological traits of weight-conscious teenagers: A comparison of eating-disordered patients and high- and low-risk groups. Adolescence 22:157-167, 1987.

32. Mitchell, J.E. Bulimia nervosa. Contemp. Nutr. 14:1-2; 1989.

33. Myburgh, K.H.; Hutchins, J.; Fataar, A.B.; Hough, S.F.; Noakes, T.D. Low bone density is an etiologic factor for stress fractures in athletes. Ann. Int. Med. 113:754-759; 1990.

34. Pasman, L.; Thompson, J.K. Body image and eating disturbance in obligatory runners, obligatory weightlifters, and sedentary individuals. Int. J. Eating Disord. 7:759-769; 1988.
35. Pomeroy, C.; J.E. Mitchell. Medical issues in the eating disorders. In: Brownell, K.D.; Rodin, J.; Wilmore, J.H.; eds. Eating, body weight and performance in athletes: disorders of modern society. Philadelphia: Lea & Febiger; 1992: 202-221.
36. Prior, J.C.; Vigna, Y.M.; Schechter, M.T.; Burgess, A.E. Spinal bone loss and ovulatory disturbances. NEJM 323:1221-1227; 1990.
37. Rippon, C.; Nash, J.; Myburgh, K.H.; Noakes, T.D. Abnormal eating attitude test scores predict menstrual dysfunction in lean females. Int. J. Eating Disord. 7:617-624; 1988.
38. Rodin, J.; Larson, L. Social factors and the ideal body shape. In: Brownell, K.D.; Rodin, J.; Wilmore, J.H.; eds. Eating, body weight and performance in athletes: disorders of modern society. Philadelphia: Lea & Febiger; 1992: 146-158.
39. Rosen, L.W.; Hough, D.O. Pathogenic weight-control behaviors of female college gymnasts. Phys. Sportsmed. 16 (#9):141-146; 1988.
40. Rosen, L.W.; McKeag, D.B.; Hough, D.O.; Curley, V. Pathogenic weight-control behavior in female athletes. Phys. Sportsmed. 14 (#1):79-86; 1986.
41. Rucinski, A. Relationship of body image and dietary intake of competitive ice skaters. J. Am. Dietet. Assoc. 89:98; 1989.
42. Schotte, D.E.; Stunkard, A.J. Bulimia versus bulimic behaviors on a college campus. JAMA 258:1213-1215; 1987.
43. Steen, S.N.; Brownell, K.D. Nutrition assessment of college wrestlers. Phys. Sportsmed. 14:100-116; 1986.
44. Steen, S.N.; Brownell, K.D. Patterns of weight loss and regain in wrestlers: has the tradition changed? Med. Sci. Sports Exerc. 22:762-768; 1990.
45. Strober, M. Anorexia nervosa: history and psychological concepts. In: Brownell, K.D.; Foreyt, J.P., eds. Handbook of eating disorders: physiology, psychology, and treatment of obesity, anorexia, and bulimia. New York: Basic Books; 1986: 232-246.
46. Sundgot-Borgen, J. Prevalence of eating disorders in elite female athletes. Int. J. Sport Nutr. 3:29-40; 1993.
47. Sundgot-Borgen, J.; Corbin, C.B. Eating disorders among female athletes. Phys. Sportsmed. 15 (#2):89-95; 1987.
48. Walberg, J.L.; Johnston, C.S. Menstrual function and eating behavior in female recreational weight lifters and competitive body builders. Med. Sci. Sports Exerc. 23:30-36; 1991.
49. Warren, M.P.; Brooks-Gunn, J.; Hamilton, L.H.; Warren, L.F.; Hamilton, W.G. Scoliosis and fractures in young ballet dancers; relation to delayed menarche and secondary amenorrhea. NEJM 314:1348-1353; 1986.
50. Weight, L.M.; Noakes, T.D. Is running an analog of anorexia?: a survey of the incidence of eating disorders in female distance runners. Med. Sci. Sports Exerc. 19:213-217; 1987.
51. Weissinger, E.; Housh, T.J.; Johnson, G.O.; Evans, S.A. Weight loss behavior in high school wrestling: wrestler and parent perceptions. Ped. Exerc. Sci. 3:64-73; 1991.
52. Wilmore, J.H.; Wambsgans, K.C.; Brenner, M.; Broeder, C.E.; Paijmans, I.; Volpe, J.A.; Wilmore, K.M. Is there energy conservation in amenorrheic compared with eumenorrheic distance runners? J. Appl. Physiol. 72:15-22; 1992.
53. Woods, E.R.; Wilson, C.D.; Masland, R.P. Weight control methods in high school wrestlers. J. Adolesc. Health Care 9:394-397; 1988.

Part V

International Perspectives: Activity, Growth, and Cardiovascular Disease

Chapter 12

Children's Cardiopulmonary Fitness and Physical Activity Patterns: The European Scene

Neil Armstrong, PhD

Are European Children and Adolescents Fit?

Cardiopulmonary fitness may be defined as the ability of the circulatory and pulmonary systems to supply fuel and to eliminate waste products during physical activity. With adults, it is widely recognized that the single best indicator of cardiopulmonary fitness is maximal oxygen uptake ($\dot{V}O_2$max), the highest rate at which an individual can consume oxygen during exercise. There is, however, a growing conviction that the appropriate term to use with children and adolescents is peak oxygen uptake (peak $\dot{V}O_2$), which represents the highest oxygen consumption elicited during an exercise test to exhaustion, rather than $\dot{V}O_2$max, which conventionally implies the existence of a $\dot{V}O_2$ plateau (8).

Data on European children and adolescents' peak $\dot{V}O_2$ have been accumulating since Åstrand's (9) classical study of Swedish children. No information, however, appears to be available on randomly selected groups of youngsters, and because volunteers are generally used as subjects, selection bias cannot be ruled out. Nevertheless, cross-sectional studies of peak $\dot{V}O_2$ have emerged from several countries including the Netherlands (25), Austria (20), France (18), the United Kingdom (8a), Czechoslovakia (36), Italy (14), Finland (39), Denmark (21), Norway (2), and Sweden (40). Longitudinal studies are rare, but data on Dutch (24), Norwegian (33), and German (33) children and Czechoslovakian boys (38) have been published.

Both cross-sectional and longitudinal studies have provided a consistent picture of a progressive rise in boys' peak $\dot{V}O_2$ from 8 to 16 years of age. With girls there is a similar but less consistent trend. From age 8 to 13 years, girls' peak $\dot{V}O_2$ appears to increase with chronological age, but several cross-sectional studies have indicated a leveling-off or even a fall in peak $\dot{V}O_2$ from 13 to 16 years of age. Rutenfranz and his associates (33), in their longitudinal studies of Norwegian girls (aged 10.3-15.2 years) and German girls (aged 12.7-15.7 years), found peak $\dot{V}O_2$ to reach its highest value at 13.3 years in Norway and at 14.7 years in Germany. Analysis of both cross-sectional and longitudinal data reveals that treadmill determined peak $\dot{V}O_2$ is about 12% higher in males than females at age 10 years (typically about 1.68 vs. 1.49 L/min), increasing to about 37% higher at 16 years of age (typically about 3.06 vs. 2.24 L/min) (8).

As most physical activity involves moving body mass from one place to another, to compare the peak $\dot{V}O_2$ of individuals who differ in body mass peak $\dot{V}O_2$ is conventionally expressed in relation to mass as mL/min · kg. When peak $\dot{V}O_2$ is expressed relative to body mass, a different picture emerges from that apparent when absolute values are used. European boys' mass-related peak $\dot{V}O_2$ appears to be fairly consistent over the age range 8 to 16 years (typically about 50 mL/min · kg), whereas girls' data demonstrate a decrease in mass-related peak $\dot{V}O_2$ with age (typically in the range 47-41 mL/min · kg). In this form of analysis girls are penalized for their greater accumulation of subcutaneous body fat during the circumpubertal years, and boys' values of mass-related peak $\dot{V}O_2$ are significantly higher than those of girls, at least from the age of 10 years.

Mass-related peak $\dot{V}O_2$ remains the most popular method of expressing children and adolescents' peak $\dot{V}O_2$ despite the fact that this type of analysis may cloud our understanding of true growth and maturational changes in peak $\dot{V}O_2$ (8). Bar-Or (10) has, however, suggested that for practical purposes there is no advantage to be gained by using other than body mass or height for growth-related comparisons. This convention will be followed for the purpose of this paper.

Bell and his associates (12) expressed the view that a lower limit of mass-related peak $\dot{V}O_2$ in the absence of other health-related problems may represent a health risk and proposed a "risk level" of 35 mL/min · kg for boys and 30 mL/min · kg for girls. These figures represent values approximately three standard deviations below the mean for European boys and two standard deviations below the mean for European girls. Kemper and Verschuur (27) analyzed data from 200 subjects who have remained in their 8-year longitudinal study of Dutch children and reported that the percentage of males at risk (<35 mL/min · kg) increased with age from 1 to 8%, and in females (<30 mL/min · kg) from 3 to 17%. The higher percentage of females was partly explained by the extra gain in body mass caused by the sex-specific increase in fat during puberty. A reworking using these criteria of Armstrong et al.'s (8a) data on 220 British children revealed that 3% of boys and 3% of girls aged 11 to 16 years could be classified as "at risk."

Bell et al. (12) also emphasized the importance of identifying "health indicators" and proposed a peak $\dot{V}O_2$ of >40 mL/min · kg for boys and >35 mL/min · kg for girls as falling into this category. Armstrong's data suggest that 90% of boys and 85% of girls can be classified as "healthy." However, the difficulties with this type of arbitrary cut-off criterion are readily apparent when one considers that others have used higher values of peak $\dot{V}O_2$ as indicative of a coronary risk factor (44).

The peak $\dot{V}O_2$ values of European children and adolescents compare favorably with the values of children from elsewhere (30). Comparison of recent data with earlier studies of similar groups of youngsters suggests that the peak $\dot{V}O_2$ of European children and adolescents has not deteriorated over the last 3 decades.

In fact, in studies using the conventional mass-related analysis, children and adolescents appear to be the fittest section of the population. This is not to say that efforts should not be made to enhance the cardiopulmonary fitness of European children and adolescents, but there is little evidence to suggest that European children and adolescents are unfit.

Are European Children and Adolescents Active?

The problems involved in monitoring children's habitual physical activity have been well-documented (35) and data must be interpreted with caution. Nevertheless, children's physical activity patterns have been studied in several European countries, largely through either self-report (questionnaires, interviews, diaries) or physiological monitoring (monitoring of heart rate and/or oxygen consumption).

Self-Report of European Children and Adolescents' Physical Activity

Surveys of children and adolescents' physical activity by self-report have been carried out in Sweden (16,17), Italy (32), Belgium (42), Finland (40a), Norway (41), Czechoslovakia (37), Germany (19), the Netherlands (15), and the United Kingdom (22,23,43). Findings have been remarkably similar, and I will use some of the more comprehensive surveys to illustrate methodology and general trends.

Engstrom (16, 17) reported results from interviewing a random selection of 1,050 girls and 1,089 boys, aged 15 years, about their sporting activities during leisure time. He followed up the study by analyzing self-report questionnaires on the same topic, which were mailed back to him by 796 of the girls and 849 of the boys 5 years later. He concluded that, although boys were on average more active than girls, the average amount of physical activity decreased during adolescence in both sexes. The Oslo Youth Study (41) illustrated the wide range of participation in physical activity by 10- to 15-year-old Norwegian children. Seventeen percent of 431 boys and 8% of 397 girls self-reported exercising daily, 64% of both genders claimed to exercise 1 to 3 times per week, but 16% of boys and 22% of girls admitted to exercising less than 2 to 3 times per month.

The Welsh Youth Health Survey (23) obtained information on the physical activity patterns of 6,581 children, aged 11 to 16 years, from 81 secondary schools in Wales. The data were collected through a series of questions concerned with physical activity and sports participation. Vigorous activity was defined as "games and sports that make you out of breath or sweat." Eighty percent of 11-year-old boys claimed to take part in vigorous activity outside school at least twice per week, but the figure fell to 70% of 16-year-old boys making the same claim. The corresponding figures for girls were 63% at 11 years and 33% at 16 years of age. More than a third of 16-year-old girls self-reported that they took part in vigorous activity once per month or less. The Welsh Heart Health Survey

(22) involved contacting a random sample of 21,000 households in Wales and asking those aged 12 to 64 years to complete a questionnaire booklet and return it by post. Almost 22,000 people replied. A "very active" classification was designed to identify people who took the type of exercise considered to reduce the risk of heart disease, and 49% of 12- to 17-year-old males and 19% of females of the same age were reported to fall into this category.

Williams (43) administered a self-completion questionnaire to 921 14- to 15-year-old English students from six schools. She reported that 60.5% of boys and 39.8% of girls participated in some form of physical activity outside school and that boys also tended to be more frequent participants. However, this investigation illustrates some of the difficulties involved in interpreting physical activity data collected in different studies. The school with the highest participation rate outside school time (72.7%) was an all-boys school, and the school with the lowest female participation rate (16%) contained a large proportion of Muslim girls who had certain restrictions placed upon their movements.

Research teams led by Saris (34) and Kemper (24) in Holland have carried out the most comprehensive longitudinal surveys of European children and adolescents' physical activity. Both surveys employed various means of assessing physical activity patterns, but only recall methods will be considered at this point. Over a 6-year period, Saris investigated the level of physical activity of more than 400 children initially 6 years of age, by collecting data biannually through questionnaires completed by teachers. Boys were shown to be more active than girls at each age studied. Kemper's study involved 159 girls and 148 boys. A standardized activity interview based on a questionnaire required the children to recall the previous 3 months. The interview was limited to activities with a minimal intensity of 4 METs, which the researchers equated to walking at 5 km/h. Total energy expenditure per week and average daily energy expenditure were estimated from the interview. In both boys and girls the total activity time >4 METs was shown to decrease gradually from the age of 12/13 years to 17/18 years. The girls reduced their weekly activity time from 9.5 to 8.0 hours per week, and the boys' weekly activity time decreased from 10.0 to 7.5 hours. Kemper and his colleagues concluded that, in general, boys and girls have a similar development with a decrease in their daily activity throughout their teens. However, boys spend more time on vigorous activities than girls do at all ages.

Physiological Monitoring of European Children and Adolescents' Physical Activity

Bedale's (11) detailed analysis of energy expenditure ("heat production") during selected activities was probably the first attempt to classify the energy expenditure of European children. Her work was, of course, limited by the available technology as she used Douglas bags to collect expired gas, which she subsequently analyzed for oxygen and carbon dioxide content using a Haldane apparatus. Bedale reported her results in terms of "total heat production in 24 h" and concluded that boys' values rose from 2,191 calories (9.16 MJ) at 8 years of age to 3,901 calories

(16.31 MJ) at 17 years of age. Girls' "heat production" increased from 2,223 calories (9.29 MJ) at 9 years of age to 3,214 calories (13.43 MJ) at 17 years of age. Although difficult to interpret, her results indicated that boys have a higher "heat production" at all ages studied.

Saris (34) developed an eight-level heart rate integrator which stored heart rates within appropriate ranges over 24 hour periods and used the instrument in a biannual analysis of 217 boys and 189 girls over a 6-year period beginning when the children were 6 years old. The Dutch children's total energy expenditure over a 24 hour period including a normal school day was calculated from their heart rate. The energy spent above 50% of maximal aerobic power was subsequently determined from individual regression equations. Saris reported that, at all ages, boys had a higher total energy expenditure and spent more energy above 50% of maximal aerobic power than girls did. This finding was in agreement with the children's class teacher's view of their physical activity levels. Kemper and Verschuur (24) used Saris's heart rate integrator to annually monitor Dutch children for 48 hours over a 4-year period. They estimated daily energy expenditure from the heart rate and either an individual regression equation or, in the case of the lower heart rate categories, a fixed value for energy expenditure of 6.0 kJ/min.kg. The daily energy expenditure of girls in relation to body mass was found to decrease from 12/13 years to 17/18 years of age. The boys' daily energy expenditure in relation to body mass was almost constant from age 12/13 years to 14/15 years and decreased at 17/18 years of age. Boys demonstrated significantly higher energy expenditures than girls at ages 13/14 years and 14/15 years.

Other investigators have made no attempt to convert heart rates to energy expenditures and have simply reported their findings as heart rate data. Seliger et al. (37) monitored the heart rates of 11 12-year-old Czechoslovakian boys for 24 hours and reported that heart rates of over 150 bpm were rare and only fleetingly encountered. They commented, "The daily activity heart rate response implied that very little circulation response was required to support the daily activity." Armstrong et al. (4) monitored the heart rates of 266 11- to 16-year-old English children over 3 weekdays from 0900 to 2100. They reported that boys spend a significantly higher percentage of their time than girls with heart rates above both 159 bpm (2.6% vs. 1.4%) and 139 bpm (6.2% vs. 4.2%). Two hundred and twelve of the children also had their heart rate monitored for 12 hours on a Saturday, and the boys were again shown to spend a significantly higher percentage of their time than girls with heart rates above 159 bpm (2.1% vs. 0.8%) and 139 bpm (5.5% vs. 2.6%). In girls, age was negatively and significantly correlated with the percentage of time spent with a heart rate >139 bpm, but in boys no relationship between age and heart rate was detected. To put the heart rate thresholds used into perspective, Armstrong noted that brisk walking at 6 km/h and jogging at 8 km/h elicited steady-state heart rates averaging 146 and 164 bpm with these students. Mean peak heart rates during treadmill running were 200 ± 8 bpm. Armstrong and Bray (6) used the same methodology to monitor 67 boys and 65 girls aged 10 years and from the same catchment area. They reported no significant differences between boys and girls in the percentage of time they spent with heart rates above 139 bpm during weekdays (9.4% vs. 8.2%) or Saturdays (5.2% vs. 6.0%). The boys, however, spent a significantly higher percentage of time with heart rates above 159 bpm during weekdays (4.5% vs. 3.5%) but not during Saturdays (1.8% vs. 1.8%).

Despite the problems involved in monitoring children's habitual physical activity, data from European countries are remarkably consistent. Significant numbers of children do not engage in appropriate physical activity, the activity level of girls (and possibly boys) appears to decrease with age, and girls are less likely to participate in high intensity activities than boys are. However, the data are difficult to interpret in detail because well-established physical activity guidelines for children and adolescents are not readily available.

Physical Activity Guidelines

Sallis convened an International Consensus Conference on Physical Activity Guidelines for Adolescents in June 1993 (33a). The consensus conference was designed to develop physical activity guidelines for adolescents (11-21 years of age) that are based on age-specific data on the effects of physical activity and to provide suggestions for implementing the guidelines in primary medical care settings. Two important recommendations emerged:

Recommendation 1:   All adolescents should be physically active daily or nearly everyday, as part of play, games, sports, work, transportation, or recreation in the context of family, school, and community activities.

Recommendation 2:   In addition to daily lifestyle activities, three or more sessions per week of activities lasting 20 minutes or more that require moderate to vigorous levels of exertion are recommended.

To examine whether European children and adolescents meet these recommendations, two recent studies will be discussed. The first study carried out on behalf of the World Health Organization (29) addresses Recommendation 1. In each of 10 European countries, target groups representative of the national population in terms of age, gender, and geographic distribution were recruited. Three age groups were targeted to simulate a longitudinal study, the median ages of which were set at 11, 13, and 15 years. Sample sizes ranged from 2,984 subjects in Austria to 6,498 subjects in Hungary. Students were asked how often per week they exercise outside school hours to the point they get out of breath or sweat. The percentages of boys and girls who exercise at least four times per week outside school are illustrated by age and participating country in Figures 12.1 and 12.2. Figures 12.3 and 12.4 illustrate the other side of the picture and show the percentages of boys and girls who exercise once a week or less by age and participating country. Taken together the figures emphasize that there are substantial differences between countries. For example, the activity levels of

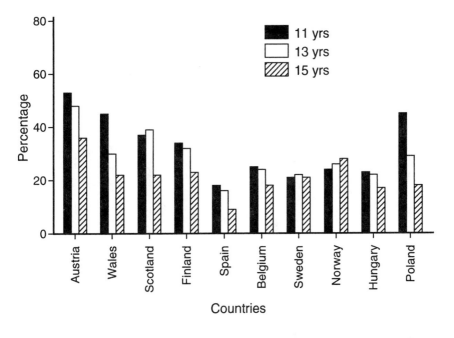

Figure 12.1. Percentage of girls who exercise at least four times a week outside school.

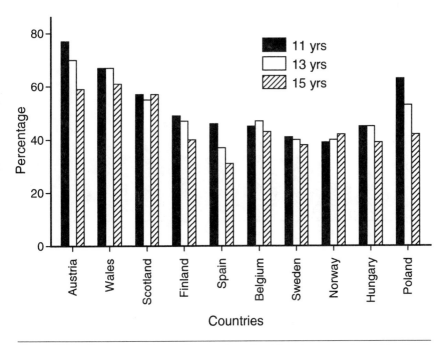

Figure 12.2. Percentage of boys who exercise at least four times a week outside school.

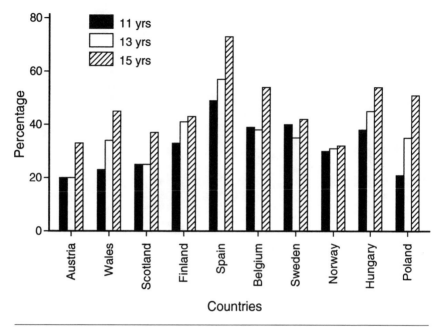

Figure 12.3.   Percentage of girls who exercise once a week or less outside school.

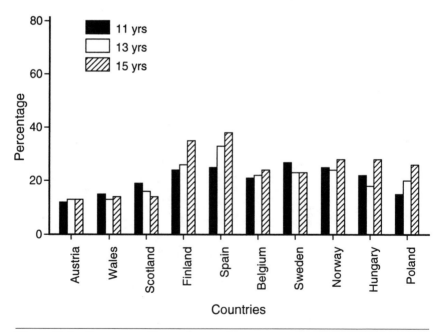

Figure 12.4.   Percentage of boys who exercise once a week or less outside school.
Note: Figures 12.1-12.4 are drawn from data in King, A.J.C. and Coles, B. (1992). The Health of
Canada's Youth. Canada Ministry of National Health and Welfare.

Spanish children appear to be significantly lower than those of, say, Austrian children. The decrease in exercise participation by age 15, especially for girls, is readily apparent and fairly consistent across countries. Norway and Sweden are exceptions as their numbers remain relatively stable or are the reverse of other countries. According to this form of analysis, fewer boys than girls appear to be inactive, but substantial numbers of both sexes fail to satisfy Recommendation 1 of the International Consensus Conference.

Armstrong's studies of British children described earlier (4,6) also considered sustained periods of moderate to vigorous levels of exertion in line with Recommendation 2 of the International Consensus Conference. Armstrong reported that 4% of 11- to 16-year-old boys and less than 1% of similarly aged girls experienced a daily 20 minute period equivalent to brisk walking (heart rate > 139 bpm). Thirty-six percent of boys and 52% of girls did not experience even a single 10-minute period equivalent to brisk walking during 3 days of 12 hour heart rate monitoring. Armstrong concluded that many children seldom experience the intensity and duration of physical activity that are believed to stress the cardiopulmonary system appropriately.

The data reviewed in this section suggest that a significant number of European children and adolescents follow sedentary lifestyles. There are substantial differences in the levels of physical activity in different countries, but trends are consistent. Boys appear to be more active than girls, particularly when vigorous activities are considered. Girls' activity levels deteriorate more than those of boys as they move from childhood through adolescence. Although data have been collected over several decades, methodological differences between studies preclude any meaningful analysis of whether European children and adolescents' habitual physical activity has declined over time.

Are Physical Activity and Cardiopulmonary Fitness Related in Children and Adolescents?

The evidence linking children and adolescents' peak $\dot{V}O_2$ to their habitual physical activity is conflicting and needs to be interpreted in the light of the problems associated with estimating levels of physical activity.

Kemper and Verschuur (26) commented that a high level of physical activity may account for the high peak $\dot{V}O_2$ values in their male population, and in a follow-up study of the same subjects, they attributed the decline in aerobic fitness to a reduction in the intensity of daily physical activity (28). Sunnegardh and Bratteby (40) reported significant correlations between peak $\dot{V}O_2$ and level of physical activity in 8-year-old boys and in 13-year-old boys and girls, but not in 8-year-old girls.

In contrast to these reports, Andersen et al. (3), on examination of their longitudinal data, concluded that peak $\dot{V}O_2$ was statistically unrelated to variations in "sport activity score." They commented, "There are sedentary, moderately active and very active children among those who are in excellent condition'' (p. 435). Saris (34) grouped preadolescents into low, middle, and high activity groups but, following an analysis of their peak $\dot{V}O_2$, he concluded that children with different levels of maximal aerobic power do not differ substantially in their daily physical activity. Armstrong et al. (5) examined the relationship between peak $\dot{V}O_2$ and habitual physical activity in 196 11- to 16-year-old students. No significant relationship was detected between peak $\dot{V}O_2$ and heart rate indicators of habitual physical activity. In a subsequent study of 96 preadolescent children, the same investigators (7) again reported no significant relationship between peak $\dot{V}O_2$ and habitual physical activity as estimated from three 12-hour periods of heart rate monitoring.

These equivocal findings are not surprising given the complexity of any relationship that may exist. Peak $\dot{V}O_2$ is a physiological variable whereas habitual physical activity is a behavior, and although it has been suggested that high levels of cardiopulmonary fitness may encourage individuals to engage in strenuous leisure-time activities, this remains to be established. The problem of comparing physical activity levels with peak $\dot{V}O_2$ is further confounded by the presence of an as yet unquantified genetic component of peak $\dot{V}O_2$ (13). However, it appears that very few European children and adolescents satisfy recommended criteria for the improvement of peak $\dot{V}O_2$ through exercise, and this may be the simple explanation for a lack of relationship between peak $\dot{V}O_2$ and habitual physical activity during childhood and adolesence.

Do Physical Activity Patterns Track From Childhood and Adolescence Into Adult Life?

The definitive study of physical activity tracking from childhood into adult life has yet to be carried out, but evidence to support the hypothesis that children's physical activity patterns persist into adult life is accumulating. Engstrom (17) interviewed more than 2,000 randomly selected Swedish 15-year-olds about their sporting activities during leisure time and followed the same group through mailed questionnaires 5, 10, and 15 years later. The results clearly indicated, ''Early experiences of physical activity are important for psychological readiness to participate in keep-fit activities in later life'' (p. 89). Kuh and Cooper (31) examined activity patterns in work and leisure in a British national sample of more than 3,300 men and women aged 36 years who were members of the 1946 national birth cohort study. Based on data collected at 13 and 36 years of age, their report stated that adolescent characteristics that were positive predictors of high sporting activity at age 36 years included above average ability at school games at age 13 years and high energy level at 13 years, as assessed by teachers.

The longitudinal findings of Engstrom (17) and Kuh and Cooper (31) were recently supported by a national survey of fitness and physical activity patterns which involved a representative sample of 6,000 English adults selected at random throughout the country (1). The results showed that 25% of the adults who were active when they were 14 to 19 years old were classified very active now, compared with only 2% classified active now who were inactive at that earlier age, thus indicating that lifelong physical activity is most likely to begin in childhood and adolescence.

Summary and Conclusions

The studies surveyed in this review indicate that although there is little evidence to suggest that European children and adolescents have low levels of cardiopulmonary fitness, sedentary lifestyles are common. Boys are more active than girls, and girls' activity levels deteriorate more rapidly than those of boys as they move from childhood through adolescence. Children's habitual physical activity does not appear to be related to cardiopulmonary fitness, but there is evidence to suggest that adult activity patterns may be established during childhood and adolescence.

Available data therefore emphasize the importance of promoting and fostering more active lifestyles during childhood and adolescence, but a number of research areas require further exploration. Groups of scholars need to collaborate to address research problems on an interdisciplinary and cross-cultural basis. Current issues in this context include the assessment and interpretation of both cardiopulmonary fitness and habitual physical activity, the effects of structured exercise programs, drop-out from exercise programs, and the determinants/correlates of habitual physical activity; all in relation to age, sex, and maturity.

References

1. Activity and Health Research. Allied Dunbar national fitness survey. London: Sports Council and Health Education Authority; 1992.
2. Andersen, K.L.; Seliger, V.; Rutenfranz, J.; Mocellin, R. Physical performance capacity of children in Norway. Part I - Population parameters in a rural inland community with regard to maximal aerobic power. Eur. J. Appl. Physiol. 33:177-195; 1974.
3. Andersen, K.L.; Ilmarinen, J.; Rutenfranz, J.; Ottman, W.; Berndt, I.; Kylian, H.; Ruppel, M. Leisure time sport activities and maximal aerobic power during late adolescence. Eur. J. Appl. Physiol. 52:431-436; 1984.
4. Armstrong, N.; Balding, J.; Gentle, P.; Kirby, B. Patterns of physical activity among 11- to 16-year-old British children. Br. Med. J. 301:203-205; 1990a.
5. Armstrong, N.; Balding, J.; Gentle, P.; Williams, J.; Kirby, B. Peak oxygen uptake and physical activity in 11 to 16 year olds. Pediatr. Exerc. Sci. 2:349-358; 1990b.
6. Armstrong, N.; Bray, S. Physical activity patterns defined by heart rate monitoring. Arch. Dis. Child. 66:245-247; 1991.
7. Armstrong, N.; Welsman, J.; Kirby, B. Daily physical activity estimated from continuous heart rate monitoring and laboratory indices of aerobic fitness in pre-adolescent children. Res. Q. Exerc. Sport. 64:(Suppl)A24; 1993.
8. Armstrong, N.; Welsman, J. Assessment and interpretation of aerobic fitness in children and adolescents. Exerc. Sports Sci. Rev. 22:435-476; 1994.
8a. Armstrong, N.; Williams, J.; Balding, J.; Gentle, P.; Kirby, B. The peak oxygen uptake of British children with reference to age, sex and sexual maturity. Eur. J. Appl. Physiol. 62:369-375; 1991.

9. Åstrand, P.O. Experimental studies of physical working capacity in relation to sex and age. Copenhagen: Munksgaard; 1952.

10. Bar-Or, O. Paediatric sports medicine for the practitioner. New York: Springer-Verlag; 1983.

11. Bedale, E.M. Energy expenditure and food requirements of children at school. London: Proceedings of the Royal Society. 94:368-404; 1923.

12. Bell, R.D.; Macek, M.; Rutenfranz, J.; Saris, W.H.M. Health indicators and risk factors of cardiovascular diseases during childhood and adolescence. In: Rutenfranz, J.; Mocellin, R.; Klimt, F., ed. Children and exercise XII. Champaign, IL: Human Kinetics; 1986: 19-27.

13. Bouchard, C.; Lortie, G. Heredity and endurance performance. Sports Med. 1:38-64; 1984.

14. Ceretelli, P.; Aghemo, P.; Rovelli, E. Morphological and physiological observations in school children in Milan. Medicina Dello Sport. 2:109-121; 1963.

15. deHass, J.H. Risk factors of coronary heart disease in children—a retrospective view of the Westland study. Postgrad. Med. J. 54:187-189; 1978.

16. Engstrom, L-M. Physical activity of children and youth. Acta Pediatr. Scand. (Supplement)283:101-105; 1980.

17. Engstrom, L-M. The process of socialisation into keep-fit activities. Scand. J. Sports Sci. 8:89-97; 1986.

18. Flandrois, R.; Grandmontagne, M.; Mayet, R.; Favier, R.; Frutoso, J. La consommation maximale d'oxygene chez le jeune francais sa variation avec l'age le sexe et l'entrainement. J. Physiol. (Paris). In: Krahenbuhl, G.; Skinner, J.S.; Kohrt, W.M. Developmental aspects of maximal aerobic power in children. Exerc. Sports Sci. Rev. 13:503-538; 1985.

19. Fuchs, R.; Semmer, N.K.; Lippert, P.; Powell, K.E.; Dwyer, J.H.; Hoffmeister, H. Patterns of physical activity among German adolescents: the Berlin-Bremen study. Prev. Med. 17:746-763; 1988.

20. Gaisl, G.; Buchberger, J. The significance of stress acidosis in judging the physical working capacity of boys aged 11 to 15. In: Lavallee, H.; Shephard, R.J., ed. Frontiers of activity and child health. Quebec: Pelican; 1977: 161-168.

21. Hansen, H.S.; Froberg, K.; Hydlebrandt, N.; Nielsen, J.R. A controlled study of eight months of physical training and reduction of blood pressure in children: the Odense school child study. Br. Med. J. 303:682-685; 1991.

22. Heartbeat Wales. Welsh Youth Health Survey 1986. (Heartbeat Report No. 5); 1986.

23. Heartbeat Wales. Exercise for Health. (Heartbeat Report No. 23); 1987.

24. Kemper, H.C.G., ed. Growth, health and fitness of teenagers. Basel: Karger; 1985.

25. Kemper, H.C.G.; Verschuur, R. Measurement of aerobic power in teenagers. In: Berg, K.; Eriksson, B.O., ed. Children and exercise IX. Baltimore: University Park Press; 1980: 55-63.

26. Kemper, H.C.G.; Verschuur, R. Maximal aerobic power. Med. Sports Sci. 20:107-126; 1985.

27. Kemper, H.C.G.; Verschuur, R. Longitudinal study of coronary risk factors during adolescence and young adulthood—the Amsterdam Growth and Health Study. Pediatr. Exerc. Sci. 2:359-371; 1990.

28. Kemper, H.C.G.; Verschuur, R.; deMey, L. Longitudinal changes of aerobic fitness in youth ages 12 to 23. Pediatr. Exerc. Sci. 1:257-270; 1989.

29. King, A.J.C.; Coles, B. The health of Canada's youth. Canada: Ministry of Health and Welfare; 1992.

30. Krahenbuhl, G.S.; Skinner, J.S.; Kohrt, W.M. Developmental aspects of maximal aerobic power in children. Exerc. Sports Sci. Rev. 13:503-538; 1985.

31. Kuh, D.J.L.; Cooper, C. Physical activity at 36 years: patterns and childhood predictors in a longitudinal study. J. Epidemiol. Comm. Health. 46:114-119; 1992.

32. Marella, M.; Colli, R.; Faina, M. Evaluation de l'aptitude physique: Eurofit, batterie experimentagle. Romes Scuola Dello Sport. In: Tuxworth, W.: 1988. The fitness and physical activity of adolescents. Med. J. Aust. 148:513-521; 1986.

33. Rutenfranz, J.; Andersen, K.L.; Seliger, V.; Klimmer, F.; Berndt, I.; Ruppel, M. Maximum aerobic power and body composition during the puberty growth period: similarities and differences between children of two European countries. Eur. J. Pediatr. 136:123-133; 1981.

33a. Sallis, J.F. (ed) Physical activity guidelines for adolescents. Pediatric Exercise Science. 6:294-463, 1994.

34. Saris, W.H.M. Aerobic power and daily physical activity in children. Meppel, Netherlands: Kripps Repro; 1982.

35. Saris, W.H.M. The assessment and evaluation of daily physical activity in children: a review. Acta Paediatr. Scand. 318:37-48; 1985.

36. Seliger, V.; Cermak, V.; Hendzo, S.; Horak, J.; Jirka, Z.; Macek, M.; Pribil, M.; Rous, J.; Skranc, O.; Ulbrich, J.; Urbanak, J. Physical fitness of the Czechoslovak 12- and 15-year-old population. Acta Paediatr. Scand. 217:37-41; 1971.

37. Seliger V.S.; Trefny, S.; Bartenkova, S.; Pauer, M. The habitual physical activity and fitness of 12-year-old boys. Acta Paediatr. Belg. 28:54-59; 1974.

38. Sprynarova, S.; Parizkova, J.; Bunc, V. Relationships between body dimensions and resting and working oxygen consumption in boys aged 11 to 18 years. Eur. J. Appl. Physiol. 56:725-736; 1987.

39. Sundberg, S.; Elovainio, R. Cardiorespiratory function in competitive endurance runners aged 12-16 years compared with ordinary boys. Acta Paediatr. Scand. 71:987-992; 1982.

40. Sunnegardh, J.; Bratteby, L.E. Maximal oxygen uptake, anthropometry and physical activity in a randomly selected sample of 8- and 13-year-old children in Sweden. Eur. J. Appl. Physiol. 56:266-272, 1987.

40a. Telema, R.; Viikari, J.; Valimaki, I.; Siren-Tiusanen, H.; Akerblom, H.K.; Uhari, M.; Dahl, M.; Fesonen, E.; Lahde, P.L.; Piet Kainen, M. Atherosclerosis precursors in Finnish children and adolescents leisure time physical activity. Acta Paediatr. Scnd. 318:169-180; 1985.

41. Tell, G.S.; Vellar, O.D. Physical fitness, physical activity and cardiovascular disease risk factors in adolescence. The Oslo Youth Study. Prev. Med. 17:12-24; 1988.

42. Weymans, M.L.; Reybrouck, T.M.; Stijns, H.J.; Knops, J. Influence of habitual levels of physical activity on the cardiorespiratory endurance capacity of children. In: Rutenfranz, J.; Mocellin, R.; Klimt, F., ed. Children and exercise XII. Champaign, IL: Human Kinetics; 1986: 149-156.

43. Williams, A. Physical activity patterns among adolescents—some curriculum implications. Phys. Ed. Rev. 11:28-39, 1988.

44. Wilmore, J.H.; Constable, S.H.; Stanforth, P.R.; Tsao, W.Y.; Rotkis, T.C.; Paicius, R.M.; Mattern, C.M.; Ewy, G.A. Prevalence of coronary heart disease risk factors in 13- to 15-year-old boys. J. Card. Rehab. 2:223-233; 1982.

Chapter 13

Cardiovascular Health Status of Latin American Children and Youth

Robert M. Malina, PhD, FACSM

Discussions of the health status of Latin American children and youth generally focus on the consequences of chronic undernutrition. In contrast, concern about risk factors for cardiovascular disease is increasingly indicated in discussions of modernization and lifestyles associated with affluence. This report considers the cardiovascular health status of Latin American children and youth. Growth status is considered where relevant, particularly in the context of obesity. With the exception of research on the aerobic fitness and performance of elite athletes in several centers, there is little research on the quantity and quality of habitual physical activity in the Latin American population.

Latin America is defined as including Mexico, Central America, and South America. The Caribbean will not be considered, although it is included in some global statistics.

Land of Contrasts

Latin America is a land of contrasts—geographic, climatic, ethnic, and economic. Most countries are within or have significant parts within the tropical zone (between the Tropics of Cancer and Capricorn). The mountain chain running from Mexico through Central America into the western part of South America includes many active volcanoes and geological faults; thus, the geology can be violent at times. The geography of Latin America is also unique in that the Andes, which cover parts of Ecuador, Peru, Bolivia, Argentina, and Chile, are the home of many inhabitants living at altitudes above 3,000 meters.

The ethnic composition of Latin America was altered with the conquest of the New World in the sixteenth century. Many areas experienced rapid depopulation, so that the resulting population is largely admixed among Amerindians, Europeans, and Africans. However, Amerindians comprise a significant percentage of the national populations of Guatemala (60%), Bolivia (59%), Peru (37%), Ecuador (34%), and Mexico (12%); their numbers are considerably smaller in the other countries (35). In addition, there has been considerable rural to urban migration over the past two decades resulting in sprawling urban slums (e.g., *favelas* in Brazil, *colonias* in Mexico) and related problems (e.g., water and sanitation, economic disparities, and so on).

In the Human Development Index (HDI), all countries of Latin America are classified as developing (in contrast to industrial). The HDI is based on indicators of longevity, education, and income: (a) life expectancy at birth, (b) two educational indicators—adult literacy and mean years of schooling, and (c) per capita purchasing power parity. It is defined as a minimal "measure of people's ability to live a long and healthy life, to communicate and to participate in the life of the community and to have sufficient resources to obtain a decent living" (64, p. 104). However, income and resources are inequitably distributed in many countries. In Brazil, for example, the richest fifth of the population has 26 times the income of the poorest fifth. Hence, when the income component of the HDI is adjusted for this disparity, the HDI of Brazil is reduced by 14%. Similar adjustments for inequitable distribution of income result in reductions of 11% in Honduras and Panama, 8% in Mexico, and smaller percentages in other Latin American countries (64).

Contrasting Health Problems

The general health status of Latin American children and youth can, to some extent, be dichotomized to reflect the two faces of malnutrition. The majority of children are reared under conditions of chronic poverty and undernutrition with associated consequences in growth, morbidity, and mortality. On the other hand, a relatively smaller number of children are reared under well-off economic and nutritional conditions with potential for development of risk factors for cardiovascular and related diseases (e.g., obesity, elevated lipids, sedentary lifestyle, and so on).

Although the percentage of chronically undernourished people (those who "did not consume enough food to maintain body weight and support light activity" over the course of a year) in Latin America has decreased from 19% in 1969-1971 to 13% in 1988-1990, the absolute number has increased from 54 to 59 million (19). When viewed as stunting (stature for age > 2 SDs below the median of U.S. reference data) (22), 26% of children 24 to 59 months of age in Latin America and the Caribbean between 1980 and 1990 are stunted. In contrast, only 5% of children 12 to 23 months of age are wasted (weight for stature > 2 SDs below the median of U.S. reference data) (65). Stunting reflects chronic undernutrition, while wasting indicates acute malnutrition. Percentages of stunted preschool children vary among countries (Table 13.1). They are higher in countries with a high indigenous population and are, in general, inversely related to the HDI and estimated per capita energy available per day in the food supply. The fact that countries with relatively high HDIs have a significant number of preschool children with stunted growth is a further indication of the economic disparities within many Latin American countries.

Chronic undernutrition increases the risk of morbidity and mortality, especially during the preschool years. Reduced body size and muscle mass are characteristic of the survivors of these rigorous selective forces and have functional consequences for strength and motor performance (29,30), aerobic power (55,56), and possibly economic productivity (23,24).

Table 13.1   Growth stunting, energy availability, and the human development index in several Latin American countries

Country	Stunting[a] (%, 1980-1990)	Energy[b] (kcal/capita)	HDI[c]
Guatemala	57	2327	0.489
Ecuador	39	2302	0.646
Bolivia	38	2096	0.398
Peru	37	2277	0.592
El Salvador	36		0.503
Honduras	34	2139	0.472
Brazil	29	2703	0.730
Colombia	23	2544	0.770
Mexico	22	3123	0.805
Nicaragua	22		0.500
Paraguay	17	2784	0.641
Uruguay	16	2746	0.881
Chile	10	2581	0.864
Venezuela	7	2534	0.824

[a]Adapted from the World Bank (65). Stunting in children 24-59 months of age. It is defined as stature for age > 2 SDs below the median of the reference data.
[b]Adapted from the Food and Agriculture Organization (18).
[c]Adapted from the United Nations Development Program (64).

Overweight and obesity are increasing in the more affluent segments of the Latin American population. Estimated prevalences are discussed later in the report.

Cardiovascular Health: General Considerations

In an attempt to estimate the burden of disease on human productivity, the World Bank (65, p. 213) has developed a statistic, the disability-adjusted life year (DALY), which "combines the loss of life from premature death in 1990 with the loss of healthy life from disability." The statistic is weighted for several factors including potential years of life lost due to a death at different ages, estimated value of a healthy year of life at different ages, estimated value of the future relative to the present (i.e., illnesses and injuries can last for years or decades), and weights for different disabilities ranging from perfect health to death. Estimated DALYs lost to different conditions in several areas of the world are shown in Figure 13.1. The overall magnitude of the burden of noncommunicable diseases, a major component of which are cardiovascular, is reasonably similar in the different regions. The burden of communicable and noncommunicable diseases in Latin America is about equal, in contrast to countries with established market economies, in which the burden of DALYs lost to noncommunicable diseases far outweighs those lost

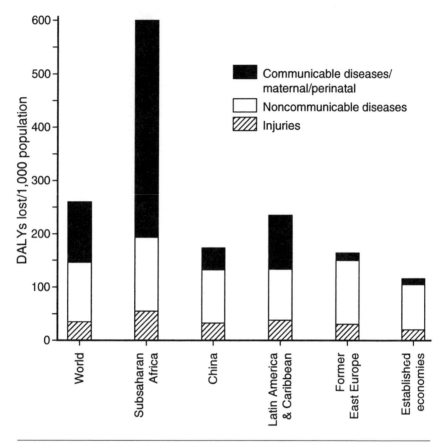

Figure 13.1. Estimated disability-adjusted life years (DALYs) lost to different conditions in several areas of the world.
Drawn from data reported by the World Bank (65).

to communicable diseases and injuries. Cardiovascular diseases account for 21.5% of DALYs lost to noncommunicable diseases in Latin America compared to 29.8% in countries with established market economies (65).

Cardiovascular diseases, often viewed as diseases of affluence, are thus a burden in Latin America. They are, however, more of a burden in the more developed Latin American countries (Figure 13.2). A relatively high HDI is associated with higher mortality from diseases of the circulatory system ($r = 0.79$) and lower mortality from communicable diseases ($r = -0.85$).

Dietary fat is a factor in cardiovascular disease. The more developed Latin American countries (higher HDIs) consume a greater percentage of energy from fat and a lesser percentage of energy from carbohydrate than lesser developed countries, and obtain a greater percentage of protein from animal sources (Figure 13.3). Relationships for energy from protein (r with HDI = 0.28) and for animal and vegetable sources of fat (r with HDI = 0.30) are not as strong.

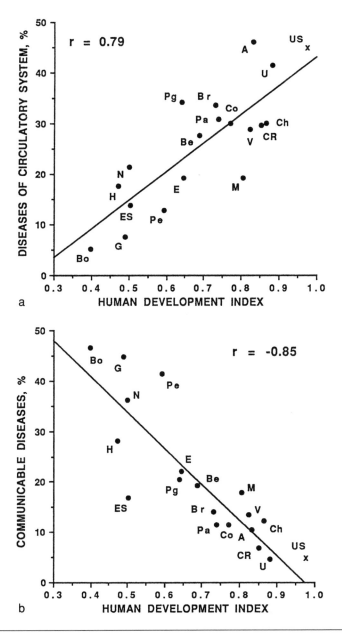

Figure 13.2. Relationship between the human development index and mortality from diseases of the circulatory system (A) and communicable diseases (B). The data for the United States (US) are not included in the calculation. Abbreviations for Latin American countries are as follows: A, Argentina; Be, Belize; Bo, Bolivia; Br, Brazil; Ch, Chile; Co, Colombia; CR, Costa Rica; E, Ecuador; ES, El Salvador; G, Guatemala; H, Honduras; M, Mexico; N, Nicaragua; Pa, Panama; Pg, Paraguay; Pe, Peru; U, Uruguay; V, Venezuela.

Drawn from data reported by the United Nations Development Program (64) and the Pan American Health Organization (44).

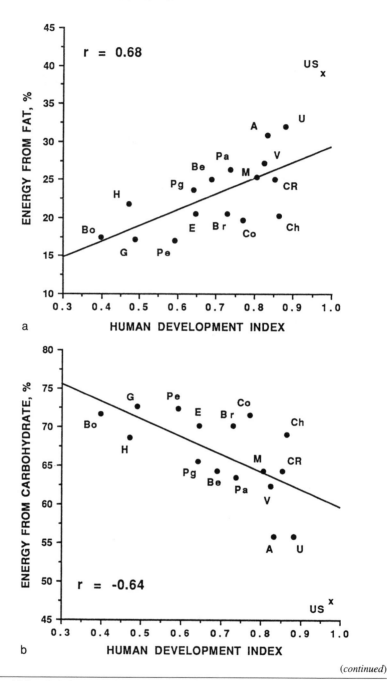

Figure 13.3.   Relationship between the human development index and estimated daily per capita energy available from fat (A) and carbohydrate (B), and the ratio of animal/vegetable protein sources (C). Abbreviations for countries are as in Figure 13.2. The data for the United States (US) are not included in the calculations.

Drawn from data reported by the United Nations Development Program (44) and the Food and Agriculture Organization (18).

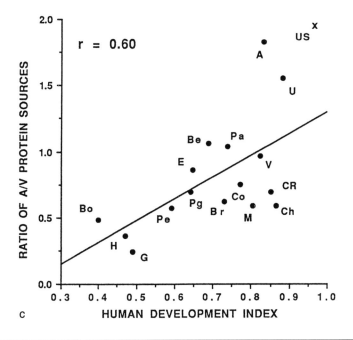

Figure 13.3. (*continued*)

Precursors of Atherosclerotic Disease

Evidence from the International Atherosclerosis Project (1960-1965) indicates that atherosclerosis begins during childhood (15,59). The coronary arteries of males 10 to 19 years of age from Chile, Costa Rica, and Guatemala show only slightly less involvement with fatty streaks than American Black and White males from New Orleans (Figure 13.4). However, fatty streak involvement is significantly greater in Blacks and Whites at older ages. Raised lesions are not common in the coronary arteries of Latin American males 10 to 19 years of age. They are apparent in a small percentage of American White males 15 to 19 years of age, and involvement with raised lesions increases sharply with age. The development of raised lesions proceeds at a slower pace in Latin American males. Corresponding comparisons of the coronary arteries of females are generally similar, with the exception of more extensive fatty streak involvement in American Blacks. Latin American females also show less involvement with raised lesions during the second and third decades. Although numbers are small, female specimens from Guatemala show no raised lesions until 35+ years of age.

In contrast to the coronary arteries, fatty streaks in the aorta do not show ethnic variation with the exception of black females. Raised lesions of the aorta also do not differ between the three Latin American and two American samples

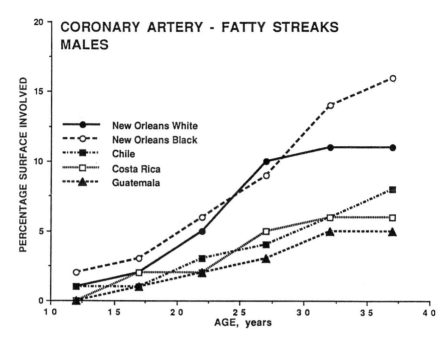

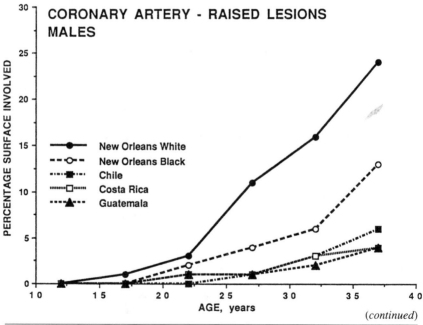

(continued)

Figure 13.4.   Percentage of the surface of coronary arteries involved with fatty streaks and raised lesions in males (this page) and females (next page) from three Latin American sites and the United States.

Drawn from data reported by Strong and McGill (59).

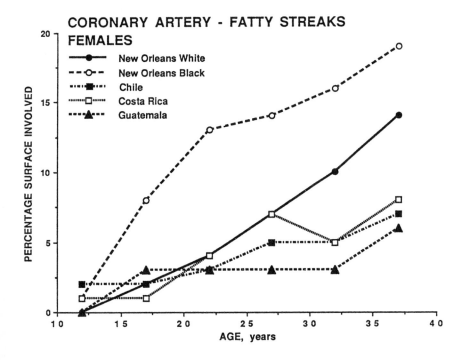

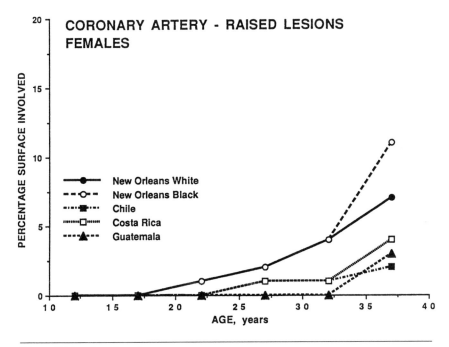

Figure 13.4.   (*continued*)

during adolescence (10-19 years). However, American Whites show greater involvement with raised lesions after about 25 years of age, males more so than females (59).

Straight lines were fitted to mean fatty streak and raised lesion involvement of the coronary arteries in two samples from the United States and ten samples from Central and South American countries (15). The age intercept for fatty streak involvement was quite similar in all samples, indicating a generally uniform timing of appearance of fatty streaks in all samples (Table 13.2). However, the slopes varied indicating differences in the rate at which fatty streaks increased with age. The slopes were generally lower in the Latin American samples compared to American Blacks and Whites. Corresponding analysis of the extent of raised lesions in the coronary arteries of males (Table 13.3) showed a younger age intercept in American Whites (17 years) compared to the other samples (21-31 years); thus, timing of raised lesion involvement occurred earlier in Whites. The estimated slopes for all Latin American samples, except Brazilian Whites, were lower than those in American males.

Autopsy evidence thus indicates the presence of atherosclerotic involvement in youth 10 to 19 years of age from several Central and South American countries. Although there is variation, it appears that the progression of fatty streaks and

Table 13.2   Regression with age (10-44 yrs) of percentage surface involved with fatty streaks in the coronary arteries in Latin American compared to New Orleans samples[a]

| Group | Males | | Females | |
	Age intercept[b]	Slope[c]	Age intercept	Slope
New Orleans				
White	11	0.36	13	0.52
Black	11	0.54	10	0.58
Mexico	11	0.26	10	0.25
Guatemala	12	0.26	13	0.28
Costa Rica	10	0.22	6	0.20
Venezuela	10	0.28	8	0.30
Colombia-Cali	11	0.34	12	0.37
Colombia-Bogota	12	0.34	12	0.34
Peru	11	0.29	6	0.25
Brazil-White	11	0.28	11	0.32
Brazil-Black	11	0.25	10	0.29
Chile	12	0.29	8	0.27

[a]Adapted from Eggen and Solberg (15).
[b]Age in years
[c]Slope in % surface per year

Table 13.3   Regression with age (25-69 yrs) of percentage surface involved with raised lesions in the coronary arteries in Latin American compared to New Orleans samples of males[a]

Group	Age intercept[b]	Slope[c]
New Orleans-White	17	0.80
New Orleans-Black	26	0.78
Mexico	24	0.31
Guatemala	26	0.29
Costa Rica	24	0.36
Venezuela	21	0.54
Colombia-Cali	23	0.33
Colombia-Bogota	29	0.33
Peru	31	0.64
Brazil-White	30	0.81
Brazil-Black	24	0.28
Chile	27	0.52

[a]Adapted from Eggen and Solberg (15).
[b]Age in years.
[c]Slope in % surface per year

raised lesions in the coronary arteries with increasing age proceeds at a slower pace in the Latin American samples. However, the autopsy data were collected in the 1960s and given changes in Latin America over the past 30 years, the extent and severity of atherosclerotic involvement in children, youth, and young adults may have changed also.

Risk Factors

Lipids

Serum total cholesterol and triglyceride levels in several samples of Latin American children and youth are summarized in Table 13.4. Assuming a normal distribution and adding one standard deviation to the means, a significant number of Venezuelan (Caracas) and Chilean (Concepcion) children and youth have total cholesterol levels >170 mg/dL and would be classified at moderate risk (60). The 75th percentiles for Chilean boys and girls, respectively, were 166 and 174 mg/dL (36). In contrast, 35% and 41% of Venezuelan boys and girls, respectively, had serum total cholesterol levels ≥160 mg/dL, described by the authors as the upper desirable limit (42). The mean total serum cholesterol of 175±34 mg/dL in 18-year-old Argentinian (Rosario) males (45) also suggests that a significant

Table 13.4   Serum cholesterol and triglyceride levels (mg/dL) in several samples of Latin American children and youth

Location	Age	n	Sex	Mean	SD
Cholesterol					
Mexico					
Huixquilucan	5-9	106	M + F	100	28
(Otomi, 20)	10-14	103	M + F	100	24
Chihuahua	5-18	118	M	115	19
(Taramuhara, 12)		104	F	117	25
Venezuela					
Caracas (42)	6-15	1385	M	153	29
		1412	F	156	29
Chile					
Concepcion (36)	6-15	326	M	146	30
		226	F	154	33
Argentina					
Rosario (45)	18	238	M	175	34
Triglycerides					
Mexico					
Chihuahua	5-18	118	M	110	51
(Taramuhara, 12)		104	F	122	48
Venezuela					
Caracas (42)	6-15	1385	M	72	31
		1412	F	78	35
Chile					
Concepcion (36)	6-15	326	M	80	35
		226	F	93	40

number have cholesterol levels that fall into the moderate and high risk categories. In contrast, serum cholesterol levels were quite low in two largely Amerindian samples from Mexico. No Taramuhara children had serum levels ≥ 160 mg/dL (12) and only 4% of the Otomi children had serum levels >140 mg/dL (20).

Data for cholesterol fractions are limited. LDL-cholesterol (LDL-C) levels in Chilean boys and girls were, respectively, 83±29 mg/dL and 89±32 mg/dL, while HDL-cholesterol (HDL-C) levels were, respectively, 46±11 mg/dL and 48±12 mg/dL (36). LDL-C >110 mg/dL is indicative of moderate risk (60), so that a significant number of children have LDL-C levels beyond this range. HDL-C levels of 49 (5-9 years) and 46 (10-14 years) mg/dL are indicative of moderate risk in white boys, and levels of 47 (5-9 years) and 45 (10-14 years) mg/dL are indicative of moderate risk in white girls (60). The median levels of Chilean boys (45 mg/dL) and girls (46 mg/dL) almost approximated these criteria. Corresponding data for 18-year-old Argentinian males, LDL-C 122±25 mg/dL and HDL-C 53±11 mg/dL, also indicate many with profiles at risk (45). Levels of LDL-C and HDL-C in a combined sample of Taramuhara boys and girls were 83±16 mg/dL and 26±9 mg/dL, respectively. These levels should be viewed in the context of their low total cholesterol and a diet that is low in cholesterol, fat, and saturated fat (12).

Serum triglyceride levels were surprisingly higher in Taramuhara children than in Chilean and Venezuelan children, and 16% of Taramuhara children had levels >150 mg/dL (12). Only small percentages of Venezuelan boys (3.3%) and girls (5.7%) had triglyceride levels ≥140 mg/dL (42), while the 90th percentiles were 122 mg/dL and 142 mg/dL, respectively, for Chilean boys and girls (36).

Serum total cholesterol and triglycerides vary with socioeconomic status (SES). Children from high SES have higher levels of total cholesterol and triglycerides, and thus present a more atherogenic profile, while low SES children have significantly lower levels (Table 13.5). Among 18-year-old Argentinian males, total cholesterol and LDL-C are especially higher in the upper SES, while the middle and lower SES samples do not differ. On the other hand, HDL-C does not differ among the three SES groups (45).

Information relating serum total cholesterol and triglycerides to other risk factors for cardiovascular disease in Latin American samples of children are not

Table 13.5 Social class variation in serum cholesterol (CH) and triglyceride (TG) levels (mg/dL) in several samples of Latin American children and youth

Location	Age	SES*	Sex	n	Mean	SD
Argentina (CH)						
Buenos Aires (9)	1-2	H	M + F	20	153	37
		M		118	138	36
		L		105	128	24
Rosario (45)	18	H	M	25	195	41
		M		104	174	28
		L		109	170	34
Guatemala (CH, 53)						
Urban	7-12	H	M + F	56	187	27
Urban		M		56	143	29
Rural		L		56	121	24
Urban		H	F	56	188	30
Urban		M		56	156	30
Rural		L		56	128	24
Venezuela (CH & TG)						
Caracas (42)	6-15	H	M + F		166 (CH)	
		L			143	
	6-15	H	M + F		80 (TG)	
		L			67	

*H, High; M, Medium; L, Low

available. Among 18-year-old Argentinian males, heavy smokers had higher total serum cholesterol and LDL-C than moderate smokers and non-smokers; the latter had the lowest lipid levels. HDL-C did not differ among the smoking groups (45). Occupational physical activity (manual vs. non-manual) did not influence lipoprotein levels in these 18-year-old males (45). Among Brazilian young adults (20-29 years), only 31% and 39% of males and females, respectively, had no cardiovascular risk factors (smoking, obesity, familial diabetes, contraceptive use in females). Of the risk factors, obesity was most related to elevated levels of cholesterol and triglycerides in both sexes (34).

Blood Pressures

Age-specific blood pressures of boys and girls 6 to 15 years of age are given in Figure 13.5, while those from studies grouping subjects across several years are shown in Figure 13.6. The Bogalusa data (mean plus two standard deviations) are used as the reference comparison. The diastolic pressure is the K4 reading, although K5 is recommended for adolescents (61). However, much of the available data from Latin America reported K4 values or did not indicate which sound was used. Blood pressures increase gradually with age and mean values for children from Mexico and Venezuela are generally at or above the Bogalusa means (Figure 13.5). Diastolic pressures for La Sabana, a black coastal community in Venezuela, are K5 readings.

Criteria used to define hypertension in the surveys of Latin American children vary. With the mean + 2 SDs as the upper limit, estimates are 1% for boys 6 to 20 years of age, 2% for girls 6 to 15 years of age, and 10% for girls 12 to 20 years of age in Mexico City (38), and 4% for boys 6 to 13 years of age and 3% for girls 8 to 14 years of age in Guadalajara (11). In the latter study, hypertension was significantly more prevalent in obese children. Using the 95th percentiles of the Bogalusa study and the Task Force on Blood Pressure Control in Children as the criteria, estimates are 10% with the former and 1% with the latter in Mexico City children 6 to 12 years of age (39). Estimates of hypertension (≥ 130 mm Hg and ≥ 84 mm Hg 6-10 years; ≥ 140 mm Hg and ≥ 90 mm Hg 11-15 years) in Venezuelan children 6 to 15 years of age are 7% in boys and 13% in girls. There were no race differences in hypertension, but the prevalence of hypertension increased with age in girls from 12% at 6 to 10 years to 16% at 11 to 15 years (41). Among Brazilian children of both sexes, estimates of hypertension (95th percentile) are 7% at 6 to 9 years and 3% at 10 to 15 years (7,8). Elevated blood pressures and higher body weights are also characteristic of the parents and siblings of the target children (7,8). Familial aggregation is also suggested among siblings in the Venezuelan black community of La Sabana (50). In contrast to limited data for children, a review of hypertension in Brazilian adults suggests higher blood pressures in blacks and mulattoes (25).

During adolescence and young adulthood, mean blood pressures of two Mestizo samples from Mexico and several samples of Amerindians are generally at or below the Bogalusa means (Figure 13.6). The three Aymara samples are from

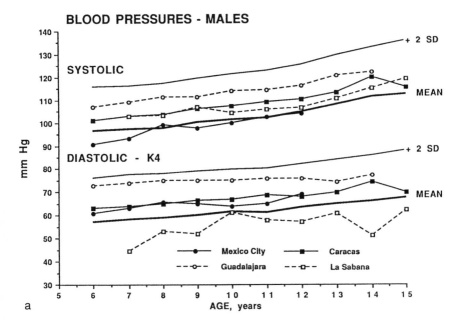

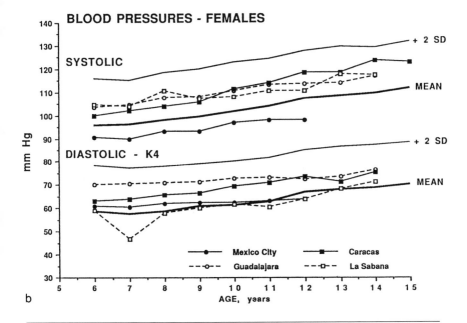

Figure 13.5. Blood pressures in males (A) and females (B) 6-15 years of age from several Latin American cities: Mexico City (38), Guadalajara (11), Caracas (41), and La Sabana (50). Bogalusa data (61) are the reference comparison. The diastolic pressure is the K4 reading.

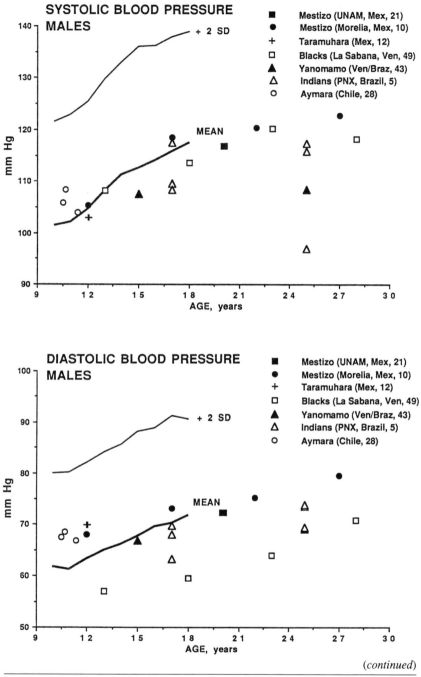

Figure 13.6. Blood pressures in adolescent and young adult males (this page) and females (next page) from several Latin American countries. Sources of the data are indicated in the figure. Bogalusa data (61) are the reference comparison. The diastolic pressure is the K4 reading.

(continued)

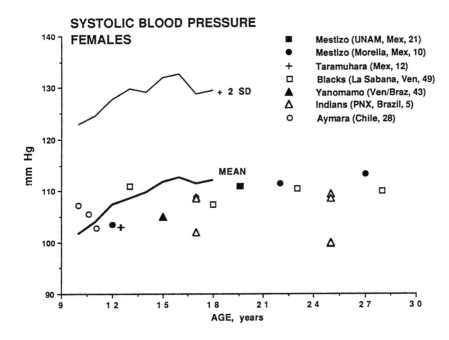

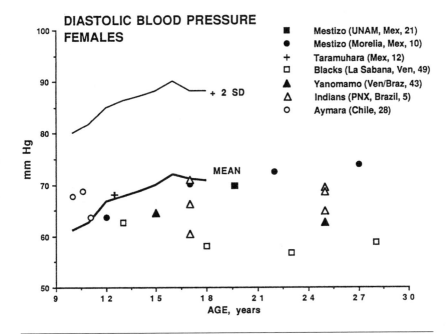

Figure 13.6.   (*continued*)

low (sea level-300 m), moderate (3,000-3,500 m), and high (4,000-4,600 m) altitudes, and differences among them are small (28). Adolescent and young adult samples of South American Indians (Yanomamo and those in the Xingu park) have especially lower blood pressures which do not appear to increase with age. These low levels suggest that hypertension is rare, perhaps reflecting their traditional diet with no salt, lower levels of stress, and a physically active lifestyle (5,43). Some evidence suggests that regular external contacts (acculturation) have no effect on blood pressures of the Yanomamo, but they are associated with increased body weight and sodium intake (32). It would be interesting to track blood pressures as acculturation continues. In contrast, modernization is associated with adult blood pressures in rural Mexico (14) and urban Brazil (13), and the estimated effect of modernization is similar to that of other risk factors (e.g., body mass index). Data on the effects of acculturation and/or modernization on blood pressures of Latin American children and youth are not available.

Among Mexican medical students 17 to 24 years of age, 85% and 81% of males and females, respectively, had one or more risk factors for arterial hypertension (21). A sedentary lifestyle was the most prevalent risk factor in both sexes (47% of males, 67% of females). Familial antecedents of hypertension were also common (34% of males, 44% of females). Other risk factors included smoking, overweight, elevated salt intake, and alcohol consumption.

Obesity

Concern for increasing prevalence of overweight and obesity in Latin American children is often expressed, but the data are limited. As with other risk factors, criteria for overweight and obesity are variable. Among 4 to 5 year olds in a private pediatric practice in Brazil (Recife), about 13% of boys and 15% of girls had a relative weight ≥111 versus local reference data (i.e., overweight) (17). Using the triceps skinfold and local reference data (90th percentile) with 5 to 12-year-old children from Argentina (Cordoba), researchers found that obesity occurred in only 2% of boys and 11% of girls (1). The prevalence of obesity increased with age, especially after 8 years in girls. Among Brazilian (Ribeirao Preto, Sao Paulo) children 7 to 11 years of age, the prevalence of obesity was greatest in the high SES and lowest in the low SES samples. Specific prevalences, however, were confounded because both local and international reference data were used. Nevertheless, when two of three criteria (weight for age, weight for stature, and triceps skinfold) were in the obese category, 38% of high SES children were obese in contrast to only 12% of middle SES children and 4% of low SES children. And within the high and middle SES groups, more boys than girls were classified as obese (4).

Using weight for stature criteria of the World Health Organization with 13 to 15 year old adolescents from Chile (Santiago), about 41% of girls and 26% of boys were classified as obese (i.e., weight for stature > 2SD), while an additional 23% of girls and 18% of boys were overweight (i.e., weight for stature > 1SD < 2SD) (37). Among small subsamples, obese girls consumed less energy than non-obese girls, while obese boys consumed more energy than non-obese boys. Non-obese boys were slightly more involved in sport activity than the obese boys (77% vs. 65%). A similar trend was apparent in girls (29% vs. 19%), but only few non-obese and obese girls were active in sport (37).

Relationships between weight and stature vary during the growth spurt so that weight for stature as an indicator of obesity has limitations at this time. In addition, possible ethnic variation in stature may influence the interpretation of weight for stature relationships. Mean/median statures and weights of representative samples of children from several Latin American countries with a high HDI (Argentina, Chile, Venezuela, Mexico) and a somewhat lower HDI (Brazil) were thus plotted relative to United States reference data (Figure 13.7). Chilean boys and girls are shorter than P 25 of the reference data throughout. Weights of Chilean girls, on the other hand, vary between P 25 and P 50, while weights of boys tend to be slightly above P 25 in childhood, at P 25 between 12 and 15 years, and below P 25 in late adolescence. Thus, it is no surprise that a significant percentage of Chilean adolescents have excess weight for stature as noted. Among the other samples compared, late adolescent statures tend to approximate P 25 of the reference data. Weights are more variable and are above P 25 in several samples. Mexican adolescent girls tend to have weights that approximate the reference median, while their statures are close to P 25; hence, they have greater weight for stature and thus many would be classified as overweight. The trend is similar for Mexican adolescent boys.

There are clear social class gradients in the growth of Latin American children and youth. As shown in Brazilian data (33), children from lower social strata are consistently shorter and lighter than those from upper social strata. Among late adolescent girls, however, upper and lower SES girls differ significantly in stature, but not in body weight. Hence, lower SES girls have, on average, greater weight for stature and a significant number are likely overweight and/or obese, which is consistent with the commonly reported trend toward greater prevalence of obesity in lower SES women. Among low-income urban adults 20-70+ years in Brazil (Rio de Janeiro), for example, about 50% of women and 35% of men were overweight (BMI $\geq$25 - 29.9 kg/m^2) or obese (BMI $\geq$30 kg/m^2) (2). On the other hand, the prevalence of overweight and/or obesity in young adults is less than when the entire adult age span is considered. Among 18- to 24-year-old Brazilians (Municipio de Araquara, Sao Paulo), only about 4% of females and 5% of males had BMIs $\geq$30 kg/m^2 (i.e., obese), while the prevalence of overweight (BMI $\geq$25-29.9 kg/m^2) was higher, 16% of females and 8% of males (27). Over the entire age span of the study, 18 to 74 years, the prevalence of overweight/ obesity increased with age.

Caution is warranted in interpreting results based on the BMI. An elevated BMI may not have the same significance as a risk factor in all populations. For example, Mexican Americans (San Antonio, Texas) do not have increased mortality even though they have, on average, significantly higher BMIs than American whites (58).

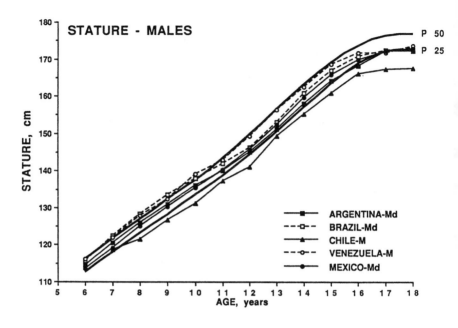

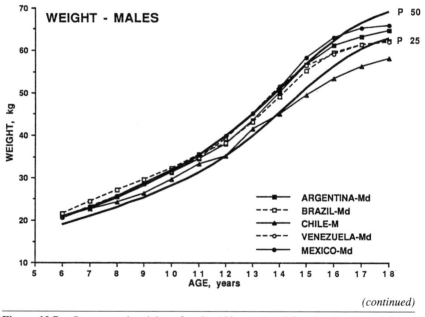

(continued)

Figure 13.7.   Statures and weights of males (this page) and females (next page) from several Latin American countries plotted relative to reference data for the United States. The reported data are means (M) or medians (Md).

The data for Mexico are from Ramos Galvan (46), while those for the other countries are reported in Eveleth and Tanner (16).

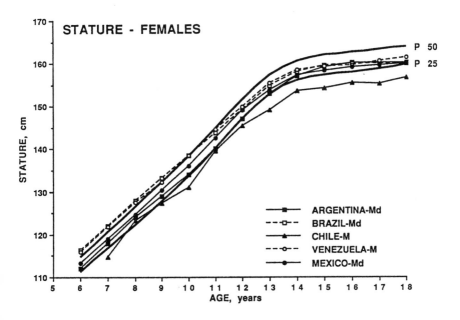

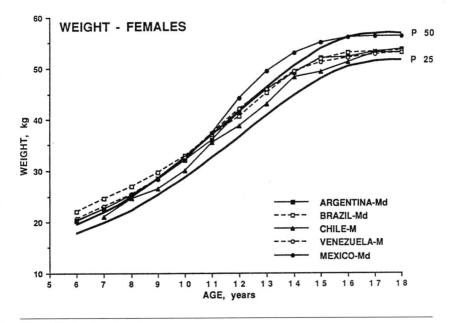

Figure 13.7.   (*continued*)

The available data on the prevalence of overweight/obesity in Latin America are largely limited to several countries. Evidence from early surveys in five South American countries in the late 1950s and early 1960s (3) suggests that the prevalence of obesity (relative weight >120) in individuals >15 years varied inversely with the prevalence of undernutrition (relative weight < 90). At the extremes, for example, the prevalences of obesity and undernutrition in Uruguay were, respectively, 30% and 9%, while corresponding figures in Ecuador were, respectively, 8% and 21%, and in Colombia were, respectively, 7% and 19% (3).

Fat Distribution

Centrally deposited fat is a risk factor for several metabolic diseases in adults. The association between relative fat distribution and risk factors for cardiovascular disease, however, is not necessarily the same in children and adults. Evidence for a representative United States sample suggests that fatness per se is a more important risk factor than relative fat distribution in children (52). Relative fat distribution, however, changes toward a more central pattern during the normal progression of puberty (31), so that relative fat distribution is significantly related to risk factors for cardiovascular disease in postpubertal adolescents (51).

Some evidence suggests a tendency toward a more central and upper body pattern of fat distribution in Latin American populations (40). Data for upper and lower SES Guatemalan children indicate relatively more fat on the trunk (subscapular skinfold) than the extremities (triceps skinfold) than U.S. reference data (26). However, other data for Guatemalan children based upon the same two skinfolds indicate little ethnic difference in upper SES Ladino and Indian children, and an ethnic difference in low SES children (6). Preferential fat loss at the triceps site associated with low SES may influence the ethnic difference. These studies are limited to the triceps and subscapular skinfolds, and additional skinfolds are necessary to better characterize subcutaneous fat distribution.

Physical Activity

Lack of physical activity is indicated as a factor associated with hypertension and obesity in adolescents and young adults (21,37), while a physically active lifestyle is indicated as a significant factor in the lower blood pressures of Brazilian Indians (5,43). Surveys of habitual physical activity of upper, middle, or low SES Latin American children and youth are not available. Studies in Guatemala have considered reduced levels of spontaneous physical activity during energy restriction in preschool children and adults and the role of activity in nutritional rehabilitation of preschool Guatemalan children (62,63), while studies in Colombia have focused on physical activity and energy expenditure in marginally undernourished children, youth, and adults (47,57; see also Spurr this volume). More recently, comparisons of activity levels of Bolivian boys in the high and low altitude paradigm have been reported (54).

Summary

The growth status of Latin American children and youth is reasonably well documented. Information on cardiovascular health status and risk factors is limited and to some extent dated. Physical activity has been approached primarily in the context of the consequences of chronic mild-to-moderate undernutrition (marginal nutritional status). Studies of cardiovascular health and physical activity need to be extended to more representative samples across the diverse economic strata. This is a complex and difficult task given the contrasts that characterize Latin America. Nevertheless, the time is ripe for systematic study as the health status of children and youth has important implications for the future in developing countries.

References

1. Agrelo, F.; Lobo, B.; Bazan, M.; Mas, L.B.; Lozada, C.; Jazan, G.; Orellana, L. Prevalencia de delgadez y gordura excesiva en un grupo de escolares de la ciudad de Cordoba, Argentina. Arch. Latinoam. Nutr. 38:69-80; 1988.
2. dos Anjos, L.A. Vigilancia nutricional em adultos: Experiencia de uma unidade de saude atendendo populacao favelada. Cad. Saude Publ., Rio de Janeiro 8:50-56; 1992.
3. Arteaga L., A. The nutritional status of Latin American adults. In: Scrimshaw, N.S.; Behar, M., eds. Nutrition and agricultural development: significance and potential for the tropics. New York: Plenum Press; 1976: 67-76.
4. Artega P., H.; dos Santos, J.E.; Dutra de Oliveira, J.E. Obesity among schoolchildren of different socioeconomic levels in a developing country. Inter. J. Obes. 6:291-297; 1981.
5. Baruzzi, R.; Franco, L. Amerindians of Brazil. In: Trowell, H.C.; Burkitt, D.P., eds. Western diseases: their emergence and prevention. London: Edward Arnold; 1981: 138-153.
6. Bogin, B.; Sullivan, T. Socioeconomic status, sex, age, and ethnicity as determinants of body fat distribution for Guatemalan children. Am. J. Phys. Anthropol. 69:527-535; 1986.
7. Brandao, A.P.; Brandao, A.A.; Araujo, E.M. The significance of physical development on the blood pressure curve of children between 6 and 9 years of age and its relationship with familial aggregation. J. Hypertens. 7 (suppl. 1):S37-S39; 1989.
8. Brandao, A.P.; Brandao, A.A.; Araujo, E.M.; Oliveira, R.C. Familial aggregation of arterial blood pressure and possible genetic influence. Hypertension 19 (suppl. II):214-217; 1992.
9. Carmuega, E. Hipercolesterolemia en la infancia: Es hora de enfrentar el desafio. Boletin de Estudios sobre Nutricion Infantil 1:26-29; 1987.
10. Chavez C., J.F.; Herrera A., J.E.; Salazar, L.A.; Vidal G., J.; Moreno R., A.; Tena M., I.; Chavez, D., R. Valores de la presion arterial en diversos grupos de poblacion urbana de la ciudad de Morelia. Arch. Inst. Cardiol. Mex. 60:577-586; 1990.
11. Cobos G., O.; Rubio S., R.; Garcia de Alba G., J.E.; Parra C., J.Z. La presion arterial en escolares de Guadalajara. Salud Publ. Mex. 25:177-183; 1983.
12. Connor, W.E.; Cerqueira, M.T.; Connor, R.W.; Wallace, R.B.; Malinow, M.R.; Casdorph, H.R. The plasma lipids, lipoproteins, and diet of the Tarahumara Indians of Mexico. Am. J. Clin. Nutr. 31:1131-1142; 1978.
13. Dressler, W.W.; dos Santos, J.E.; Gallagher, P.N.; Viteri, F.E. Arterial blood pressure and modernization in Brazil. Am. Anthropol. 89:398-409; 1987.
14. Dressler, W.W.; Mata, A.; Chavez, A.; Viteri, F. Arterial blood pressure and individual modernization in a Mexican community. Soc. Sci. Med. 24:679-687; 1987.

15. Eggen, D.A.; Solberg, L.A. Variation of atherosclerosis with age. Lab. Invest. 18:571-579; 1968.

16. Eveleth, P.B.; Tanner, J.M. Worldwide variation in human growth (2nd edition). New York: Cambridge University Press; 1990.

17. Ferreira, O.S.; Filho, P.N.B.; Charifker, H.; Coelho, E.F.; Lima, G.M.S.; Alves, J.G.B. Sobrepeso em criancas atendidas em um consultorio pediatrico privado do Recife. Pediatria (S. Paulo) 6:69-73; 1984.

18. Food and Agriculture Organization. Food balance sheets. Rome: Food and Agriculture Organization of the United Nations; 1991.

19. Food and Agriculture Organization. World food supplies and prevalence of chronic undernutrition in developing regions as assessed in 1992. Rome: Food and Agriculture Organization of the United Nations; 1992.

20. Golubjatnikov, R.; Paskey, T.; Inhorn, S.L. Serum cholesterol levels of Mexican and Wisconsin schoolchildren. Am. J. Epidemiol. 96:36-39; 1972.

21. Guemez S., J.C.; Moreno A., L.; Kuri M., P.; Argote R., A.; Leonel, A.A.; Mendez V., R.; Ramos V., E. Estilo de vida y antecedentes familiares y personales patologicos relacionados con hipertension arterial en estudiantes de la facultad de medicina de la U.N.A.M. Arch. Inst. Cardiol. Mex. 60:283-287; 1990.

22. Hamill, P.V.V.; Drizd, R.A.; Johnson, C.L.; Reed, R.D.; Roche, A.F. NCHS growth charts for children, birth-18 years, United States. Vital and Health Statistics, Series 11, No. 165; 1977.

23. Immink, M.D.C. Energy intake and productivity of Guatemalan sugarcane cutters: an empirical test of the efficiency wage hypothesis. Part I and Part II. J. Develop. Econ. 9:251-271, 273-287; 1981.

24. Immink, M.D.C.; Viteri, F.E.; Flores, R.; Torun, B. Microeconomic consequences of energy deficiency in rural populations in developing countries. In: Pollitt, E.; Amante, P., eds. Energy intake and activity. New York: Liss; 1984: 355-376.

25. James, S.; de Almeida-Filho, N.; Kaufman, J.S. Hypertension in Brazil: a review of the epidemiological evidence. Ethnic. Dis. 1:91-98; 1991.

26. Johnston, F.E.; Bogin, B.; MacVean, R.B.; Newman, B.C. A comparison of international standards versus local reference data for the triceps and subscapular skinfolds of Guatemalan children and youth. Hum. Biol. 56:157-171; 1984.

27. Lolio, C.A.; Latorre, M. do R.D. de O. Prevalencia de obesidade em localidade do Estado de Sao Paulo, Brasil, 1987. Rev. Saude Publ., S. Paulo 25:33-36; 1991.

28. Makela, M.; Barton, S.A.; Schull, W.J.; Weidman, W.; Rothhammer, F. The Multinational Andean Genetic and Health Program. IV. Altitude and the blood pressure of the Aymara. J. Chron. Dis. 31:587-603; 1978.

29. Malina, R.M. Physical activity and motor development/performance in populations nutritionally at risk. In: Pollitt, E.; Amante, P., eds. Energy intake and activity. New York: Liss; 1984: 285-302.

30. Malina, R.M. Growth of Latin American children: socioeconomic, urban-rural and secular comparisons. Rev. Brasil. Cienc. Moviment. 4:46-75; 1990 (June).

31. Malina, R.M.; Bouchard, C. Subcutaneous fat distribution during growth. In: Bouchard, C.; Johnston, F.E., eds. Fat distribution during growth and later health outcomes. New York: Liss; 1988: 63-84.

32. Mancilha C., J.A.; Lima, J.A.C.; Carvalho, J.V.; Marcilio de S., C.A. Blood pressure is directly related to the degree of acculturation among primitive Yanomamo Indians. Circulation 72 (suppl. III):296; 1985 (abstract).

33. Marques, R.M.; Marcondes, E.; Berquo, E.; Prandi, R.; Yunes, J. Crescimento e desenvolvimento pubertario em criancas e adolescentes brasileiros. II. Altura e peso. Sao Paulo: Editora Brasileira de Ciencias; 1982.

34. Martins, I.S.; Gomes, A.D.; Pasini, U. Niveis lipemicos e alguns fatores de risco de doencas cardiovasculares em populacao do municipio de Sao Paulo, SP, (Brasil). Rev. Saude Publ., S. Paulo 23:26-38; 1989.

35. Mayer, E.; Masferrer, E. La poblacion indigena de America en 1978. Am. Indigena 39:217-337; 1979.

36. Milos G., C.; Casanueva E., V.; Campos G., R.; Cid C., X.; Silva F., V.; Rodriguez Y., W.; Rodriguez C., M.S. Factores de riesgo de enfermedad cardiovascular en una poblacion de escolares chilenos: I parte: Lipidos sericos en 552 ninos y adolescentes de 6-15 anos. Rev. Chil. Pediatr. 61:67-73; 1990.

37. Montecinos G., M.; Araya H., P.; Cabrera C., M.; Cisternas M., P.; Molina Y., J.C.; Montero L., S.; Rodriguez A., J.; Trujillo N., C. Prevalencia de obesidad y de algunos factores asociados en una poblacion escolar adolescente. Bol. Hosp. San Juan de Dios 33:225-231; 1986.

38. Moragrega, J.L.; Mendoza A. Cifras de tension arterial en la infancia y la adolescencia en Mexico. Arch. Inst. Cardiol. Mex. 51:179-184; 1981.

39. Moreno A., L.; Kuri M., P.; Guemez S., J.C.; Villazon S., S. Tension arterial en escolares de la ciudad de Mexico: Importancia de las tablas de valores normales. Bol. Med. Hosp. Infant. Mex. 44:389-395; 1987.

40. Mueller, W.H. The biology of human fat patterning. In: Norgan, N.G., ed. Human body composition and fat distribution. Wageningen, The Netherlands: Stichting Nederlands Instituut voor de Voeding; 1986: 159-174.

41. Munoz, S.; Munoz, H.; Zambrano, F. Blood pressure in a school-age population: distribution, correlations, and prevalence of elevated values. Mayo Clin. Proc. 55:623-632; 1980.

42. Munoz, S.; Munoz, H.; Zambrano, F.; Gueron, N. Serum cholesterol and triglyceride levels in a school-age population: distribution, correlation, and prevalence' of high values. Arch. Intern. Med. 141:24-29; 1981.

43. Oliver, W.J.; Cohen, E.L.; Neel, J.V. Blood pressure, sodium intake, and sodium related hormones in the Yanomamo Indians, a ''no salt'' culture. Circulation 52:146-151; 1975.

44. Pan American Health Organization. Health statistics from the Americas. Washington, D.C.: Pan American Health Organization, Scientific Publication No. 537; 1991.

45. Poletto, L.; Pezzotto, S., Morini, J. Blood lipid associations in 18-year-old men. Rev. Saude Publ., S. Paulo 26:316-320; 1992.

46. Ramos Galvan, R. Somatometria pediatrica estudio semilongitudinal en ninos de la ciudad de Mexico. Arch. Invest. Med. 6 (suppl. 1):83-396; 1975.

47. Reina, J.C.; Spurr, G.B. Daily activity level of marginally malnourished school-aged girls: a preliminary report. In: Pollitt, E.; Amante, P., eds. Energy intake and activity. New York: Liss; 1984: 263-283.

48. Rodriguez, A. Factores que influyen sobre la presion arterial en la poblacion infantil de La Sabana, D.F. Acta Cient. Venezolana 30:175-182; 1979.

49. Rodriguez, A. La presion arterial en los habitantes de La Sabana, D.F.: Algunas variables determinantes. Acta Cient. Venezolana 31:53-61; 1980.

50. Rodriguez L., A. Familial aggregation of differences in blood pressure readings between two consecutive examinations. Acta Cient. Venezolana 34:353-359; 1983.

51. Sangi, H.; Mueller, W.H. Which measure of body fat distribution is best for epidemiologic research among adolescents? Am. J. Epidemiol. 133:870-883; 1991.

52. Sangi, H.; Mueller, W.H.; Harrist, R.B.; Rodriguez, B.; Grunbaum, J.G.; Labarthe, D.R. Is body fat distribution associated with cardiovasacular risk factors in childhood? Ann. Hum. Biol. 19:559-578; 1992.

53. Scrimshaw, N.S.; Balsam, A.; Arroyave, G. Serum cholesterol levels in school children from three socio-economic groups. Am. J. Clin. Nutr. 5:629-633; 1957.

54. Slooten, J.; Kemper, H.C.G.; Post, G.B.; Lujan, C.; Coudert, J. 24-hours heart rate measurement in 10-12 year old Bolivian boys living at low and high altitude. Ped. Exerc. Sci. 5:473; 1993 (abstract).

55. Spurr, G.B. Nutritional status and physical work capacity. Yrbk. Phys. Anthropol. 26:1-35; 1983.

56. Spurr, G.B. The impact of chronic undernutrition on physical work capacity and daily energy expenditure. In Harrison, G.A.; Waterlow, J.C., eds. Diet and disease in traditional and developing societies. Cambridge: Cambridge University Press; 1990: 24-61.

57. Spurr, G.B. Physical activity and energy expenditure in undernutrition. Prog. Food Nutr. Sci. 14:139-192; 1990.

58. Stern, M.P.; Patterson, J.K.; Mitchell, B.D.; Haffner, S.M.; Hazuda, H.P. Overweight and mortality in Mexican Americans. Inter. J. Obes. 14:623-629; 1990.

59. Strong, J.P.; McGill, H.C., Jr. The pediatric aspects of atherosclerosis. J. Atheroscler. Res. 9:251-265; 1969.

60. Strong, W.B.; Dennison, B.A. Pediatric preventive cardiology: atherosclerosis and coronary heart disease. Pediatr. Rev. 9:303-314; 1988.

61. Task Force on Blood Pressure Control in Children. Report of the second task force on blood pressure control in children—1987. Pediatrics 79:1-25; 1987.

62. Torun, B. Incremento de la actividad fisica mediante mejoria del estado nutricional. Arch. Latinoam. Nutr. 19:308-326; 1989.

63. Viteri, F.E.; Torun, B. Nutrition, physical activity, and growth. In: Ritzen, M.; Aperia, A.; Hall, K.; Larsson, A.; Zetterberg, A.; Zetterstein, R., eds. The biology of normal human growth. New York: Raven Press; 1981:265-273.

64. United Nations Development Program. Human development report 1991. New York: Oxford University Press; 1993.

65. World Bank. Investing in health: world development indicators (World Development Report 1993). New York: Oxford University Press; 1993.

Chapter 14

A North American Perspective on Physical Activity Research in Children and Adolescents

James F. Sallis, PhD

Concepts from the field of behavioral epidemiology are used to organize a summary of pediatric physical activity research focusing on studies from North America. In traditional epidemiology, the distribution and etiology of diseases are studied. In behavioral epidemiology, the distribution and etiology of behaviors that are believed to be linked with health are studied.

Ideally, research in behavioral epidemiology follows a sequence of three phases. In phase 1, associations of the behavior in question with health outcomes are examined to determine the health benefits and risks of the behavior. If the behavior is found to be related to important health outcomes, then the focus changes and the behavior becomes the dependent variable rather than the independent variable. In phase 2, the goal is to learn about the distribution and etiology of the behavior itself. In physical activity research, questions such as these are asked: How active are children? and What factors influence activity level? If the influences, or determinants, of the behavior can be identified, these factors can be modified in attempts to change the behavior in phase 3. Thus, studies of behavior change interventions constitute phase 3 behavioral epidemiology. In concept, each phase provides useful information for the next phase.

In the field of child physical activity, research is ongoing in all three phases, though it is most advanced in phase 1. In this chapter, I have briefly summarized each phase of behavioral epidemiology research related to child and adolescent physical activity, emphasizing North American studies. Key research issues are identified.

Phase 1: The Association Between Physical Activity and Health Indicators

Studies linking physical activity in childhood with health indicators provide information used to set priorities for physical activity research and intervention efforts by health professionals, policy makers, and other researchers. Understanding the health-related effects of physical activity in children is complicated by the number of physiological systems that are affected. Physical activity may be related to a number of chronic diseases and acute conditions, and the strength of association is likely to vary for different conditions.

Physical activity may affect both the current and future health of children and adolescents (4). Any effects on infectious diseases, mood or other psychological states, or musculoskeletal injuries are considered relevant to morbidities in childhood. However, more attention has been paid to the potential for physical activity in youth to inhibit the development of chronic diseases, such as cardiovascular diseases (CVD). This concern has led to studies of the association between childhood physical activity and physiological risk factors for CVD, such as serum lipids, blood pressure, obesity, and cardiovascular fitness. Because skeletal development in youth is believed to be related to risk for osteoporosis in later life, the effects of physical activity on skeletal health has become an active area of study.

Recently, studies on the association between physical activity and seven health outcomes were reviewed for the adolescent age group, defined as ages 11 to 21 years. The results of the International Consensus Conference on Physical Activity Guidelines for Adolescents (41) are summarized. The review papers were written by pairs of leading scientists who identified the highest quality studies and summarized their findings at a conference in San Diego, California, in June 1993. The goal was not only to determine whether an association existed between physical activity and the health outcome, but also to recommend an amount of physical activity that would be expected to lead to an improved level of the health outcome in question. For some health outcomes, the research was not sufficient to support specific recommendations.

Cardiovascular fitness is a predictor of total mortality in adults, and it may mediate several health effects in adults and youth (27). The association between physical activity and cardiorespiratory fitness has been frequently studied in adolescents, and fitness is influenced by numerous other factors. Reported associations varied widely, but the typical correlation was approximately .20, accounting for only 4% of the variance. Thus, in the studies to date, physical activity has been definitely related to fitness in adolescents, but the association is weak. The intensity of physical activity required to increase cardiovascular fitness in adolescents is probably higher than in adults.

It is likely that risk of osteoporosis in later life could be reduced by enhancing peak bone mass through physical activity in adolescence (3). Approximately 20 studies of varying designs were reviewed, and active adolescents showed evidence of better bone health than more sedentary peers at most of the bone sites examined. For skeletal health it was recommended that weight-bearing activities that work all large muscle groups be done on a frequent basis. Individual bones must be stressed to promote greater mass, so a variety of activities were needed for overall bone health. The duration of the activity, however, did not seem as important as the frequency. Both vigorous aerobic activities and anaerobic activities, such as resistance training, appeared to be effective in increasing bone mass.

Studies of the association between physical activity and adiposity in adolescents were conflicting, in part because some studies assessed physical activity behavior and others estimated energy expenditure, which is confounded with body size (6). Physical training in the general adolescent population can lead to a modest reduction in body fat and a small increase in fat free mass. Physical activity programs for the obese were most successful when the intervention continued for more than 1 year and when lifestyle activities were emphasized over regimented activities. Reductions in body fat due to physical activity in the obese were modest. The minimum activity dose could not be determined for either obese or non-obese adolescents, but the combination of calorie restrictions and almost daily physical activity are probably needed for meaningful decreases in adiposity in adolescents.

There are many mechanisms by which physical activity could reduce blood pressure, and many studies have been conducted with adolescents (1). Both observational and intervention studies indicated that the association between resting blood pressure and physical activity was either very weak or nonexistent in the general population of adolescents. Thus, normotensive adolescents were unlikely to reduce their blood pressure further through physical activity. For adolescents at or above the 90th percentile for age and sex, studies consistently found physical activity effective in reducing blood pressure. While the reductions were clinically meaningful, "normal" blood pressures were not attained, on average. Elevated blood pressures can be decreased in adolescents by exercising at 60% of maximum heart rate for at least 30 minutes three times per week. At least 3 months of training were required for a detectable effect.

In adults, an association between physical activity and HDL-cholesterol has been found with relative consistency, but in adolescents the studies have mixed results (2). Experimental studies with adolescents in the general population did not show increased HDL-cholesterol after training, but observational studies generally found significant associations. As with blood pressure, the association between physical activity and HDL-cholesterol in adolescents was weak. A few studies of obese adolescents and adolescents with family histories of heart disease found that physical activity was effective in increasing HDL-cholesterol in these high-risk groups.

One of the surprises of the consensus conference was the comparatively strong evidence linking physical activity with psychological health in adolescents (8). About 12 studies examined the association in general population samples using the most valid available measures of depression, anxiety/stress, and self-esteem/self-concept. Most of the studies showed significant associations, and the average effect size of .40 indicated a moderate-strength relationship. Several randomized trials suggested that significant psychological benefits were obtained by clinically "normal" adolescents after 10 to 15 weeks of training at 70% of maximum heart rate for 20 minutes three times per week. There were too few studies on clinical samples of adolescents to support any conclusions on the effect of physical activity on clinical disorders.

One of the concerns about promoting physical activity was that an increase in musculoskeletal injuries could be a negative side effect. While injuries are the most frequent cause of death in adolescence, physical activity and sports account for only about 5% of mortality from injuries (23). Musculoskeletal injuries during the growing years were of concern, because damage to the growth plates in long bones could have permanent effects. However, growth plate injuries were rare. No data could be found on rates or risk factors for recreational injuries in adolescents. Injury rates for high school and college team sports suggested that football and wrestling may be among the most risky sports. The available data on the risk for injuries due to physical activity in adolescents were inadequate to support further conclusions.

Physical Activity Guidelines for Adolescents

Based on the systematic review of the literature on the health effects of physical activity among adolescents, two physical activity guidelines were developed.

> *Guideline 1:* All adolescents should be physically active daily or nearly every day, as part of play, games, sports, work, transportation, recreation, physical education, or planned exercise, in the context of family, school, and community activities.
>
> Adolescents should do a variety of physical activities as part of their daily lifestyles. These activities should be enjoyable, involve a variety of muscle groups, and include some weight bearing activities. The intensity or duration of the activity is probably less important than the fact that energy is expended and a habit of daily activity is established. Adolescents are encouraged to incorporate physical activity into their lifestyles by doing such things as walking up stairs, walking or riding a bicycle for errands, having conversations while walking with friends, parking at the far end of parking lots, or doing household chores. (41)

There was considerable discussion of the need to quantify the amount of time for daily activity, but the data did not support a specific recommendation. However, the U.S. National Health Promotion and Disease Prevention Objectives (48) and the guidelines from the U.S. Centers for Disease Control and American College of Sports Medicine (9) recommend 30 minutes per day of physical activity, and this is a reasonable minimum for adolescents as well.

> *Guideline 2:* In addition to daily lifestyle activities, three or more sessions per week of activities lasting 20 minutes or more at a time, that require moderate to vigorous levels of exertion, are recommended.
>
> Moderate to vigorous activities are those that require at least as much effort as brisk or fast walking. A diversity of activities that use large muscle groups are recommended as part of sports, recreation, chores, transportation, work, school physical education, or planned exercise. Examples include brisk walking, jogging, stair climbing, basketball, racquet sports, soccer, dance, swimming laps, skating, strength (resistance) training, lawn mowing, strenuous housework, cross country skiing, and cycling. (41)

There is specific evidence in adolescence that this level of physical activity enhances psychological health, increases cardiorespiratory fitness, and may increase HDL-cholesterol. The two primary guidelines apply to the general population of adolescents. However, some subgroups, such as the obese and those with elevated blood pressure, can be expected to obtain additional benefits from regular physical activity. These guidelines also apply to adolescents with physical impairments or other needs, but specific subgroups may require special assistance to become more active.

One of the critical limitations of this literature is that few studies investigated the types and amounts of physical activity that were needed to produce health benefits in adolescents. More specific dose-response information is needed so that studies of physical activity determinants and interventions can examine the types of activity most closely associated with health outcomes. For several of the health outcomes reviewed for the conference, few studies of the relationship with physical activity in adolescence could be found, yet many other suspected health effects have not been investigated at all. Thus, there is a need to diversify phase 1 studies. Another critical gap in the literature is that the health effects of physical activity on younger children are poorly understood. Studies are needed across the entire child and adolescent age range. The SCAN projects (Studies of Children's Activity and Nutrition) in the United States are providing information on the health effects of physical activity in preschool children (12,17).

In summary, physical activity has important effects on physical and psychological health in adolescents. Through its effects on risk factors for CVD and osteoporosis, physical activity in adolescence has the potential to reduce risk for these adult diseases. It is reasonable to conclude that physical activity is an important health-related behavior in adolescence, so it is justified to consider phase 2 and phase 3 behavioral epidemiology studies.

Phase 2: Distribution and Etiology of Physical Activity in Youth

Descriptive Epidemiology of Physical Activity in Youth

Problems in measuring physical activity in children and adolescents constrain the ability to describe types and amounts of physical activity in populations of young people. In a recent review of the descriptive epidemiology of physical activity in children aged 6 to 18 years, nine studies that examined at least two age groups were located (36). Only four of the studies were from North America, and three of the four studies with objective measures were European. Though these studies do not permit accurate estimates to be made of levels of physical activity, they do permit comparisons by age and sex.

Two conclusions can be drawn from these results. First, males were consistently more active than females. Self-report measures suggested males were 14% more active, while objective measures (primarily heart rate monitoring) indicated a 23% difference between sexes.

The second conclusion was that physical activity declined during childhood and adolescence, and the decline was greater in females. Though studies varied in their estimates, the average decline in physical activity was 2 to 3% per year for males and 3 to 7% per year for females. These data suggest that during the school ages of 6 to 18, boys decrease their activity by at least 24% and girls decrease their activity by at least 36%. Interventions appear to be needed to halt the age-related decline in physical activity, especially among girls.

Pate, Long, and Heath (30) reviewed recent data and estimated how many adolescents were meeting the physical activity guidelines. The various studies reported means ranging from 30 to 120 minutes in some type of physical activity per day. Therefore, the majority of adolescents, perhaps as many as 80%, appeared to be active at least 30 minutes per day.

Guideline 2 calls for more structured moderate to vigorous physical activity three or more times per week. National data from the U.S. indicate that three-quarters of boys and fewer than half adolescent girls meet this criterion. Interventions to promote regular moderate to vigorous physical activity in adolescents are needed, but further descriptive data are required for younger children.

Determinants of Physical Activity in Youth

Explaining variation in human behavior is inherently interesting, so studying the determinants of physical activity has value as basic science. This research also has practical value. The applied goal of research to identify influences on, or determinants of, physical activity is to discover the mechanisms by which the behavior is controlled. The assumption is that when those mechanisms are known, they can be targeted for change through intervention programs. If the determinants are altered, then the behavior should change. To be effective, interventions must change the most powerful determinants.

Because of the unlimited number of potential influences on children's physical activity, it is essential to start with a conceptual framework. An array of theories and models to explain physical activity have been used as the basis of determinants research (10,19). An adequate model must be broad, because significant associations have been found between physical activity and biological factors, psychological factors, social and cultural factors, and physical environment factors. These studies have recently been reviewed (42).

Biological factors that have been associated with physical activity in children include heredity (32), sex, and obesity. Sex differences in activity level have been most thoroughly studied, but it is not known whether the primary mechanism for the boys' higher activity levels is biological, such as motor skills, or due to differences in socialization.

A wide array of psychological variables have been examined for associations with physical activity. Because of the cognitive demands of the self-report measures, most of this research has been conducted with adolescents. Personality traits are unrelated to physical activity level or sports participation. Knowledge of the health effects of physical activity is also unrelated to the behavior (29), which implies that interventions based on providing information will be ineffec-tive. Attitudes or beliefs about the effects of physical activity are usually associ-ated with the behavior, but the strength of the relationship is weak to moderate.

Three types of psychological variables are consistently and strongly related to physical activity in adolescents. First, self-efficacy, or specific ratings of confi-dence to participate in physical activity, is one of the few variables of any kind to prospectively predict physical activity in adolescents (33). Second, ratings of intentions to be active are associated with actual physical activity (15). Third, perceptions of specific barriers to activity, such as time constraints, are related to participation (47). Because it appears adolescents can identify levels of personal confidence and intentions to be active and can even specify the factors that prevent them from being more active, these psychological variables may have applications in interventions. Based on ratings of self-efficacy, behavioral inten-tions, and barriers, a tailored plan could be developed to meet the personal needs of the adolescent.

Social and cultural factors are expected to play key roles in youth physical activity, but research is just starting to investigate the strength of social influences. Though Anglo-American children have been found to be more physically active than Mexican-American (25) and African-American children (16), it is likely that these apparent ethnic differences actually reflect socioeconomic differences (16). Family influences on children's physical activity have been the most fre-quently studied social factors. Most studies show that family members, especially parents, influence children's activity levels through verbal encouragement (21), modeling of physical activity (26), constraining activity through rules (40), and supportive actions such as transporting children to places where they can be active (37). There are probably other mechanisms of family influence, but developmental theory posits that by adolescence, peers are more important influences on most behaviors than parents. Peer influences on physical activity, however, have been inadequately studied, and this is a high priority for continued work.

Factors in the physical environment are believed to be strong influences on children's physical activity, but there is little documentation of such effects. As expected, there are seasonal variations in physical activity (35), and children appear to be more active on the weekends when they are not sitting in school most of the day (43). The single strongest correlate of physical activity in young children is time spent outdoors (20,40), and access to play spaces is also related to amount of physical activity (40). Television viewing is widely believed to inhibit children's physical activity, but in most studies, viewing time is unrelated to habitual activity levels (34). More studies are needed of the environmental constraints and resources that influence children's ability to be active.

Research on the distribution and determinants of physical activity in youth is not very advanced. The lack of valid and practical measures of physical activity in youth is a major limitation in this research. However, new national surveillance efforts, such as the Youth Behavioral Risk Factor Surveillance System (22), will greatly improve the descriptive epidemiology of youth physical activity, despite problems in the accuracy of the measures. One of the challenges for the future is to obtain data on physical activity patterns across the entire age range of childhood and adolescence. In the determinants area, improved conceptual models of influences on physical activity are needed, and age-appropriate measures of hypothesized determinants must be developed and evaluated for children and adolescents. Physical activity determinants studies should focus on modifiable variables so the results are relevant for intervention development.

In summary, epidemiologic data suggest that most adolescents do some physical activity each day, but there is a need for most adolescents to increase their moderate to vigorous intensity activities. The research on determinants of physical activity in children and adolescents demonstrates that biological, psychological, social, and physical environmental variables are all important. Many of the identified influences are potentially modifiable. If there is no single major determinant of children's physical activity, it follows that effective interventions to promote children's activity will need to take several factors into consideration. No single strategy is likely to be successful. Program designers must consider how to promote children's confidence in their ability to be active, reduce perceived barriers, enhance social support from family and friends, and provide easy access to environments and programs that facilitate physical activity, while providing particular assistance to girls and the economically disadvantaged. How well have intervention designers met these challenges?

Phase 3: Promoting Physical Activity in Youth

Development of effective interventions for promoting physical activity in children and adolescents must begin with a clear conceptualization of desired outcomes. The available epidemiologic data suggest that most adolescents are meeting Guideline 1, which relates to doing some physical activity nearly every day. The intervention goal in this case is to ensure that this guideline continues to be met by most adolescents. Many adolescent females are not meeting Guideline 2 concerning three sessions per week of moderate to vigorous physical activity. Therefore, interventions are most needed to increase the proportion of adolescents who meet Guideline 2. Because of the age-related decline in activity, it can be assumed that more children than adolescents are meeting the guideline, but the exact percentages are unknown. Interventions are needed in adolescence to increase moderate to vigorous physical activity and/or in childhood to prevent the age-related decline to activity levels that do not meet Guideline 2.

The immediate goal of increasing moderate to vigorous physical activity among youth is justified because it will provide health benefits. However, the possibility that physical activity programs in youth could enhance the likelihood of maintaining regular activity through adulthood has more public health significance because of the close association of physical activity with CVD morbidity and mortality in adulthood. The goal of promoting the maintenance of physical activity is difficult, but intervention developers must start working toward this goal.

Principles of community interventions for health promotion (7,18) suggest that multi-site, multi-level programs are needed. Some programs provide information and skills to individuals and groups, while others foster environmental change by working with policy makers and community leaders. Three sites for interventions to promote youth physical activity are considered; schools, community settings, and primary health care. Parents and families can be involved in programs at any or all of these settings. Interventions in all sites need to address as many of the biological, psychological, social, and physical environmental factors that influence physical activity as appropriate.

Any serious effort to increase physical activity in children and adolescents must include a school component. The personnel and physical resources devoted to school physical education, while not satisfactory to many, are still extensive. The current challenge is to halt the deterioration of those resources and use the existing resources more effectively. Research that demonstrates behavioral, psychological, physiological, and academic benefits of improved physical education may play a role in increasing administrative support for quality physical education.

Observational studies demonstrate that physical education classes include limited opportunities for physical activity (14,44). The typical curriculum emphasizes sports skills more than activities that promote health-related fitness (38), so the curricula must be reformed. Interested professional groups have reached a consensus that school physical education should adopt health-related physical activity goals and prepare students for lifelong activity (38). Several studies have shown that active physical education leads to important physiological changes, while classroom-based educational programs typically do not result in physical activity or fitness improvements (42). However, no study has yet demonstrated maintenance of physical activity, so a combination of physical education and behavioral training in the classroom may be needed.

There is a clear need for staff development programs for both classroom teachers and physical education specialists to train them to provide students with more physical activity, in an enjoyable context, and to effectively implement new health-related curricula. Structured training programs with on-site follow-up have been shown to improve the teaching of both classroom teachers (24) and physical education specialists (45).

Two large studies are testing contemporary school-based physical activity promotion programs for elementary students. The acronym *SPARK* describes the project goals of Sports, Play, and Active Recreation for Kids. The SPARK curriculum combines a physical education program that promotes activity with a classroom-based self-management program that teaches behavior change skills relevant to generalizing and maintaining regular physical activity (39). There is some parent participation in the self-management program. Implementation by trained classroom teachers is compared to implementation by physical education specialists (24).

The second program is the Child and Adolescent Trial for Cardiovascular Health (31). CATCH is a multi-risk factor program that targets physical activity, dietary habits, and smoking. It is being conducted in four locations in the United States. Depending on the school district, either classroom teachers or physical education specialists are trained to implement the physical education curriculum. The classroom curriculum includes a physical activity component, and a strong parent involvement program is being evaluated.

Both of these studies include assessments of physical activity, physical fitness, and psychosocial variables believed to mediate changes in physical activity. Skills training in physical education is designed to enhance self-efficacy, and enjoyment of physical activity is stressed as a means of changing attitudes. Social factors are modified through self-management in SPARK and through parent involvement in CATCH. The physical environment is changed primarily through alterations in the physical education curriculum.

Children obtain the majority of their physical activity through organized activities outside school (35), so community organizations are already playing a role in promoting physical activity. However, the goals are to increase the time devoted to physical activity in youth programs and to increase the number of young people who participate. Though youth sports organizations are particularly relevant for present purposes, YMCAs, YWCAs, boys' and girls' clubs, scout groups, religious organizations, and social service agencies could also participate in the effort to increase children's physical activity. There is a special role for parks and recreation departments at all levels of government, because low income children must rely on public facilities and programs. No studies could be located that promoted physical activity in children or adolescents by intervening with community organizations.

A recent paper considered the role that primary health care providers could play in promoting physical activity in youth (11). Though there is virtually no research evaluating primary care interventions for this purpose, providers have the opportunity to intervene in several ways. Physical activity assessment and counseling should be considered part of an overall program for health maintenance. Primary care providers are expected to be highly credible sources of social influence regarding health matters such as physical activity. It is realistic for physicians, nurses, and other primary care providers to assess patients' physical activity patterns on a periodic basis and provide brief counseling that is appropriate to each patient's needs. Primary care providers are well suited to deliver counseling that is consistent with the health status of the patient, if there are illnesses or disabilities to be considered. Health professionals can also be effective advocates for physical activity programs in schools and community organizations. The ability of health professionals to be effective change agents for their patients and in their communities now needs to be evaluated.

Parents can be involved in interventions in all settings, and several studies have evaluated family-based programs. When parents were trained to consistently reinforce their children's physical activity, the programs were highly successful. In studies of low-fit (46) and obese children (13), parents were given intensive instruction and support in reinforcing children, and the results were impressive. However, when programs have been attempted with healthy families using less intensive behavior change methods, family interventions have not been effective (5,28). Thus, one generalization that can be derived from both the school-based and family-based interventions is that when children are essentially required to be active as part of physical education classes or by their parents, children receive the benefits of increased physical activity. However, when educational or behavior change programs do not require physical activity, they have been consistently ineffective. Efforts to generalize and maintain physical activity in children and adolescents have not been effective, so more work is needed in this area.

Conclusion

Concepts from behavioral epidemiology were used to organize a discussion of the status of research on physical activity and health in children and adolescents. Phase 1 research indicated that physical activity provides important health benefits for adolescents, and the positive effects far outweigh the risks. More research is needed on the effects of physical activity on children. Physical activity's effects on CVD risk factors may have some implications for prevention of CVD in adulthood, but there is no direct evidence to support this hypothesis. The data were sufficient to support specific guidelines for physical activity for all adolescents.

Phase 2 research showed that most children and adolescents were meeting the first guideline related to some physical activity nearly every day. Because of an age-related decline in physical activity during childhood and adolescence, which is particularly steep for females, many adolescents are not meeting the second guideline of participating in moderate to vigorous physical activity at least three times per week.

The influences on physical activity in youth are poorly understood, but it is known that numerous biological, psychological, social, and physical environment factors are important. Many of the influences that have been identified are modifiable, so this information can be used to guide the design of intervention programs.

Few systematic attempts to promote physical activity in youth have been evaluated. The studies to date show that when physical activity is required in school physical education or by parents trained in behavior modification, physical activity increases and physiological changes are seen. However, purely educational programs are not effective, and generalization outside school or maintenance beyond the end of the intervention has not been convincingly demonstrated. These results suggest that more sophisticated behavior change programs are needed. Furthermore, the only effective method of increasing children's physical activity is to require it, although promoting active lifestyles by enhancing intrinsic motivation would be preferable. The health benefits of physical activity in youth, however, may justify external control of physical activity until more effective methods of teaching children to manage their own physical activity are demonstrated.

References

1. Alpert, B.S.; Wilmore, J.H. Physical activity and blood pressure in adolescents. Ped. Exerc. Sci. 6:361-380; 1994.
2. Armstrong, N.; Simons-Morton, B. Physical activity and blood lipids in adolescents. Ped. Exerc. Sci. 6:381-405; 1994.
3. Bailey, D.A.; Martin, A.D. Physical activity and skeletal health in adolescents. Ped. Exerc. Sci. 6:330-347; 1994.
4. Baranowski, T.; Bouchard, C.; Bar-Or, O.; Bricker, T.; Heath, G.; Kimm, S.Y.S.; Malina, R.; Obarzanek, E.; Pate, R.; Strong, W.B.; Truman, B.; Washington, R. Assessment, prevalence, and cardiovascular benefits of physical activity and fitness in youth. Med. Sci. Sports Exerc. 24:S237-S247; 1992.
5. Baranowski, T.; Simons-Morton, B.; Hooks, P; Henske, J.; Tiernan, K.; Dunn, J.K.; Burkhalter, H.; Harper, J.; Palmer, J. A center-based program for exercise change among black-American families. Health Educ. Quart. 17:169-196; 1990.
6. Bar-Or, O.; Baranowski, T. Physical activity, adiposity, and obesity among adolescents. Ped. Exerc. Sci. 6:348-360; 1994.
7. Bracht, N., ed. Health promotion at the community level. Newbury Park, CA: Sage; 1990.
8. Calfas, K.J.; Taylor, W.C. Effects of physical activity on psychological variables in adolescents. Ped. Exerc. Sci. 6:406-423; 1994.
9. Centers for Disease Control and Prevention. Prevalence of sedentary lifestyle: behavioral risk factor surveillance system, United States, 1991. Morbid. Mortal. Weekly Rep. 42:576-579; 1993.
10. Dishman, R.K.; Dunn, A.L. Exercise adherence in children and youth: implications for adulthood. In: Dishman, R.K., ed. Exercise adherence: Its impact on public health. Champaign, IL: Human Kinetics; 1988: 155-200.
11. DuRant, R.H.; Hergenroeder, A.C. Promotion of physical activity among adolescents by primary health care providers. Ped. Exerc. Sci. 6:448-463; 1994.
12. Eck, L.H.; Klesges, R.C.; Hanson, C.L.; Slawson, D. Children at familial risk for obesity: an examination of dietary intake, physical activity, and weight status. Internat. J. Obesity 16:71-78; 1992.
13. Epstein, L.H.; Wing, R.R.; Koeske, R.; Ossip, D.J.; Beck, S. A comparison of lifestyle change and programmed aerobic exercise on weight and fitness changes in obese children. Behav. Ther. 13:651-665; 1982.
14. Faucette, N.; McKenzie, T.L.; Patterson, P. Descriptive analysis of nonspecialist elementary physical education teachers' curricular choices and class organization. J. Teaching Phys. Educ. 9:284-293; 1990.
15. Godin, G.; Shephard, R.J. Psychosocial factors influencing intentions to exercise of young students from grades 7 to 9. Res. Q. Exerc. Sport 57:41-52; 1986.
16. Gottlieb, N.H.; Chen, M. Sociocultural correlates of childhood sporting activities: their implications for heart health. Soc. Sci. Med. 21:533-539; 1986.
17. Gutin, B.; Basch, C.; Shea, S.; Contento, I.; DeLozier, M.; Rips, J.; Irigoyen, M.; Zybert, P. Blood pressure, fitness, and fatness in 5- and 6-year-old children. J. Am. Med. Assoc. 264:1123-1127; 1990.
18. King, A.C. Community intervention for promotion of physical activity and fitness. Exerc. Sport Sci. Rev. 19:211-259; 1991.
19. King, A.C.; Blair, S.N.; Bild, D.E.; Dishman, R.K.; Dubbert, P.M.; Marcus, B.H.; Oldridge, N.B.; Paffenbarger, R.S.; Powell, K.E.; Yeager, K.K. Determinants of physical activity and interventions in adults. Med. Sci. Sports Exerc. 24:S221-S236; 1992.
20. Klesges, R.C.; Eck, L.H.; Hanson, C.L.; Haddock, C.K.; Klesges, L.M. The effects of obesity, social interactions, and the physical environment on physical activity in preschool children. Health Psychol. 9:435-449; 1990.

21. Klesges, R.C.; Malott, J.M.; P.F. Boschee; Weber, J.M. The effects of parental influences on children's food intake, physical activity, and relative weight. Internat. J. Eating Disord. 5:335-346; 1986.

22. Kolbe, L.J. An epidemiological surveillance system to monitor the prevalence of youth behaviors that most affect health. Health Educ. 21:44-48; 1990.

23. Macera, C.; Wooten, W.J. Epidemiology of sports and recreation injuries among adolescents. Ped. Exerc. Sci. 6:424-433; 1994.

24. McKenzie, T.L.; Sallis, J.F.; Faucette, N.; Kolody, B. Effects of a curriculum and inservice program on the quantity and quality of elementary physical education classes. Res. Q. Exerc. Sport 64:178-187; 1993.

25. McKenzie, T.L.; Sallis, J.F.; Nader, P.R.; Broyles, S.L.; Nelson, J.A. Anglo- and Mexican-American preschoolers at home and at recess: activity patterns and environmental influences. J. Develop. Behav. Pediat. 13:173-180; 1992.

26. Moore, L.L.; Lombardi, D.A.; White M.J.; Campbell, J.L.; Oliveria, S.A.; Ellison, R.C. Influence of parents' physical activity levels on activity levels of young children. J. Pediatr. 118:215-219; 1991.

27. Morrow, J.R.; Freedson, P.S. Relationship between habitual physical activity and aerobic fitness in adolescents. Ped. Exerc. Sci. 6:315-329; 1994.

28. Nader, P.R.; Sallis, J.F.; Abramson, I.S.; Broyles, S.L.; Patterson, T.L.; Senn, K.; Rupp, J.W.; Nelson, J.A. Family-based cardiovascular risk reduction education among Mexican- and Anglo-Americans. Fam. Comm. Health 15:57-74; 1992.

29. O'Connell, J.K.; Price, J.H.; Roberts, S.M.; Jurs, S.G.; McKinley, R. Utilizing the health belief model to predict dieting and exercising behavior of obese and nonobese adolescents. Health Educ. Q. 12:343-351; 1985.

30. Pate, R.R.; Long, B.J.; Heath, G. Descriptive epidemiology of physical activity in adolescents. Ped. Exerc. Sci. 6:434-447; 1994.

31. Perry, C.L.; Stone, E.J.; Parcel, G.S.; Ellison, R.C.; Nader, P.R.; Webber, L.S.; Luepker, R.V. School-based cardiovascular health promotion: the child and adolescent trial for cardiovascular health (CATCH). J. School Health 60:406-413; 1990.

32. Perusse, L.; Tremblay, A.; LeBlanc, C.; Bouchard, C. Genetic and familial environmental influences on level of habitual physical activity. Am. J. Epidemiol. 129:1012-1022; 1989.

33. Reynolds, K.D.; Killen, J.D.; Bryson, S.W.; Maron, D.J.; Taylor, C.B.; Maccoby, N.; Farquhar, J.W. Psychosocial predictors of physical activity in adolescents. Prev. Med. 19:541-551; 1990.

34. Robinson, T.N.; Hammer, L.D.; Killen, J.D.; Kraemer, H.C.; Wilson, D.M.; Hayward, C.; Taylor, C.B. Does television viewing increase obesity and reduce physical activity? Cross-sectional and longitudinal analyses among adolescent girls. Pediat. 91:273-280; 1993.

35. Ross, J.G.; Dotson, C.O.; Gilbert, G.G.; Katz, S.J. After physical education . . . Physical activity outside of school physical education programs. J. Phys. Educ. Recreat. Dance 56(1):35-39; 1985.

36. Sallis, J.F. Epidemiology of physical activity and fitness in children and adolescents. Crit. Rev. Food Sci. Nutr. 33:403-408; 1993.

37. Sallis, J.F.; Alcaraz, J.E.; McKenzie, T.L.; Hovell, M.F.; Kolody, B.; Nader, P. Parent behavior in relation to physical activity and fitness in 9-year-old children. Am. J. Dis. Child. 146:1383-1388; 1992.

38. Sallis, J.F.; McKenzie, T.L. Physical education's role in public health. Res. Q. Exerc. Sport 62:124-137; 1991.

39. Sallis, J.F.; McKenzie, T.L.; Alcaraz, J.E.; Kolody, B.; Hovell, M.F.; Nader, P.R. Project SPARK: effects of physical education on adiposity in children. Ann. N.Y. Acad. Sci. 699:127-136; 1993.

40. Sallis, J.F.; Nader, P.R.; Broyles, S.L.; Berry, C.C.; Elder, J.P.; McKenzie, T.L.; Nelson, J.A. Correlates of physical activity at home in Mexican-American and Anglo-American preschool children. Health Psychol. 12:390-398; 1993.

41. Sallis, J.F.; Patrick, K. Physical activity guidelines for adolescents: consensus statement. Ped. Exerc. Sci. 6:302-314; 1994.
42. Sallis, J.F.; Simons-Morton, B.G.; Stone, E.J.; Corbin, C.B.; Epstein, L.H.; Faucette, N.; Iannotti, R.J.; Killen, J.D.; Klesges, R.C.; Petray, C.K.; Rowland, T.W.; Taylor, W.C. Determinants of physical activity and interventions in youth. Med. Sci. Sports Exerc. 24:S248-S257; 1992.
43. Shephard, R.J.; Jequier, J.C.; LaVallee, H.; LaBarre, R.; Rajic, M. Habitual physical activity: effects of sex, milieu, season, and required activity. J. Sports Med. Phys. Fitness 20:55-66, 1980.
44. Simons-Morton, B.G.; Taylor, W.C.; Snider, S.A.; Huang, I.W. The physical activity of fifth-grade students during physical education. Am. J. Public Health 83:262-265; 1993.
45. Simons-Morton, B.G.; Parcel, G.S.; Baranowski, T.; Forthoffer, R.; O'Hara, N.M. Promoting healthful diet and physical activity among children: results of a school-based intervention study. Am. J. Public Health 81:986-991; 1991.
46. Taggart, A.C.; Taggart, J.; Siedentop, D. Effects of a home-based activity program: a study with low-fitness elementary school children. Behav. Modif. 10:487-507; 1986.
47. Tappe, M.K.; Duda, J.L.; Ehrnwald, P.M. Perceived barriers to exercise among adolescents. J. School Health 59:153-155; 1989.
48. U.S. Department of Health and Human Services. Healthy people 2000: national health promotion and disease prevention objectives. DHHS Pub. No. (PHS) 91-50212. Washington, DC: U.S. Government Printing Office; 1991.

Chapter 15

The Canadian Inuit: Studies of a Population Undergoing Rapid Acculturation

Roy J. Shephard, MD, PhD, DPE, and Andris Rode, PhD

A substantial proportion of the Canadian Inuit are now concentrated in the major urban center of Iqualuit, formerly known to southerners as Frobisher Bay. This has become the administrative headquarters and air transportation hub for the eastern arctic. However, traditional Inuit culture was based on much smaller settlements, often only 100 people. These were geographically and even genetically isolated from each other, making it difficult to describe the Inuit as a single group. The present paper offers a 20 year panorama of physical activity, growth, and cardiovascular health of young Inuit living in one of the more isolated settlements, Igloolik (69°40'N; 81°W), a small island near the tip of the Melville Peninsula. At the beginning of our observations (in 1969-70) there were 533 inhabitants, and the population has approximately doubled over the two subsequent decades.

The settlement was one of three circumpolar communities selected for study by the International Biological Program (IBP) in the mid-1960s (6,18). The overall philosophy of the IBP was that specialized populations such as the !Kung bush-dwellers and circumpolar Inuit were rapidly becoming acculturated to the dominant societies of urban civilizations, but that there was still a brief opportunity to collect benchmark data on traditional lifestyles and to determine how adaptation to a variety of physically challenging habitats had been achieved (25). The three circumpolar communities (Upernavik, Greenland; Igloolik, N.W.T.; and Wainwright, Alaska) were chosen as representative of progressive stages in acculturation. More recently (11) this data has been supplemented by repeat observations in Igloolik (1979-80, 1989-90) and by parallel observations on nGanasan and Dolgans living in the Volochanka region of Russia (14). All five of the circumpolar populations that we have studied have a distant common ancestry in outer Mongolia, but they have lived in relative isolation in their present communities for perhaps 800 years.

Activity, Growth, and Cardiovascular Health in 1969-70

Sociocultural Status

The initial physiological studies of Igloolik were undertaken in 1969-70 (7). Acculturation had already begun by the time that the IBP study was launched.

The last Inuit family had moved from tents and igloos into a permanent prefabricated bungalow, built by the Federal government, in the winter of 1969-70. A small airstrip had been built, and in good weather light aircraft were flying a Class C service one to two times per week from Iqualuit. An eight-grade school had been established in the village, and there was a choice of an Anglican or a Roman Catholic church to attend. Some 500 dogs were still kept by local hunters, but about 30 families had already purchased snowmobiles, and some 20 boats had been equipped with outboard motors. A substantial number of the men in the village were still hunting regularly for meat, fish, eggs, and furs, but two stores were providing 60 to 70% of the food energy requirements of the community.

Activity Patterns

As might be expected from the extremes of climate encountered in the Igloolik region, patterns of physical activity showed a tremendous seasonal variation (5). No one month could be considered representative of the whole year.

Children spent much of their leisure time playing the traditional Inuit games and learning tasks important to their later survival, such as ice fishing and handling miniature dog teams (4,17). In the summer months of perpetual daylight, such activities continued for much of the night. A weekly cinema show in the village hall offered further suggestions for active play, as the children mimicked the strange exploits of cowboys and Indians. Older children were frequently absent from school, as they accompanied their fathers on hunting trips.

Activities around the village demanded a high level of energy expenditure for much of the year. In winter and spring, walking was over deep snow drifts, encumbered by heavy clothing, and in summer there were rough, rocky hills to climb in search of birds' eggs. Many of the older girls added to their basic energy expenditure the cost of carrying a younger brother or sister on their backs throughout the day in the traditional *amauti*.

During the spring and early summer months, entire families migrated to their favorite hunting areas on Baffin Island or the mainland. There, they pursued communal activities related to the harvesting of seals and caribou, including butchering meat and preparing skins. Television had not reached the village. We did not make any direct measurements of daily energy expenditures on the children, but our impression (substantiated by data collected on their parents) was that it was high (5).

Growth Patterns

Growth patterns in 1969-70 were assessed by both cross-sectional data and by semi-longitudinal measurements repeated after the elapse of one year. We attempted to determine the breakpoints for the growth curves by the fitting of polynomials to the semi-longitudinal data (8), although the number of data points was rather limited for this purpose. We estimated that the maximal growth in height was reached at 13.3 years in the boys, with no clear maximum in the girls. Corresponding values for body mass were 13.8 and 12.8 years.

Because the girls continued to perform hard physical work during their adolescence, they not only became taller, but also had a greater leg strength than the boys between 11 and 14 years of age.

Cardiovascular Health

Before we consider details of physical growth and cardiovascular health in 1969-70, it is important to underline constraints of sampling and measurement technology which have marred much circumpolar research, as in studies of other remote and inaccessible locations.

Population Sampling

Published reports commonly describe findings on a convenience sample of perhaps 10 young and 10 older adults. No effort is made to establish the total population from which subjects have been drawn, and no tests are made to assess whether the selected individuals are representative of the community under study (18). A priori, it seems likely that there will be a bias toward the inclusion of people who are the most acculturated, speak the most English, and have had the greatest contact with urban civilization. In a locale such as Igloolik, where the traditional Inuit are frequently absent from the village on long hunting trips, there will be an active exclusion of such families from the sample, unless investigators live in the village for a long period and make systematic attempts to recruit such people.

Studies that focus on fitness and exercise testing also tend to attract the healthier members of the community, whereas studies with a medical focus recruit those with chronic disease. Remote communities sometimes have a high prevalence of conditions such as tuberculosis, with potential adverse effects on many facets of cardiorespiratory function. For these reasons, some early studies concluded that the North American Inuit did not have a particularly high level of cardiorespiratory fitness (20).

We were able to attract some 85% of children and adolescents over the age of 10 years to our study, a much larger sample of Inuit children than had ever been evaluated. Despite relatively complete sampling of the villagers in all age groups, the findings for adults at least showed some evidence of biased averages relative to data collected by medical investigators during the same year (18); the medical team saw a larger proportion of the older adults with advanced tuberculosis and fewer of the fit individuals. Nevertheless, the percentage recruitment was age-related, at least for the physiologists, and selective sampling was a much smaller problem in children than in older adults.

Test Methodology

A second reason why some authors have reported normal or low fitness scores among the Inuit is the use of an inadequate test methodology. Sometimes there has been insufficient motivation to all-out effort. Many tests of cardiorespiratory function require all-out physical effort, and such intensive, competitive activity is a foreign concept to the Inuit culture of cooperation and patience in the face of adverse conditions. Sometimes observers have had difficulties in communicating test requirements. Functional testing cannot be conducted satisfactorily through an interpreter, but many investigators have failed to master sufficient Inuktittuk or other local dialect to enable them to communicate procedures to the volunteers. Sometimes the equipment has been inadequate because it is a costly undertaking to fly the equipment of a modern laboratory, including the necessary voltage and frequency stabilizers, to a remote settlement. Finally, there have been attempts to transpose concepts originally developed in urban settings to the interpretation of data collected in remote areas. For example, height or body mass standardization is usual when interpreting cardiorespiratory data in urban children (19). However, heights differ between the Inuit and southern Canadians. The adult height of the Igloolik population is some 10 cm shorter than that of Torontonians (13), and the leg length of the Igloolik population is a little shorter in relation to trunk length. Furthermore, older adolescents and young adults commonly develop a 3 to 5 cm shortening of stature, apparently because the vertebral column is compressed by the repeated operation of high-speed snowmobiles for long distances over very rough terrain (23). Because the skeletal muscles are well developed, they may account for an increased proportion of the total body mass (20), thus invalidating the usual calculations of ponderal index. Skinfold equations developed on urban populations also give poor predictions of body density and body fat content (14); the greater muscularity and lesser calcification of the bones reduces the overall density of the lean tissue compartment in the Inuit, and a higher proportion of the body fat also seems to be carried internally (21). Finally, because of the Inuit's lack of familiarity with bicycles, the mechanical efficiency of such exercise may be less than is assumed in the norms associated with such testing in an urban environment (9).

Cardiorespiratory Fitness

The skinfold thicknesses of the Inuit, as measured by Lange calipers, were much less than that of the population in southern Canada in 1969-70—indeed, in the younger children, there was almost no subcutaneous fat after allowing for the thickness of a double fold of skin (7). The children were, nevertheless, well-nourished and had normal hemoglobin levels. However, the findings must be interpreted with some caution, because our studies with deuterated water suggested that the proportion of internal fat was greater than that of the population in urban societies (21).

Aerobic power was predicted generally from the performance of a progressive double step submaximal test (15) using a computerized version of the Åstrand nomogram (16). Oxygen consumption was measured directly (to avoid problems from an atypical mechanical efficiency), and in a proportion of subjects the assumptions inherent in the Åstrand nomogram were verified by direct maximal testing. The results showed extremely high average aerobic powers, particularly in the boys, throughout childhood and adolescence (7). We took the unusual precaution of making a biological calibration of our equipment and procedures, using a panel of southern Canadians who had also been tested in our Toronto laboratories, so that the findings could not be dismissed as arising through a technical aberration (18). In contrast to many white populations, the maximal oxygen intake (expressed in ml/[kg · min]) remained relatively stable at a high level into adulthood. The gender difference of about 25% was, nevertheless, at least as large as the gender difference in urban settings.

Quadriceps extension strength was measured by a Clark cable tensiometer system, commencing at a joint angle of 120°. Norms for this procedure depend greatly upon details of technique, but the values we obtained were greater than what we would have observed in children of the same age in Toronto. In contrast, handgrip force, measured with a Stoelting dynamometer, was unremarkable.

Lung volumes were well up to expected norms for urban societies. When cross-sectional data were plotted as a power function of stature, exponents for $FEV_{1.0}$ were close to 3.0, but those for FVC substantially exceeded 3.0 (10). Regrettably, cigarette smoking began early in adolescence; 50% of the boys were smoking regularly by the age of 15 to 16 years, and 50% of the girls were smoking regularly by 13 to 14 years (10).

Details about the prevalence of other cardiac risk factors during the 1970s remain sketchy and are drawn mainly from other traditional Inuit communities (1). Blood pressures tend to be low, and the adults rarely have heart attacks (although this is due in part to early deaths from accidents, other forms of violence, and infectious disease). The traditional diet contains large quantities of unsaturated fish oils (3), and the serum lipid profile compares favorably with that found in white Europeans (1) and Inuit who have moved to Montreal (2).

Physical Activity, Growth, and Cardiovascular Health in 1979-80 and 1989-90

Sociocultural Change

Many indigenous societies have witnessed a resurgence of pride in their cultural heritage over the past 2 decades. In some instances, this has precluded further scientific study of the community concerned. Thus, we have greatly appreciated the willingness of the Igloolik Hamlet Council to continue their generous support of our investigations. In 1979-80 we tested 75% of inhabitants between the ages of 10 and 20 years, and in 1989-90 we tested 76% of the male inhabitants under the age of 20 years, but only 49% of females in the same age bracket.

Despite a strong and growing ethnic pride over the two decades of study, the process of acculturation to the attitudes, habits, and behaviors of southern Canada has developed rapidly in the Canadian arctic. The Igloolik airstrip now boasts landing lights and a small terminal building, with 12 Schedule B flights each week to 6 destinations in the eastern arctic. Satellites provide the villagers with instant access to worldwide TV and telephone communication. The majority of children and young adults now have a substantial English vocabulary, and nearly every family has a relative or a friend who is living in the "outside" world. Many members of the community fly south regularly to visit such contacts, and pupils from the Igloolik school have paid an educational visit to Toronto.

Activity Patterns

Housing now provides hot and cold running water, indoor sanitation, a refrigerator, and an electric stove, which eliminate certain household chores such as the carrying of ice and sewage. Mechanization of the village has proceeded apace. By 1990 the village boasted 165 snowmobiles, a taxi service, 9 private cars and trucks, 78 all-terrain vehicles, 216 bicycles, and 90 motorboats. Because of the power of most snowmobiles and motorboats, hunting grounds that previously had been a day or more's journey away could now be reached in a few hours. The inhabitants even made short trips within the village in powered vehicles. However, because of the high price of gasoline, the majority of food was purchased at the village store with only occasional supplementation by hunting.

Other influences further modified community patterns of physical activity. The replacement of dog teams greatly reduced the heavy physical work demanded of older adolescent males in butchering, burying, and digging up 50 to 60 kg "sausages" of seal and walrus meat to feed the dogs. The boycott of seal fur trading also almost eliminated the work undertaken by females in the preparation of such skins for sale.

The school had been extended to 12 grades, restricting the ability of adolescents to accompany their parents on hunting trips. The village was equipped with a large recreation hall including an indoor swimming pool, and a full-size indoor skating rink and curling rink were almost ready for use. A regulation-size basketball court also was available at the school. School staff offered programs of indoor soccer, floor hockey, basketball, and volleyball throughout the academic year.

The government of the Northwest Territories made periodic efforts to foster traditional Inuit games, but recreation was increasingly sought in the pursuits of southern Canada. In the late 1970s, a few television and videocassette players appeared in the village, and a large public lending library began operations. By 1990, Igloolik had cable TV; 134 of 139 households had at least one TV set, and 81 households also had a video player. Combined, the two main stores in the village had sold more than 100 Nintendo machines. Many children and adolescents now allocated several hours per day to these passive pursuits, particularly in the winter months.

Growth Patterns

In 1969-70, a cross-sectional analysis of statures had suggested that there was a rapid secular trend to an increase of adult height, perhaps amounting to as much as 3 cm/decade (18). However, to our surprise, when the same adults were reevaluated in 1979-80 and 1989-90, their heights had decreased by 3 to 5 cm. In some instances, comparative chest radiographs were available, and it was possible to show that the change had arisen from a shortening of the vertical axis of the spine, as seen in PA radiographs (23). The immediate cause was thought to be repeated snowmobile trauma, although it was less clear whether the underlying pathology was an increased thoracic kyphosis, a compression of the intervertebral discs, or an actual vertebral collapse. Before the age of puberty, children showed a continuing trend to an increase of stature, but in the older adolescents (who were the most aggressive operators of snowmobiles and all-terrain vehicles) the secular trend was reversed.

From 1978-79 to date, we have collected measurements of height, body mass, skinfold thicknesses, and grip strengths on all school students three times per year. This has allowed us to apply more sophisticated statistical modeling techniques to data individually synchronized in terms of peak height velocities. This approach has shown a peak height velocity at age 12.1 years in the boys and 10.6 years in the girls, with little inter-cohort difference over the 12 years of observation. The peak velocity of body mass was seen at 13.8 years in the males and 14.6 years in the females. The age of peak height velocity is relatively young, although there have been other suggestions of early puberty in groups of oriental origin (Malina: Personal communication).

The skinfold readings of the boys showed a small prepubertal surge, and as might be expected, the girls developed a large and continuing increment at puberty. In both sexes, there was a systematic secular trend to an increase of skinfold readings from 1970 to 1980. Grip strength showed a sharp pubertal rise in the boys, although there was a trend to slightly lower values in later cohorts. Girls showed little pubertal increase of grip strength.

Cardiovascular Health

The measures of skinfold thickness, predicted aerobic power, and muscle strength adopted in 1969-70 were reapplied in 1979-80 and in 1989-90; we were particularly fortunate that the same investigator was able to apply the same test procedures using the same equipment throughout (11).

Skinfold readings had increased somewhat by 1980, but showed a larger rise in 1990 (Figure 15.1). By this time, the average values (8-10 mm in boys, 10-20 mm in girls) were at least as great as in southern Canada, and some of the Inuit children and adolescents were developing substantial obesity.

The predicted aerobic power (Figure 15.2) demonstrated a parallel decrement, but average values still remained somewhat higher than values for sedentary individuals in southern Canada.

Age-adjusted knee extension strength decreased in both sexes over the 2 decades, but (perhaps because of the local muscular demands of controlling high-speed snowmobiles) grip strength was unchanged.

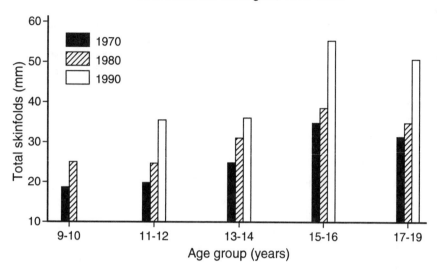

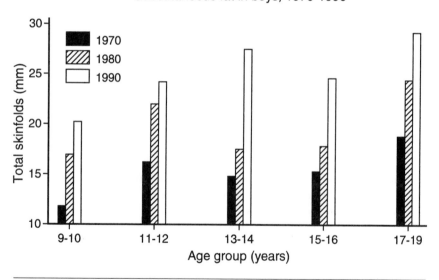

Figure 15.1. Changes in skinfold readings with acculturation to a sedentary lifestyle. Cross-sectional data showing sum of triceps, subscapular, and suprailiac skinfolds for Inuit children of Igloolik, measured in 1970, 1980, and 1990.
Source: Rode & Shephard, 1992.

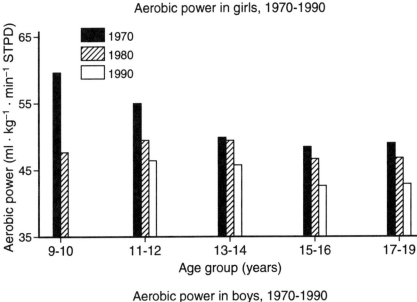

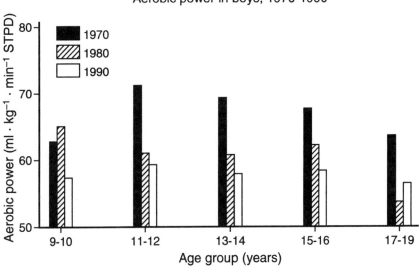

Figure 15.2.   Changes in aerobic power with acculturation to a sedentary lifestyle. Cross-sectional predictions of maximal oxygen intake (ml/[kg.min]) for Inuit children of Igloolik tested in 1970, 1980, and 1990.
Source: Rode & Shephard, 1992.

Lung volumes showed a small increment over the 20 years, in part because the younger children of 1990 were a little taller than their peers of 1970. The logarithmic exponent governing the relationship of lung volumes to height showed no substantial change over the two decades. The percentage of regular smokers had increased among the young females, but in the male subjects the age-specific prevalence of smoking was greatest in 1980, and had declined somewhat by 1990.

Future Prospects for the Circumpolar Inuit

Sociocultural Change

The adoption of southern Canadian attitudes, habits, and behaviors, already well-advanced, will probably continue in Canadian Inuit communities such as Igloolik. One attempt of a few families to return to a more traditional nomadic lifestyle was quickly abandoned in favor of the comforts of the modern settlement. Although the fertility rate is now lower than a decade ago, it seems likely that the village population (which doubled from 1970 to 1990) will further expand. This will place further pressure on the game reserves of the area and will inhibit a return to subsistence hunting. Lack of employment will continue to plague the community, despite attempts to expand traditional crafts such as soapstone carving and to initiate orchestrated hunting excursions for wealthy southerners. As in other indigenous communities, drug abuse, alcoholism, and suicide will continue to be major causes of concern.

Currently, such issues pose a larger threat to life than the risk of cardiovascular disease, although the experience of other indigenous communities suggests that unless current trends in habitual physical activity are reversed, gross obesity, diabetes, an adverse lipid profile, and a high risk of cardiovascular disease may not be many years distant.

In terms of prevention, it is plainly not possible to advocate a community-wide return to traditional hunting and trapping, and our studies of modern-day hunters show that villagers who have persisted with such activities are now somewhat more obese than other members of the community (11). Instead, the new generation must learn a concept that is largely foreign to the Inuit culture: the deliberate pursuit of active physical leisure in a recreation center offering competitive sports and games.

A cross-sectional comparison of young males who are active in such programs with young males who are not, suggests that community sport may be an effective tactic for conserving traditional fitness (12). Those who follow such pursuits have, in general, conserved the low levels of subcutaneous fat, the high aerobic power, and the strong leg muscles that were characteristic of the Inuit children tested in 1970. It is tempting to infer causality, but there is some possibility that a part of their advantage is due to competitive selection (22). In particular, the active individuals are substantially taller than the sedentary population. Thus, longitudinal experiments are needed to check how much of the apparent benefit is program related.

Comment

The experiments that have been described illustrate many of the challenges faced in making international comparisons of physical activity patterns, growth rates, and cardiovascular health between remotely located indigenous populations. Because of relatively complete sampling, the use of standard IBP methodology, and the biological calibration of both equipment and procedures, the findings from Igloolik can be accepted with much more confidence than some published reports. On the other hand, the settlement is still sufficiently isolated, both genetically and socioculturally, that the results cannot necessarily be extrapolated to other populations of Inuit living in larger centers such as Iqualuit. Moreover, given the pace of change in Igloolik, the situation of children in that community also will alter radically over the next decade.

The changes in hunting patterns and general mechanization of life within the village have undoubtedly been important influences for the older adolescents, but for the younger children the primary cause of a deteriorating physical condition has been the advent of television and video games. It has long been suspected that the 20 to 30 hours per week that urban children devote to such pursuits is bad for their cardiovascular health, but this is one of the few instances where there has been opportunity to document the impact of such technology upon the physical condition of a whole generation of children.

The patterns of social change documented in Igloolik find their parallel in many other indigenous communities and developing nations. From the Indian reservations of Canada to the indigenous populations of the South Pacific, acculturation is associated with obesity, diabetes mellitus, and poor cardiovascular health. It is hard to know the most effective measures to reverse this trend. Plainly, we cannot ban television and video games. One possible remedy may lie in a change of the school curriculum. The issue here is not so much an insistence upon required physical education as upon the development of better role models. Currently, the person to emulate is the overweight white entrepreneur. But the Inuit could, and probably should, be taught that their distinctive heritage has been maintained over the centuries by a superior level of physical fitness. It was this that allowed them to colonize the difficult habitat of the circumpolar territories. It could be emphasized further that those participating in the village sport programs have conserved a large part of their heritage of physical fitness. Interest in developing fitness for winter survival could possibly be fostered by programs such as Outward Bound for the current generation of students. Finally, as in urban centers, the fitness of many students could probably be improved if the school buildings were moved 2 to 3 km from the village, with walking as the sole means of reaching this destination.

Conclusions

Over the past 20 years, the Inuit children of Igloolik, like their parents, have lost the high level of cardiorespiratory fitness which once distinguished them from southern Canadians. In older adolescents, a decreased participation in hunting expeditions is a factor, but in young children the arrival of television and video games seems largely responsible. A minority of children who participate in local sports programs have conserved high fitness levels. Methods of encouraging the remainder of the young villagers to greater physical activity are discussed.

Acknowledgments

This research was supported in part by research grants from Health & Welfare, Canada (NHRDP) and Canadian Tire Acceptance Limited and by training grants from the Department of Indian and Northern Affairs. We are also grateful to J. MacDonald, coordinator of the Igloolik Research Center, and to W. Slipchenko, director, Circumpolar Affairs, Government of the Northwest Territories, for their enthusiastic support of this project.

References

1. Bang, H.O.; Dyerberg, J.; Hjorne, N. Investigation of blood lipids and food composition of Greenlandic Eskimos. In: Shephard, R.J.; Itoh, S., eds. Circumpolar health. Toronto: University of Toronto Press; 1976: 141-145.
2. Carrier, R.; Landry, F.; Potvin, R.; Bouchard, C. Comparisons between athletes, normal and Eskimo subjects from the point of view of selected biochemical parameters. In: Taylor, A.W., ed. Training: scientific basis and application. Springfield, IL: C.C. Thomas; 1972: 180-185.
3. Draper, H.H. Nutritional research in circumpolar populations. In: Shephard, R.J.; Itoh, S., eds. Circumpolar health. Toronto: University of Toronto Press; 1976: 120-129.
4. Glassford, G. Games of the traditional Canadian Eskimo. Proceedings of first Canadian symposium on the history of sport and physical education. Edmonton, Alberta: University of Alberta; 1970: 133-152.
5. Godin, G.; Shephard, R.J. Activity patterns of the Canadian Eskimo. In: Edholm, O.; Gunderson, K., eds. Human polar biology. London: Heinemann Publications, 1973: 193-215.
6. Milan, F., ed. The human biology of circumpolar peoples. London: Cambridge University Press; 1980.
7. Rode, A.; Shephard, R.J. Cardio-respiratory fitness of an Arctic community. J. Appl. Physiol. 31:519-526; 1971.
8. Rode, A.; Shephard, R.J. Growth, development and fitness of the Canadian Eskimo. Med. Sci. Sports. 5:161-169; 1973.
9. Rode, A.; Shephard, R.J. On the mode of exercise appropriate to a "primitive" community. Int. Z. Angew. Physiol. 31:187-196; 1973.
10. Rode, A.; Shephard, R.J. Pulmonary function of Canadian Eskimos. Scand. J. Resp. Dis. 54:191-205; 1973.

11. Rode, A.; Shephard, R.J. Fitness and health of an Inuit community: 20 years of cultural change. Ottawa: Circumpolar and Scientific Affairs; 1992.
12. Rode, A.; Shephard, R.J. Acculturation and loss of fitness in the Inuit. Arctic Med. Res. 52:107-112; 1993.
13. Rode, A.; Shephard, R.J. Secular and age trends in height of adults among a Canadian Inuit community. Arct. Med. Res. 53:18-24; 1994.
14. Rode, A.; Shephard, R.J. Prediction of body fat content in an Inuit community. Am. J. Hum. Biol. 6:249-254; 1994.
15. Shephard, R.J. The prediction of ''maximal'' oxygen consumption, using a new progressive step test. Ergonomics. 10:1-15; 1967.
16. Shephard, R.J. Computer programmes for the solution of the Åstrand nomogram. J. Sports Med. Phys. Fitness. 10:206-210, 1970.
17. Shephard, R.J. Sport for youth: the Eskimo approach. Br. J. Sports Med. 7:315-316; 1973.
18. Shephard, R.J. Human physiological work capacity. London: Cambridge University Press; 1978.
19. Shephard, R.J. Physical activity and growth. Chicago: Yearbook Publishers; 1982.
20. Shephard, R.J.; Rode, A. Fitness for arctic life: the cardio-respiratory status of the Canadian Eskimo. In: Edholm, O.; Gunderson, E.K., eds. Human polar biology. London: Heinemann Publications; 1973: 216-239.
21. Shephard, R.J.; Hatcher, J.; Rode, A. On the body composition of the Eskimo. Europ. J. Appl. Physiol. 10:1-13; 1973.
22. Shephard, R.J.; Lavallée, H.; LaRivière, G. Competitive selection among age-class ice-hockey players. Br. J. Sports Med. 12:11-13; 1978.
23. Shephard, R.J.; Goodman, J.; Rode, A.; Schaefer, O. Snowmobile use and decrease of stature among the Inuit. Arct. Med. Res. 38:32-36; 1984.
24. Shephard, R.J.; Rode, A.; Guthrie, B. A mixed longitudinal study of the growth and development of Canadian Inuit children. Paper presented at Canadian Association of Sport Sciences, Saskatoon, October, 1992.
25. Weiner, J.S. Proposals for international research. Human adaptability project- document 5. London: UK Royal Anthropological Institute; 1964.

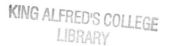

About the Editors

Cameron J.R. Blimkie, PhD, is an associate professor in the Department of Kinesiology and an associate member in the Department of Pediatrics at McMaster University, Toronto. For more than 20 years he has focused his teaching and research on the physiological aspects of the exercising child.

Dr. Blimkie's membership with the European Group of Pediatric Work Physiology (EGPWP) and the North American Society for Pediatric Exercise Medicine (NASPEM) led to his involvement as coorganizer and cohost of the first joint meeting of NASPEM and EGPWP in 1993. He is the Vice President of Education and Programs for the Canadian Society of Exercise Physiology (CSEP), as well as an active and longtime member of the American College of Sports Medicine (ACSM) and the Ontario Association of Sport and Exercise Science.

Dr. Blimkie is a widely published author and contributor to many scholarly publications. A past member of the editorial board for the Canadian Journal of Applied Sport Science, he now is on the editorial board for *Pediatric Exercise Science* and is a frequent reviewer for other journals.

Oded Bar-Or, MD, is a professor of pediatrics and Director of the Children's Exercise and Nutrition Centre at McMaster University, Toronto.

An ACSM board member since 1989, Dr. Bar-Or chairs ACSM's ad hoc committee on pediatric exercise. He also is a member of the Canadian Medical Association, the Ontario Medical Association, CSEP, and NASPEM. Dr. Bar-Or served two years as vice president of ACSM, was president of the Canadian Association of Sports Sciences (the former name of CSEP) from 1987 to 1988, and was president of the International Council for Physical Fitness Research.

Internationally known for his contributions to the growing discipline of pediatric exercise science, Dr. Bar-Or has written extensively for many scholarly publications. He also has been a coeditor and editorial board member of many journals, including the *Journal of Sports Medicine and Physical Fitness, Sports Medicine, Medicine and Science in Sports and Exercise, Pediatric Exercise Science, Journal of Basic and Clinical Physiology & Pharmacology,* and *Clinical Journal of Sports Medicine.*